Language and Deafness

Language and Deafness

Stephen P. Quigley
Peter V. Paul

University of Illinois at Urbana—Champaign

SINGULAR PUBLISHING GROUP, INC.
SAN DIEGO, CALIFORNIA

SINGULAR PUBLISHING GROUP, INC.
4284 41st Street
San Diego, California 92105

Library of Congress Cataloging in Publication Data

Quigley, Stephen Patrick, Language and deafness.

  Bibliography: p.
  Includes index.
  1. Children, Deaf—Education. 2. Children, Deaf—Language. 3. Deaf—Means of communication—Study and teaching. 4. Children, Deaf—Education—United States.
  I. Paul, Peter V. WV 100 I33]
HV2471.Q52   1984   371.91'2   83-26144
ISBN 0-933014-14-7

Printed in the United States of America

NWST
/AEG 5389

For Ruth and Mary Beth and Linda

CONTENTS

5 Written language, 141

6 Bilingualism and English as a second language, 165

7 Assessment and language instruction, 199
by Barry W. Jones, Ph.D.

Preface

The present state of the education of deaf children can be characterized as one of creative confusion. Creative is an appropriate term because the present ferment in the field seems likely to lead to significant changes, which might also be significant advances. Confusion is also an appropriate term since no strongly research supported directions for educational practice have yet emerged from the ferment. Most of the ferment centers around the languages and the communication modes that should be used initially with deaf infants and children. This book attempts to define the problems and prospects of those languages and communication modes, to discuss elements of the present creative ferment in these areas, to present and discuss much of the data based research findings pertaining to them, to synthesize the findings and those from other areas (such as bilingualism and English as a second language [ESL]), and to present some conclusions.

The book is seen as being useful to anyone seeking an in-depth introduction to language development in deaf children, but particularly to student teachers and clinicians and practicing teachers and clinicians who bear most of the responsibility for fostering that development both directly and in their training and counseling of parents. The book has much more detail on language than is common in beginning texts, but that is because the authors believe that teachers and clinicians must have a great deal of detailed knowledge about language and communication to promote, through naturally oriented practices, the initial language development of deaf children; and to direct, through analytically oriented practices, more structured development at later ages if the naturally oriented practices do not produce adequate language development. As Russell, Quigley, and Power (1976) have claimed: "It is probably a fair analogy to state that teachers of deaf children should be expected to know as much about language as a teacher of chemistry is expected to know about chemistry" (p. xi). This is not so that teachers can teach language didactically but in order that they have the knowledge and skills to structure situations and construct materials that will allow language to develop in a natural manner or, when necessary, in a more structured manner.

Both natural and structured approaches are seen as playing a role in the language development of deaf children. The preferred approach is the natural approach, in which language is acquired (or absorbed) unconsciously by the child through fluent communicative interaction with the parents in infancy and early childhood and later with teachers. Unfortunately, this early natural development does not always take place (in fact, it rarely takes place), and at some point many teachers feel the need to use more structured approaches to language development. It follows from this, that teachers and clinicians must be familiar with both approaches and know when to use each.

The statement that early language development requires fluent communicative interaction between child and parents and child and teacher raises immediately the question of communication modes, the form in which parent, teacher, and child will communicate. Here again, as with language approaches, no absolute position is taken in the book. All major approaches are described and explored. It is recognized and stated that it is not possible to examine the language development of deaf children apart from the specific communication mode through which it was developed. With hearing children, language is acquired through speech, and spoken language is the primary language on which the secondary language forms of reading and writing are based. Individual variations in IQ, socioeconomic status, educational opportunities, and other factors might alter the degree of language mastery by individual hearing children, but they will not alter the form. All variations are variations on the same basic form, spoken language.

With deaf children the situation is quite different. Any of several communication modes or forms might be used early with them, and language development can be discussed only in relation to the particular form used. That approach is followed here, particularly in chapter 3 on Primary Language Development and in the concluding chapter. The major communication forms that can be used with deaf children are referred to throughout the book as oral English (OE), manually coded English (MCE), and American Sign Language (ASL). These are described in chapter 1 on Definitions and Historical Perspectives. Pidgin sign English (PSE) is categorized here as a form of MCE, but it can be regarded also as a separate form. MCE systems are contrived systems (contrived usually by hearing people) which attempt in various ways to conform signs and fingerspelling to the structure of English. PSE is a linguistically natural language form developed from interaction or interfacing of the visual ASL with the oral OE.

As with language approaches, it follows from the variety of communication modes and the present support that exists for each, that teachers and clinicians who work with deaf children need to be conversant with, and fluent in, all of them. And since the secondary language forms of reading and writing, at least in our present state of knowledge, have to be related to the child's primary language, teachers and clinicians need to understand the implications of each primary language form (OE, MCE, ASL) for the development of reading and written language. If OE is used exclusively with a deaf child, then perhaps the methods of teaching reading to hearing children (which assume the existence of a spoken language) can be used with that child; but if ASL is the child's primary language, then it is likely that other methods of teaching reading must be sought.

In addition to being skilled in the various language approaches (natural and structured) and the various communication forms (OE, MCE, ASL) that are used with deaf children, teachers and clinicians need to be highly knowledgeable in the language and communication development of hearing children. It is important also that they be familiar with the special problems and techniques used in language development with certain other special populations, especially problems and techniques in bilingualism and the teaching of English as a second language (ESL). All of this amounts to a great deal of knowledge and skill in a large number of areas, but it is difficult to see how a teacher of deaf children can be fully competent without all of it.

This book treats, though only to limited extents, each of these areas of knowledge and skill. References are provided throughout where the reader can obtain more detailed information on the major topic discussed in each chapter. In most chapters, the topic of the chapter (e.g., reading) is discussed first in relation to the hearing population. This is in accord with the stated position that the language development of deaf children can best be examined and understood in the context of language development in general. Each chapter topic is then discussed in relation to deaf children as defined in chapter 1 and some conclusions and possible applications are presented.

Chapter 1 provides definitions of important terms and historical perspectives on important issues and topics. One of the most neglected issues in the education of deaf children is the differentiation of children who are deaf (visually oriented for purposes of communication even with the best amplification) from those who are hard of hearing (at least partially auditorily oriented). An attempt is made to do this in chapter 1. In that chapter also, definitions are provided for the various language and communication approaches used with deaf children. Then the historical paths of the various language and communication approaches are traced in an effort to show that most of the present approaches (with the exception of such relatively recent technological advances as amplification) have very long histories. This should not be surprising. The formal teaching and tutoring of deaf children has almost a 400-year history and has involved many very intelligent people. In that lengthy period, it is likely that every conceivable approach has been tried. The fact that none has prevailed, and dissension still reigns, indicates that there is as yet no one "true path" in the education of deaf children.

Chapter 2 deals with language and cognition. Again the topic is discussed in terms of hearing individuals and then in relation to deaf individuals. The position is taken that language is a subset of cognitive abilities and that adequate language development requires adequate cognitive development. It is also accepted that soon after language begins to develop, language and cognition become almost inseparable. Symbolic mediation is discussed in this chapter; the forms of internalized language used by hearing and by deaf individuals as mediators of thought and of the secondary language forms of reading and writing.

Chapter 3 presents current theories of language and traces the development of primary language in hearing and in deaf individuals. As previously stated, the language development of deaf children must be examined in relation to the communication form through which it was developed and given expression. This is done in chapter 3, with development being discussed within the communication forms of OE, MCE, and ASL. Some implications of the various forms for the later development of reading and written language are discussed. The lack of research based data is stressed.

Chapter 4 presents considerable information on the reading of hearing and of deaf children; chapter 5 similarly treats written language. The original intent had been to treat these two topics in a single chapter to emphasize their close relationship and the primacy of reading, but the large amount of material available dictated separate chapters. It is recognized, and expounded in the book, that skilled development of reading and written language requires adequate development of a primary language, which in turn is dependent on adequate cognitive development, which in its turn is dependent on early fluent communication between parent and child. But the development of literacy is the road to learning and is the primary responsibility of teachers, clinicians, and the schools. Other aspects of the deaf child's development certainly are important. But the failure to develop literacy cannot be compensated for by the promotion of cultural identity or the development of a positive self-image, important as those might be. In fact, it is doubtful that an adult who is semiliterate or illiterate for all practical purposes can have a very positive self-image or find much satisfaction or reward in cultural identity.

Chapter 6 deals with the processes and problems, theories and practices, of bilingualism and the development of English as a second language with minority-culture hearing children, and relates these areas analogically to the language development of deaf children. This is likely to be an area for much fruitful exploration and research with deaf children during the decade of the 1980s. Some of the problems and some of the possible programs and procedures that could be tried with deaf children, based on research with minority culture hearing children, are discussed. It is emphasized that successful bilingual and ESL programs seem to require that the child come to the program with at least one language already reasonably well established. That, of course, is not the case with many deaf children who often enter school and preschool programs without any well-developed first language. (Some deaf children of ASL-using deaf parents might be exceptions to this). This reinforces the importance of the family, or some substitute, providing the deaf child with a primary language in infancy and early childhood through some fluent form of communication.

Chapter 7 treats language assessment and some of the major methods used in language development and instruction. Some material in these areas is also presented, where appropriate, in other chapters and much of the other material could have been similarly treated. It was considered convenient for students and teachers, however, to have a separate chapter on these important areas. The material on instructional approaches is related back to the historical treatment of earlier approaches in chapter 1.

In the final chapter (8), some general summation of the book's topics is provided and some implications for present and future educational practices with deaf children are discussed. If there is a general focus, or unifying theme to the book, it is provided by chapter 8 and this Preface. The theme is simply that there is as yet no data based justification for any communication and language approach as the sole means of developing language in deaf children. The teacher and the clinician must master a variety of language approaches (from natural to analytic) and communication forms (e.g., OE, MCE, ASL) to function effectively with a range of deaf children. Fortunately, teachers and clinicians are usually more eclectic and more pragmatic than many textbook writers. They are usually willing to try new approaches on the basis of logical and theoretical arguments, but are also ready to abandon them if they do not seem to work.

A companion text to the present book, *Reading and Deafness* by Cynthia M. King and Stephen P. Quigley, will be published soon by the same publisher. The topics of the two books, language and reading, are obviously closely related, and the use of a single publisher allows for some overlap of content without the authors having to go through a frustrating rewriting exercise to say the same thing in different words in two different books so as not to violate copyrights held by two different publishers. A major difference between the two texts is that *Reading and Deafness* will provide both a knowledge base and instructional techniques on its topic whereas *Language and Deafness* deals primarily with a knowledge base and treats instructional techniques only generally. This is because the wider scope of the present book makes inclusion of detailed material on instruction impractical. A special chapter on assessment and instruction has been provided for the present book by Barry W. Jones, and a related text on instructional processes and techniques in language development is tentatively planned.

The authors are indebted to many persons for assistance in the preparation of this book. A major debt is acknowledged to the many teachers, clinicians, researchers, and thinkers who provided most of the material on which the book is based. Some, but certainly not all, of this debt is acknowledged by appropriate citation and referencing of the more than 500 authors whose work was used in preparation of the text. Grateful acknowledgment is also made to the graduate students who aided in locating and abstracting the works of those many authors: Jean Andrews, Cheryl Bolebruch, Cynthia King, John-Allen Payne, Stephanie Quigley, Lou Reeves, Marilyn Salter, and Pam Stuckey. And finally, the major and indispensible assistance provided by Ruth Quigley in all phases of the planning, preparation, and completion of the manuscript is gratefully acknowledged and lovingly appreciated.

Stephen P. Quigley

chapter 1

Definitions and historical perspectives

In this chapter, definitions of various terms are given along with a brief history whose purpose is to provide perspective for the present status of language development and instruction with deaf children.

DEFINITIONS

Deafness

Basically, for the purposes of this book, a child is considered deaf if hearing impairment is so great, even with good amplification, that vision becomes the child's main link to the world and main channel of communication. This is vague and is, of course, of little use in diagnosing deafness. A considerable body of evidence (see Ling, 1976; Conrad, 1979), however, indicates that the shift from audition to vision as the main channel of communication occurs at about 90 dB for many children.

For communication purposes, hearing is usually measured across a range of frequencies from 125 to 8000 Hz with measurement being on a logarithmic unit, the decibel (dB). Hearing threshold level (HTL) is graphed on an audiogram by plotting an individual's response threshold for each measured frequency. Any significant deviation (15–20 dB or more) of an individual's hearing threshold level at any frequency from the zero threshold on the audiogram represents a hearing impairment. The zero, or normal, threshold is a statistically defined average measured for each frequency on a large sample of the normal hearing population (ANSI, 1969). This threshold is represented by zero (0 dB) at each frequency on the audiogram—a straight line.

Hearing impairment is a generic term covering all degrees and types of hearing loss, with deafness, for the purposes of this book, being the extreme degree of impairment (90+ dB). Hearing threshold level on the audiogram can be measured from − 10 to 110 dB. Degree of hearing impairment is often represented as the average of the HTL for the three frequencies considered to be most important for the reception of speech: 500, 1000, and 2000 Hz. Thus, an individual with HTLs of 55 dB at 500 Hz, 60 dB at 1000 Hz, and 65 dB at 2000 Hz is considered to have a 60-dB hearing loss or impairment. Degree of impairment is the primary descriptive variable for the hearing-impaired individual or group.

Along with degree of hearing impairment, age at onset of hearing impairment is generally considered of major significance in defining deafness. Although a child who suffers a 100-dB sensorineural hearing impairment at 6 years of age has the same *degree* of impairment as a child who suffers a 100-dB impairment prior to birth, the language and communication consequences (and many other consequences) are much different. The child of 6 will have established an auditory based internalized language system developed through aural/oral communicative interaction with the parents and others in response to basic and derived needs. In the typical situation, the child born deaf will reach the age of 6 with very little of the cognitive performance and linguistic proficiency of the other child. So, age at onset of hearing impairment is a critical factor in relation to language development. In this book, the critical age at onset of hearing impairment has been set at 2 years. Although, ideally, children with normal hearing until 2 years of age should have some aural/oral communicative and language advantage over children born deaf, extensive statistical data and practical experience indicate this is not usually the case. Given the present limitations in the service system for hearing-impaired children, any such advantage usually is lost, and the child deafened at 2 years and the child born deaf tend to be indistinguishable educationally by Age 6. In fact, 2 years is probably a conservative level for the age at onset criterion.

Other important descriptive variables are etiology and type of hearing impairment and hearing status of the hearing-impaired individual's parents and siblings. Etiology is important because as many as 25 percent of what we define here as the population of deaf children might have complicating factors such as visual problems, retardation, and cerebral palsy resulting from such etiologies as anoxia and maternal rubella (Vernon, 1969). Type of hearing impairment refers to the site of the lesion or damage, to whether the impairment is conductive, sensorineural, mixed, or central in nature. In conductive impairment, usually only the conductive mechanism of the outer and middle ear is involved. Hearing impairment typically is moderate and often is fully treatable medically or by amplification (hearing aids). Sensorineural hearing impairment results from damage to the sensory mechanism of hearing which is located in the inner ear. It is usually medically irreversible and is only partly helped by amplification. Combinations of conductive and sensory impairment are known as mixed hearing impairment. Central hearing impairment results from damage to the auditory cortex or to the auditory nerve that transmits sensory information from the inner ear to the auditory cortex. Hearing status of parents and siblings (especially parents) is an important variable because it can influence the form of language and communication to which the deaf child is exposed in infancy and early childhood. Deaf parents usually (although not always) use American Sign Language (ASL) or (less commonly) coded English (MCE) with their deaf children.

Obviously, many factors interact with degree of hearing impairment, such as IQ, socioeconomic status, and so forth. Given certain advantages, a child with hearing impairment in excess of 90 dB might function as a hard-of-hearing rather than as a deaf child. Similarly, given certain disadvantages, a child with hearing impairment of less than 90 dB might function communicatively and otherwise as a deaf rather than as a hard-of-hearing child. The 90-dB criterion is offered only as a rough guide to where deafness might typically begin on the hearing threshold continuum. Some classifications of hearing impairment consider deafness as being as low as 70 dB on the hearing threshold level scale and some as high as 105 dB. Given the present state of knowledge, 90 dB is offered here as the most defensible criterion.

Although all of these variables are important to an understanding of deafness, classification systems usually are based only on HTL or HTL and age at onset. Classifications can be found in various sources (e.g., Davis & Silverman, 1978). Table 1 shows one which is based on degree of hearing impairment or HTL and which also lists some of the language and communication effects and educational needs resulting from the various levels of impairment (Bernero & Bothwell, 1966). Of the five categories in this classification, only the fifth (and to a much lesser extent the fourth) is considered in this book. Available statistics (Karchmer, Milone, & Wolk, 1979) indicate there are about 54,000 students in identifiable school programs who roughly match these two categories, with most being in the fifth category.

The population with which this book is concerned is the 50,000 or so children who have hearing threshold levels of 90 dB or greater and in whom the hearing impairment was present by the age of 2 years. However, the literature on the language and communication development problems of deaf children does not fall into this neat classification. Some of the studies used in the present book refer, in the original work, only to deaf children without descriptive data on hearing threshold level or age at onset. In other studies, children listed as deaf include some with hearing threshold levels as low as 60 dB. This is a matter for concern. The importance of hearing to language development is so powerful that even small amounts of residual hearing, especially when amplified, can make great differences in children's aural/oral language comprehension and use. So, while this book is concerned with the language development and problems of deaf children, the definition of deafness remains somewhat vague. It is probably best to state simply that deaf children are those whose hearing impairment is so great, even with good

Table 1. Relationship of degree of handicap to educational needs*

DEGREE OF HANDICAP	EFFECT OF HEARING LOSS ON UNDERSTANDING OF LANGUAGE AND SPEECH	EDUCATIONAL NEEDS AND PROGRAMS
SLIGHT 16 to 29 dB (ASA) or 27 to 40 dB (ISO)	May have difficulty hearing faint or distant speech. Will not usually experience difficulty in school situations.	May benefit from a hearing aid as loss approaches 30 dB (ASA) or 40 dB (ISO). Attention to vocabulary development. Needs favorable seating and lighting. May need lip reading instruction. May need speech correction.
MILD 30 to 44 dB (ASA) or 41 to 55 dB (ISO)	Understands conversational speech at a distance of 3–5 feet (face-to-face). May miss as much as 50% of class discussions if voices are faint or not in line of vision. May exhibit limited vocabulary and speech anomalies.	Child should be referred to special education for educational follow-up if such service is available. Individual hearing aid by evaluation and training in its use. Favorable seating and possible special class placement, especially for primary children. Attention to vocabulary and reading. May need lip reading instruction. Speech conservation and correction, if indicated.
MARKED 45 to 59 dB (ASA) or 56 to 70 dB (ISO)	Conversation must be loud to be understood. Will have increasing difficulty with school situations requiring participation in group discussions. Is likely to have defective speech. Is likely to be deficient in language usage and comprehension. Will have evidence of limited vocabulary.	Will need resource teacher or special class. Special help in language skills, vocabulary development, usage, reading, writing, grammar, etc. Individual hearing aid by evaluation and auditory training. Lip reading instruction. Speech conservation and speech correction. Attention to auditory and visual situations at all times.

Table 1. (Cont'd)

DEGREE OF HANDICAP	EFFECT OF HEARING LOSS ON UNDERSTANDING OF LANGUAGE AND SPEECH	EDUCATIONAL NEEDS AND PROGRAMS
SEVERE 60 to 79 dB (ASA) or 71 to 90 dB (ISO)	May hear loud voices about one foot from the ear. May be able to identify environmental sounds. May be able to discriminate vowels but not all consonants. Speech and language defective and likely to deteriorate. Speech and language will not develop spontaneously if loss is present before 1 year of age.	Will need full-time special program for deaf children, with emphasis on all language skills, concept development, lip reading and speech. Program needs specialized supervision and comprehensive supporting services. Individual hearing aid by evaluation. Auditory training on individual and group aids. Part-time in regular classes only as profitable.
EXTREME 80 dB or more (ASA) or 91 dB or more (ISO)	May hear some loud sounds but is aware of vibrations more than tonal pattern. Relies on vision rather than hearing as primary avenue for communication. Speech and language defective and likely to deteriorate. Speech and language will not develop spontaneously if loss is present before 1 year.	Will need full-time in special program for deaf children, with emphasis on all language skills, concept development, lip reading and speech. Program needs specialized supervision and comprehensive supporting services. Continuous appraisal of needs in regard to oral and manual communication. Auditory training on group and individual aid. Part-time in regular classes only for carefully selected children.

*Bernero, Raymond J., and Bothwell, Hazel "Relationship of Hearing Impairment to Educational Needs," Illinois Department of Public Health and Office of the Superintendent of Public Instruction, 1966.

amplification, that vision serves as their main channel of communication. Such children are likely to be naturally inclined to use visual/manual modes of communication rather than aural/oral modes.

Language

Language has been defined as "a code whereby ideas about the world are represented by a conventional system of signals for communication" (Bloom & Lahey, 1978, p. 4). Spoken words, grammatically structured, form the conventional systems of signals used in most human languages. Many deaf people, however, use a system (or systems) of conventionalized movements, also grammatically structured, as their means of communication. In the United States, and much of Canada, this form of communication is known as American Sign Language (ASL). Sign languages used in other countries also use "motion in space" as their means of communicating, but there can be variations among the sign languages just as there are variations among spoken languages (Stokoe, 1971, 1972). Sign languages seem to meet the requirements of language as defined by Bloom and Lahey (1978), and it can be shown that they meet the requirements of other popular definitions as well. In addition, sign languages have served the communicative needs of deaf people for recorded centuries, and it is a reasonable speculation that they have so served as long as there have been deaf people. Thus, any comprehensive text on language and deafness must treat sign languages as well, and as equally, as spoken and written languages.

Most hearing children seem typically to acquire language almost by osmosis. They acquire it through apparently effortless interaction with a language model (usually the mother) in infancy and early childhood. If an infant has an intact sensory system, no substantial intellectual or cognitive deficits, is exposed to a stimulating environment, and has verbal parents who provide a warm and accepting atmosphere and communicate easily and fluently with the child in response to the child's needs, an auditory based language system will be acquired by the child in an apparently effortless fashion. When these conditions are met, the typical hearing child will then readily develop cognitive abilities and linguistic abilities through which the secondary language forms of reading and writing can later be developed.

Many of the factors in these statements on the early cognitive and linguistic development of hearing children apply also to deaf children. As Quigley and Kretschmer (1982) have stated:

> Development of the deaf child's (and, in fact, of any child's) educational potential requires an early environment that provides a wealth of stimulating and relevant learning experiences that are made meaningful for the child through interaction with other people by means of a fluent and intelligible communication system. Fluent communication is particularly important in

infancy and early childhood when the parents or parent surrogates are the principal figures in the child's life. (p. xi)

It should be noted that no restriction of communication to an aural/oral mode is made or implied in this quote just as the Bloom and Lahey definition of language had no stated or implied restriction to spoken languages. Thus, American Sign Language fits the Bloom and Lahey conception of language (as it would fit many other recent conceptions), and the visual/manual mode of communication fits the Quigley and Kretschmer requirement for a fluent and intelligible communication system. The major difference between the deaf and the hearing infant is that the typical aural/oral mode of developing an initial language system has been massively disrupted in the deaf child by damage to the hearing mechanism. It follows that some major choices must be made as to how to foster cognitive and linguistic development in the deaf infant and young child.

There is a choice to be made between two modes of communication, oral and manual, and between two languages, English and American Sign Language. These two communication modes and two languages can be combined to form a variety of communication and language systems for use with deaf children. Definitions of these systems can be found in Caccamise and Drury (1976) and Quigley and King (1982). There is not complete agreement in the field about some of the definitions; the ones used here are based on Quigley and King (1982).

Communication systems

The various language and communication systems in use with deaf children can be grouped in three general categories: American Sign Language, manually coded English, and oral English.

American sign language

Rainer, Altschuler, and Kallman (1969) estimated that approximately 75% of deaf American adults use American Sign Language. In actuality, it probably is safe to speculate that almost all deaf persons in the United States and most of Canada use ASL to communicate with each other and with hearing persons who know the language, and that many of those deaf people regard ASL as their native language. ASL is manual communication (primarily hand and arm shapes, positions, and movements) in the form of signs used as a language with a grammatical structure different from the structures of spoken languages. Instead of speech sounds being used as a conventional system of signals, signs are used for the same purpose. Although a few researchers have questioned whether ASL is a bona fide language (Schlesinger & Namir, 1978), most researchers in the field present evidence for its status as a genuine language (Friedman, 1977; Klima & Bellugi, 1979; Siple, 1978; Stokoe, 1960; Wilbur,

1979). There is still question, however, whether it has the characteristics to function as well as do spoken languages for educational and similar purposes. If it is lacking in this respect, however, (and it might not be) it is not necessarily due to any lack as a language. ASL has often been repressed, or at least discouraged, in the educational system and thus has not been free to flower and evolve as have spoken languages.

Although most deaf people use ASL, only a small portion of them acquire it from their parents in infancy and early childhood in the natural, interactive manner in which hearing children absorb spoken language from hearing parents. Only about 3 or 4% of deaf children are born to two deaf parents and fewer than 10% are known to have at least one deaf parent (Rawlings & Jensema, 1977). Obviously, in the typical situation, hearing parents of deaf children do not know ASL. And not all deaf children of deaf parents are exposed to ASL as it has been defined here. Some deaf parents use oral English with their deaf children (Corson, 1973) and others use some variety of manually coded English (Brasel and Quigley, 1977). Thus, only a small percentage of deaf children acquire ASL naturally in infancy and early childhood. Most deaf children learn it from deaf peers who learned it from deaf parents or other deaf peers. This acquisition usually takes place during school years, well after the infant and early childhood years when language is usually and easily acquired.

Manually coded English

Perhaps the most common form of manually coded English is the form where signs are simply produced in English order, without the English inflectional system, and where finger spelling is used for words or concepts which do not have sign equivalents. This is used by many hearing people who know a large number of signs but do not know the structure of sign language and by many deaf people to communicate with such people. It is also used by some highly educated deaf people as an initial language to develop English in their deaf children (Brasel & Quigley, 1977).

There are two ways in which manually coded English systems can be used with deaf children. First, they can be used as the initial communication system between parent and child so that manually coded English becomes the deaf child's initial language. Since the structure (syntax) of this system conforms reasonably well to the structure of spoken and written English, manually coded English presumably can provide a base for the development of reading and writing. Also, since it uses the semantic aspects (signs) of American Sign Language, it can be used as a base for later learning ASL. Second, manually coded English can be used as a bridge from ASL to English for deaf children whose initial language is ASL. In all cases, proponents of the use of manually coded English with deaf children seem to base their claims for its superiority on the fact that it uses the manual communication (signs) of deaf people but conforms to the syntactic structure (syntax) of the language of the general society. This presumably will make the learning of reading easier. There is, however, no substantial research support for these contentions and it might be that they contain a large element of rationalization. A major reason for the continuing popularity of manually coded English, and for the recent great surge in the development and educational use of such systems, is possibly that, when it becomes evident that some form of manual communication needs to be used with many deaf children, manually coded English systems are much easier for hearing teachers, parents, and others to learn and use than is American Sign Language.

In addition to this "naturally" evolved form of manual English, there are a number of invented or contrived systems that have been used with deaf children. Six of the best known invented systems of manual English are described here and other definitions can be found in Caccamise and Drury (1976). The systems differ primarily in how closely they approximate, or claim to approximate, the structure (syntax) of English and in the devices they use to attain this approximation.

Finger spelling. Finger spelling is a means of representing the 26 letters (and also the arabic numerals) of written English by a one-to-one correspondence between the written letters and hand and figure configurations and movements representing the letters (and numerals). This enables one to write English in the air with hand configurations and movements similar to writing on paper with the written alphabet. Two important distinctions between the two forms of writing should be noted. First, alphabetic writing is more-or-less permanent and thus is available for reading at whatever speed the reader chooses and also for rereading as often as desired. Finger spelling is as transitory visually as the speech signals are auditorially. Second, writing is presented spatially, whereas finger spelling, like speech, is presented serially in time. Finger spelling is more analogous to words presented tachistoscopically, one letter at a time, than it is to printed text. This second distinction could mean that, despite the apparent visual similarity of finger spelling and writing, they are processed in quite different ways by the central nervous system. Some studies of this matter are discussed in the chapter dealing with cognitive development.

Linguistics of visual English (LOVE).   This is a system of signs designed for use with preschool and kindergarten deaf children. The signs are supposed to parallel speech rhythm (i.e., a three-syllable word is represented by a three-movement sign). The signs of LOVE bear less resemblance to ASL signs than do the signs of other manually coded English systems. Materials for the system are difficult to find and it is little used now. More detail on it can be found in an article on sign systems by Bornstein (1973).

Seeing essential English (SEE I). This was one of the first of several manual English systems that were developed during the 1960s in response to the apparent lack of success in day programs with purely oral programs. Rather than accepting American Sign Language or the general system of manually coded English used by deaf people and in many residential schools, several innovators devised systems based apparently on two premises: (1) Signs, as gross movements, are more easily read and more easily made by deaf children than speech sounds or finger spelling; and (2) since English is the general language of the United States, deaf children should acquire it as their first language and therefore manually coded English systems should be devised that conformed in detail to written English. SEE I was such a system and was reported by Anthony (1966). It uses ASL signs and signs invented to represent both root words and the inflectional system of English in order to approximate closely the syntactic structure of English.

The system classifies English words into three groups: (1) basic words, (2) compound words, and (3) complex words. The basic words consist of whole word forms or root words. There is not a one-to-one correspondence between English words and signs, so SEE I established three criteria to determine which of several possible signs would be selected for association with a particular word: meaning, spelling, and sound. A single sign is used when any two of the three criteria are the same for two or more English words. For example, the English word *right* has three common meanings (correct, direction, privilege), but the *spelling* and *sound* are the same for the word regardless of which meaning it is conveying. Therefore, SEE I uses a single sign to represent all meanings. Compound words, such as *butterfly*, are signed using the ASL signs for the separate morphemes (the sign for *butter* followed by the sign for *fly*). Markers were devised to represent the English inflectional system and the signs are presented in English word orders. Words that have no ASL sign equivalents are finger spelled (Quigley & King, 1982).

Signing exact English (SEE II). This system is similar to SEE I in many respects but differs in a few important ways, particularly in the treatment of compound and complex words. SEE II classifies English words into three groups as does SEE I: basic, compound, and complex. It also uses the same two-out-of-three (spelling, sound, and meaning) criteria for selection of sign–word associations. The major difference between the two systems is in what constitutes a root word and how compound and complex words are formed. SEE I creates a number of complex words such as *interview* by affixing inflections to root words such as *view,* and treats compound words such as *butterfly* as two root words and uses the signs for each, *butter* and *fly*. This obviously results in sign sequences that are ludicrous in ASL and to people who use ASL. SEE II attempts to remedy this by treating such words as root words and using the single ASL signs for them. In their basic text on the system, Gustason, Pfetzing, and Zawolkow (1975) estimate that SEE II employs approximately 70 affixes and is composed of 61% ASL signs, 18% modified ASL signs, and 21% newly invented signs.

Signed English. This system is a semantic representation of English devised by Bornstein (1973, 1974) to cover the syntax and vocabulary commonly used with deaf children between the ages of 1 and 6 years. ASL signs are used in English word order with 14 sign markers added to represent a portion of the English inflectional system. A dictionary and a number of story books have been produced in which the signs of the system are associated with the printed words of the story in order to teach reading. Finger spelling is used for some words for which signs do not exist. According to Quigley and King (1982) this system remains closer to the ASL use of signs than any of the preceding systems.

Pidgin sign English. This is the use of ASL signs in English word order but with limited use of the English inflectional system. It can vary from signs in strict English order with words being finger spelled for which signs are not available to some forms in which aspects of ASL grammar, such as sign space, pluralization, and directionality, are used. This system is used by well-educated deaf people when they wish to approximate English for communicating using signs and finger spelling (Bragg, 1973).

Although the manually coded English and ASL systems presented here have been discussed as discrete entities, there is frequent borrowing among systems. In addition, many signs have evolved that are used in local communities for specific purposes and do not have national recognition or usage. Also, most manually coded English systems are used in combination with aural/oral communication and are used most frequently as teaching procedures. The combination of finger spelling and speech is known as the *Rochester method* after the Rochester School for the Deaf where it has been used since 1878. The combination of signs, finger spelling, and speech in English word order is known as the *simultaneous method*.

Oral English

This is English in oral form as used among hearing speakers of the language. Two methodologies used with deaf children that rely solely on oral communication are the *aural/oral method* and the *acoupedic (or unisensory) method*. The *aural/oral method* uses speech and speechreading (lipreading) for communication between child and teacher or child and parent and assigns major emphasis to the early and consistent use of high-quality amplification and auditory training (Ling & Ling, 1978). The *acoupedic method* is similar to the *aural/oral method* except that speechreading is minimized and major emphasis is placed on amplification and auditory training in order to utilize as fully as possible the varying amounts of residual hearing that most deaf children have (Pollack, 1964). In both methods, aural development and speech development are seen as the foundations of verbal learning which will allow primary (spoken) and secondary (reading) language forms to develop in similar, although perhaps slower, manner as in hearing children.

Cued speech. This is probably best considered as a separate approach to developing communication and language in deaf children. It involves manual representation of phonetic elements of speech that are not readily visible for speech reading. Eight handshapes are used in four positions to represent those phonetic elements and thus to make speech fully visible for speech reading. The system was deliberately constructed in such a way that it could not function alone as a manual system of communication (Cornett, 1967, 1969).

Another term in common usage today is *total communication* (Denton, 1970). This has been presented as a system and as a philosophy which advocates the use of any and all means of communication by and with deaf children. It could include any or all of the systems that have been presented here.

Language development systems

In addition to using a variety of communication systems with deaf children, teachers have also used a variety of systems or approaches for developing language. Most of the language development approaches can be classified in two major categories: the natural approaches and the structural approaches.

Natural Approaches

The natural approaches treat language holistically and attempt to parallel the ways in which hearing children acquire language. The deaf child is encouraged to acquire language inductively through constant exposure to appropriate language patterns in situations that are structured on the basis of the child's needs and interests. The approach is exemplified by the work of several persons: Friedrich Moritz Hill in Germany in the early and mid-1800s; Mildred Groht in the United States in the early and mid-1900s; and Van Uden in the Netherlands in the 1970s and the present period (Bender, 1960).

Structural approaches

The structural approaches treat language atomistically and analytically and emphasize knowledge of its structure—of the parts and how the parts are related. Attention is focused on parts of speech and syntactic rules and on the students learning these through drills, formal instruction, and a strictly sequenced curriculum. Exemplars of this approach have been de l'Épeé and Sicard in France in the latter half of the 18th century, Clerc and Gallaudet in the United States in the first half of the 19th century, and Edith Fitzgerald in the United States in the first half of the 20th century (Bender, 1960).

Actually, most programs for deaf students probably use elements of both the natural and the structural approaches. Very structured instruction was typical in schools in Europe and the United States until the early part of the 20th century. This might have been due to the fact that the natural approaches (the mother method) were seen as more suited to developing language in infancy and early childhood, whereas most deaf children, until recent decades, did not enter school until 6 years of age or older. There seems still to be a tendency to use developmental techniques (natural approaches) with deaf infants and very young children and to shift more to direct instruction (structural approaches) by age 8 or 10.

HISTORICAL PERSPECTIVES

This is only a brief historical review of the various communication and language systems that have been used with deaf children. Its purpose is to provide perspective to approaches in vogue today by relating them to their historical predecessors. To use an overworked phrase, "What's past is prologue." A better sense of what is being done today, and what perhaps needs to be done in the future, can be gained by a knowledge of what has gone before. Detailed historical accounts of the education of deaf children have been provided by Bender (1960), DeLand (1931), Farrar (1923), Moores (1978), Nelson (1949), and Davis and Silverman (1978). An excellent, detailed, and historically treated presentation of language and communication approaches up to the 1960s has been provided by Schmitt (1966). Some of his material is incorporated in this chapter and is updated to the present decade.

Europe: to 1700

Up to the mid-1700s schools did not generally exist for the education of deaf children, but many deaf children were taught individually or in very small groups by private tutors. Usually, these were children of wealthy and noble families. Some accounts of the communication and language approaches used with these children have been provided in the historical sources previously listed. The first formal instruction seems to have taken place in Spain under the tutelage of the monk Ponce de Leon (1520–1584). From what sketchy accounts are available, de Leon apparently used oral communication and a structural approach to language development. He began with writing (students were older children) by teaching associations of referents (objects, etc.) with their written word. A vocabulary was developed in this way and worked into sentences by formal grammatical instruction. Speech was taught through articulation of written words and the curriculum progressed from language and communication to academic subjects.

Ponce de Leon was followed in Spain by Juan Pablo Bonet (1579–1620). Bonet used a method which proceeded from finger spelling to the articulation of sounds, syllables, and words and to eventual reading and writing. He placed great emphasis upon logical, sequential development of grammar, including formal learning of the parts of speech and memorization of word inflections (Schmitt, 1966). Thus, the communication approach was finger spelling and speech (manual and oral) and the language approach was structural. The combination of finger spelling and speech used by Bonet is a direct precursor of the Rochester method in the United States in the late 1800s and of what has been called neo-oralism in the Soviet Union in the 1950s. The one-handed manual alphabet used by Bonet and described in his book (the first published book on educating deaf children), *The Simplification of Sounds and the Art of Teaching the Dumb to Speak* (Bonet, 1620), is directly related to the one-handed manual alphabet used in the United States today. In contrast, a two-handed alphabet was developed in England, and is still used there and in many of England's former colonies.

John Wallis (England; 1616–1703) and George Dalgarno (England; 1626–1687) were major 17th century figures in England in the education of deaf children. Both used a writing and manual approach to communication but differed in their language approaches. Wallis used a structural approach, beginning with building a vocabulary of word listings according to parts of speech and then relating words through formal grammatical instruction. Dalgarno favored a more natural approach to language. He recommended that the child's mother develop receptive language through the constant use of finger spelling, and he advocated that language be learned through practical use and direct experience. Formal grammar was not used until connected language was well established (Schmitt, 1966).

Europe: The 1700s and 1800s

General, widespread education of deaf children began in the 18th century with the establishment of the first public school in Paris in 1755 by the Abbé Charles Michel de l'Épeé. This century also saw the beginning of the controversy between "French Method" manualists as exemplified by de l'Épeé in France and the "German Method" oralists as exemplified by Samuel Heinicke in Germany. In practice, neither country was wholly one or the other.

In language instruction the structural approaches prevailed. In Holland, John Amman (1669–1724) began by teaching the names of objects and lists of various parts of speech. Later, he developed the vocabulary and parts of speech into connected sentences and larger language units. Samuel Heinicke (1729–1790), in Germany, also used a formal analytical approach to language development, while maintaining strict adherence to speech and speechreading for communication. The prominent 18th century figures in England were Thomas Braidwood (1715–1806) and Henry Baker (1698–1774) who attempted to keep their methods of instructing deaf children secret, but who were reported to use oral communication and structural language approaches (Schmitt, 1966).

The dominant figure of the 18th century was the Abbé de l'Épeé (1712–1789) in France. The Abbé first used the signs of deaf people as the language of instruction. He later developed this language into a sign system to approximate the vocabulary and syntax of the French language. This involved creating signs for words and signs and other devices to function for inflections, tenses, articles and other grammatical parts of French. This system was continued and elaborated by the Abbé Sicard (1742–1822), de l'Épeé's successor, who also compiled an elaborate dictionary of signs. The great similarities between this approach and the modern day approaches in the United States of conforming sign language to the structure of English (LOVE, SEE I, SEE II) are obvious.

De l'Épeé's language instruction used structural approaches. He put little emphasis on original composition and conversation, apparently believing it more within the deaf student's capabilities to memorize sentences for the student's needs and wants. Sicard followed de l'Épeé's methods but put more emphasis on original language. Sicard's methods have been described by one of his prized pupils, Laurent Clerc, (Clerc, 1851). "After the students had learned to sign simple sentences, their language was further developed by use of Sicard's 'theory of ciphers,' a device consisting of five numbered columns: 1. Nominative case; 2. Verb; 3. Objective case; 4. Prepositions; 5. Object of the preposition" (Schmitt, 1966). As will be seen later, this is similar to the Fitzgerald key, which was widely used in the United States during the early and mid-20th century and is still in use. Schmitt points out that the predominantly grammatical (structural) orientation of the 19th century was evidenced by Clerc's complaint that of the 44 verb inflections and modes, each containing affirmative, negative, and interrogative forms, most deaf children were able to "rehearse" only 15 to 20.

Although the structural approach to language was dominant in the 18th and 19th centuries, some notable attempts were made to use a more natural approach. Jacob Pereire (1715–1780) in France, Joseph Watson (1765–1829) in England, and Guilio Tarra in Italy (1832–1899) emphasized the need to develop language in a natural fashion and related to the child's needs through meaningful situations. The teaching of grammar to deaf students was deemphasized by these teachers. This did not mean, however, a deemphasis of grammatical knowledge by the teacher of deaf children. As stated by Guilio Tarra, the teacher should be acutely aware of grammar but should not "inflict it on the feeble understanding" of the students. This is in line with the approach of the present book where it is posited that teachers of deaf children should be extremely knowledgeable about many aspects of communication and language (including grammar) in order to be able to construct situations and materials which will foster the natural development of language in deaf children, without directly teaching the mechanics or metalanguage to the children.

The most influential advocate of the natural approach to language in the latter part of the 19th century was Friedrich Moritz Hill (1805–1874) in Germany. He attempted, by his "mother's method," to parallel the way in which the hearing child naturally absorbs language from conversational interaction with the parents, usually the mother. Hill used conversational oral language in the early stages of instruction and developed reading and writing later. He believed that deaf children could be motivated to learn language by perceiving its usefulness as a means to satisfying their needs.

A climactic event in the 19th century in the communication and language approaches used with deaf children was the historic International Congress at Milan in 1880, presided over by Guilio Tarra. The members of the Congress strongly endorsed the use of oral approaches in communication and natural approaches in language development with deaf students. As Schmitt (1966) concludes, "Most countries were swift to adopt oral methods and educators became increasingly interested in the natural approach to language."

The United States: The 1800s

The formal education of deaf children in the United States is considered to have begun with the establishment of a residential school, (now the American School for the Deaf) in Hartford, Connecticut in 1817 by Thomas Hopkins Gallaudet. Gallaudet had visited the Braidwoods in England to acquire a knowledge of their methods. He did not succeed in this due to the secrecy maintained by the Braidwoods and their opposition to Gallaudet's intent to learn manual as well as oral methods of educating deaf children. Gallaudet then met with Sicard, who was traveling in England with one of his star pupils, Jean Massieu, and accepted an invitation to study at the school in Paris. Having learned the methods instituted there by de l'Épeé and Sicard, Gallaudet returned to the United States, bringing with him a deaf teacher and former student at the Paris school, Laurent Clerc. Thus began two traditions that have distinguished American education of deaf children from European systems—manual communication and deaf teachers.

Language approaches

Gallaudet and Clerc also brought to the United States the structural approaches to language development that were used in the Paris school. Clerc's methods of language instruction have previously been described. These structural approaches and manual communication reigned supreme in the United States until the establishment of the Clarke School for the Deaf in Northampton, Massachusetts in 1867 and the establishment of what is now known as the Lexington School for the Deaf in New York City shortly thereafter. In fact, manual communication and the structural teaching of language were dominant in the education of deaf children in the United States for almost a century. Oral methods of communication began with the Clarke School for the Deaf in 1867 but did not gain much ground until after the International Congress at Milan in 1880 and the establishment of day schools about 1869 and day class programs about the turn of the century. Day schools and day classes were almost completely oral until the late 1960s and early 1970s.

During the 19th century, various symbol systems and diagrams were devised to assist in language instruction with deaf children, and such devices have continued to play a significant role in structural approaches to language teaching. According to Schmitt (1966), the first such symbol system was devised by Barnard in 1836. It consisted of six simple straight-line and curved-line symbols that represented word relationships that were "substantive, attributive, connective, or showed assertion, influence, or time" (Nelson, 1949). In the 1870s, Richard Storrs devised 47 "Storrs' symbols" for use in the study of grammar. These symbols could be written above the words in a sentence to indicate such things as parts of speech, person, gender, tense, type, degree, and various inflections. The Wing's symbols (Wing, 1887) came next and consisted of letters, numbers, and other symbols placed above words to represent their forms and functions in a sentence. The eight "essential symbols" were

S = subject; V = verb (with three modifications of the V to specify the verb as transitive, intransitive, or passive); O = object; AC = adjective complement; N = noun and pronoun complement. The system also included numbers from 1 to 7 for modifying forms, six connective symbols, and 14 special symbols for such things as verb tense, types of objective cases, and other grammatical relations. These symbols are still in use in a few schools in the United States. Two other visual display and diagram systems were constructed by McKee (1895) and Robinson (1898). Neither of these devices was adopted by other educators and they have only historical interest. The most widely known and used visual system is the Fitzgerald key (Fitzgerald, 1929) which belongs to the 20th century.

Along with the various visual symbol systems for use in the structural teaching of language, a number of curricula, texts, and readers oriented to the structural approach also appeared in the 19th century. The language textbooks of Peet (1869, 1870) were widely used. These books began by establishing a 50-word vocabulary in writing and finger spelling. The books then progressed through a series of lessons devoted to vocabulary, phrase, and sentence building. Sentences began with present tense verbs and progressed to the other tenses. In general, language was introduced in a systematic and orderly fashion and in small steps. Other reading and language texts produced during the 19th century are listed in Nelson (1949).

Although grammaticism dominated language instruction with deaf children in the United States during the 19th century, there were supporters of the natural approaches also. The foremost of these was David Greenberger (1878, 1879), principal of what is now known as the Lexington School for the Deaf in New York City. This school, through the efforts of Greenberger and later of Mildred Groht, became the seat of what is now known as the natural method (Groht, 1958). Greenberger opposed memorization of sentences and of language rules and principles and urged the teaching of language in context and in natural and meaningful situations. A similar approach was advocated by Alexander Graham Bell (Bell, 1883), but Greenberger must be considered the chief advocate and developer in the United States of the "mother's method" of the German, Friedrich Moritz Hill.

Communication approaches

Although this brief history of the 1800s indicates that considerable interest and activity in language development and teaching took place in that century, American educators were also occupied with debates on communication methods. Not all educators in the early part of the century agreed with Thomas Hopkins Gallaudet and Laurent Clerc on the merits of signs. Even when signs were the accepted mode of communication, there were disagreements about the type of signs to be used (Keep, 1853). But the sign based methods of the school at Hartford, Connecticut dominated public and private residential schools throughout most of the century.

The oral methods introduced at the Clarke School for the Deaf in 1867 and shortly thereafter at what is now the Lexington School for the Deaf exerted their major influence on the programs of day schools and day classes for deaf children. The first day school was the Horace Mann School for the Deaf established in Roxbury, Massachusetts in 1869. Other day schools were gradually established in major population centers and around the turn of the 20th century day class programs began. Day programs flourished mightily in the 1940s and 1950s, and by the mid-1960s surpassed the residential schools in enrollment of deaf children.

The United States: The 1900s

Language approaches

According to Schmitt (1966), the most widely used language device during the early 1900s was the *five slate system* devised by Katharine Barry (Barry, 1899). This system was a structural approach to language and was related to Sicard's "theory of ciphers." The five slates provided deaf children with a fixed, visible sentence skeleton into which simple language could be fitted with parts of a sentence related to each of the five slates: subject, verb, object of the verb, preposition, and object of the preposition. Sentences and language principles were sequenced in order of increasing difficulty to form a complete plan for language development.

During the early decades of the present century, educators continued to produce language texts to fit the needs of deaf children. A major event was the production of a widely used four-volume series of language practice books by Croker, Jones, and Pratt (1920, 1922, 1928). Each book contained a series of four-page weekly lessons consisting of (1) a story with new vocabulary and examples of the language principle to be developed, (2) practice in writing questions (to given answers) and formal review drills on previous materials, (3) questions to be answered by the student, and (4) exercises based on the new language principle being taught. The selections ranged from very short, simple stories in the beginning book to simplified versions of classics in the fourth book. The language principles are presented in sequenced cumulative fashion. Not only were the books widely used in the 1920s, they still are used in a number of programs today, 60 years after their first publication. These books are the forerunners of special materials being prepared for deaf children in the present time.

Another major event in the early 1900s was the development of the Fitzgerald key by Edith Fitzgerald as described in her book, *Straight Language for the Deaf,* published in 1929. This has been probably the most widely used device for the structural teaching of language to deaf children. The key consists of six columns headed by interrogative words and symbols indicating parts of speech and sentence functions: (1) subject (who:, what:); (2) verb and predicate words; (3) indirect and direct objects (what:, whom:); (4) phrases and words telling where; (5) other phrases and word modifiers of the main verb (for:, from:, how:, how often:, how much:, etc.); (6) words and phrases telling when. The key can be used to build language in deaf children starting with very simple sentences that will use only two or three of the columns such as who: what: (subject), and = (verb) and working up to compound and complex sentences. Connective symbols are supplied for constructing compound sentences. The key is still used in many programs in the United States.

The natural approach in the 1900s is exemplified by the book, *Natural Language for Deaf Children* by Mildred Groht (Groht, 1958). Groht is an ardent and articulate advocate of the approach used in the Lexington School for the Deaf since the time of Greenberger in the 1870s. Language is considered, in this approach, to be a means to an end rather than an end in itself; as something that is developed and acquired rather than taught and learned. Groht discusses and explains many principles for developing language rather than teaching it. Some of these principles are (1) vocabulary and connected language must be supplied according to the child's needs rather than according to rigid lists of words and language principles; (2) natural language is acquired by repetition in meaningful situations rather than by drill and textbook exercises; (3) language use is best taught through conversation and discussion, written composition of many kinds, and through academic and skill areas of the curriculum; (4) when language principles need to be taught they should be introduced incidentally in natural situations, then explained by the teacher in a real situation, then practiced by the children through use of games, questions, stories, and conversations. The emphasis in this approach is on providing meaningful language repetitively in a variety of natural situations so as to enable students to unconsciously induce language principles rather than being taught them. It should be noted that, although language principles and structure are not taught to the children, the *teacher* must know a great deal about language structure and language principles in order to devise the situations for successful teaching of language by this approach. Some form of the natural approach to language development is widely used in programs for deaf children today.

Recent times

Language approaches

During the past 20 years, the decades of the 1960s and 1970s, there have been new developments in the natural approaches, the structural approaches, and the development of special language and reading materials for deaf children. The book, by A. van Uden, *A World of Language for Deaf Children,* (1977) continues and expands the natural approach to language development. It incorporates findings from the vast amount of psycholinguistic research conducted in the 1960s and 1970s as a result of the revolution in linguistic thinking produced by the publications of Noam Chomsky, *Syntactic Structures* (1957) and *Aspects of the Theory of Syntax* (1965). In *Sentences and other Systems* Blackwell, Engen, Fischgrund, and Zarcadoolas (1978) applied the linguistic research resulting from Chomsky's work to constructing a patterned-sentence language curriculum for deaf children which continues the structural approach. A national survey by King (1983) showed that the *Apple Tree* program (Anderson, Boren, Caniglia, Howard, & Krohn, 1980), is apparently the most widely used structural program at present in the United States. Quigley and a group of colleagues applied the linguistic developments of the 1960s and 1970s to constructing a syntax test (Test of Syntactic Abilities; Quigley, Steinkamp, Power, & Jones, 1978), language materials (*The TSA Syntax Program;* Quigley & Power, 1979), and a reading series (*Reading Milestones;* Quigley & King, 1981, 1982, 1983, 1984) for deaf children, thus continuing the development of special materials.

These, and other, developments of recent times will be presented in more detail in various chapters. They are mentioned here to show that there are several threads running through the evolution of language development and instruction with deaf children from the earliest to the most recent times. These threads are (1) natural approaches to language development, which emphasize development of language in meaningful situations based on needs and interests of the child and involving fluent communicative interaction in some form between the child and a language model, (2) structural approaches to language which involve more direct teaching of the form and structure of language to the child, and (3) development of special language materials and curricula for deaf children.

Communication approaches

Until the late 1960s and early 1970s, day schools and day classes were almost exclusively oral as were a number of private residential schools. The oral approach of the 19th century became the aural/oral approach of the 20th century with the advent of, and rapid improvements in, electronic amplification. In addition to using the speech and speech reading of the oral method and the developing devices for amplification, the aural/oral methods used the auditory training methods developed by Urbantschitz in Austria and elaborated in the United States by Goldstein who established the Central Institute for the Deaf in St. Louis, Missouri in 1914. An offshoot of the aural/oral methods was the acoupedic (or unisensory) method which emphasized the use of audition and deemphasized the use of vision in the early education of deaf children (Pollack, 1964).

During the early and mid-1900s, aural/oral methods were used in most day school and day class programs and in a number of private residential schools. In these programs, deaf children were usually discouraged from using manual communication in any form. Most public residential schools also used aural/oral methods with young children; however, many of these schools continued to use manual communication, in some form, with older children and permitted free use of manual communication by all children and by school personnel outside of the classrooms. This pattern of communication approaches with deaf children continued in the United States until about 1970.

The great increases in financial support and public and governmental interest in general education during the 1960s spilled over into special education, including the education of deaf children. Dissatisfaction was expressed with the low literacy levels that prevailed among deaf children and, in the spirit of the times, there was renewed interest in research and in trying new methods. A pioneering publication, *Sign Language Structure: An Outline of the Visual Communication Systems of the American Deaf*, by Stokoe (1960), pointed the way to renewed interest and study in American Sign Language. Coupled with the vast increase in research in linguistics and psycholinguistics resulting from the publications of Chomsky (1957, 1965), Stokoe's work led to an influx of linguists into research on ASL. In addition to Stokoe's outstanding contributions (1960, 1971, 1972), there are now a dozen or more recent books on the grammar and teaching of ASL, a considerable body of research literature in professional journals, courses in a number of linguistics departments, and a cadre of linguistic and psycholinguistic researchers in a number of universities with major interest in ASL. There is growing interest and support for the concept of developing ASL as the first language of deaf children and developing English along with it in some form in a bilingual situation or developing English later as a second language. There will be more on this in other chapters of this book.

Along with the resurgence of American Sign Language, the 1960s and 1970s witnessed the development of several systems of manually coded English, some of which are now widely used with deaf children in the United States. It has been estimated that about 65% of deaf children in this country are now taught with some combination of manual and oral communication (Jordan, Gustason, & Rosen, 1976). The effect has been greatest in day programs where instruction by manually coded English now prevails. The various forms of manually coded English have been defined previously and will be discussed in other chapters.

PRESENT STATUS OF LANGUAGE PERFORMANCE

In spite of almost 200 years of effort in the United States and more than 300 in Europe, only limited success has been achieved in developing language in deaf children to the extent where it serves as an adequate vehicle for educational development. This is best typified by performance on reading achievement measures and written language samples. It will be recalled that, in the Preface, these two variables were identified as criteria against which the success of educational programs for deaf children could be measured. Detailed information on the performance of deaf children on these and other aspects of language performance will be discussed in various chapters. The goal here is simply to give an idea of the present status of language performance of deaf children.

Reading

Some of the earliest work on reading assessment was done by Pintner and Patterson (1916) in the early part of the present century. They found in several national studies that the median scores of deaf students at any age on reading measures never reached the median for 8-year-old hearing children. The most recent national study (Trybus & Karchmer, 1977) showed essentially the same level of performance almost exactly 60 years later. Trybus and Karchmer found, for a stratified, random sample of 6,871 deaf students, that the median reading score at age 20 years and older was a grade equivalent of 4.5. Only about 10% of the students in the best reading group (18 years of age) could read at or above the eighth-grade level. In later chapters it will be documented that a similar level of reading performance is typical of deaf students in other countries and of deaf adults.

Syntax

Performance on measures of syntax tends to be indicative of the structure of the internalized language with which the subject is operating and to be reflected in reading and written performance. Quigley and a group of colleagues studied the comprehension of various syntactic structures by a stratified, random sample of approximately 450 deaf students in the United States and found that 8-year-old hearing children could outperform the average 18-year-old deaf student. When given such sentences as these:

Passive	The boy was helped by the girl.
Relative	The boy who kissed the girl ran away.
Complement	The boy learned the ball broke the window.
Nominal	The opening of the door surprised the cat.

the deaf students often comprehended them as the following:

The boy helped the girl.

The girl ran away.

The boy learned the ball.

The door surprised the cat.

It was also found, from analysis of a reading series, that these deaf students, even at 18 years of age, had considerable difficulty understanding syntactic structures that appeared in the very beginning reading books (Quigley, Wilbur, Power, Montanelli, & Steinkamp, 1976).

Written language

Probably the best single indicator of a deaf child's command of English is the quality of the child's spontaneously produced written language, but there are no good, valid, and reliable techniques for assessing this. The following samples, however, are "typical" of the performance of deaf students. Age, gender, and HTL are given after each sample.

> The girl said give the dog into the bread. The Father he go to the far. Father and Mother Wait for you the dog. We go to the park the famils show she is paly with the dog. The boy said help please. The grandpa he hepl is little boy he afriad show. The grandpa is can hepl. The little boy he cry. [10 year old female, better ear average 110 + dB (ASA) deaf prior to 2 years of age]

> The children have a picnic in the park. Mother take false glass and put on the table. The girl gave the dog some bread or meat. She like the dog. Then we drive to anywhere. The children in and watch the front to watch to the people. The boy saw the dog. The dog barked to him. The dog wanted in the car and play with children. The father mother and sister was happy to see dog. The boy hold the dog. He licked him. He laughed and laughed to him. Again, we went to the picnic to the park, and so they plan the food on the table. The children played a baseball game. Mother cook the hamburge on the fire. She looked the girl how to doing it. We have lot of fun. They liked another place to the park. [14 year old female, better ear average 100 + dB (ASA), deaf prior to 2 years of age]

> On this spring, the family went on a picnic. The young boy named was Bobby, and his sister named was Betty, Her mother and betty fixed the meat and cheese in the sandwich, and to the bag, then they put the bag into the basket. His father and Bobby pick up the blanket, baseball, gloves, ball, bat, and other thing, and his father took them, and he carried to his car.

> When they left from house, and Bobby asked to father that he wants his dog can go with them, and his father said "no." Then they went out and Bobby was very sad because his dog stayed here. Then his father drove the car, and through the town, and his mother said that she wants his dog go with them to a picnic, and his father said "OK," then they returned to his house. Bobby was happy because the dog can go with us, and he carried his dog to the car. [18 year old male, better ear average 100 + dB (ASA), deaf prior to 2 years of age]

Thus, it can be seen that the present situation for reading is one of low performance on standard reading tests, with large numbers of deaf students never reaching the level of functional literacy (fourth-grade reading level). Even lower performance is indicated when specific aspects of reading, such as syntax, are assessed. Studies of written language show similar low levels of attainment. It seems apparent that many deaf children neither read nor write the English language even adequately, and this is reflected in low educational performance in general.

SUMMARY AND CONCLUSIONS

Communication approaches

Although the emphasis in this book is on language and its development in deaf children, language is inextricably linked with communication and so communication forms must receive attention also. The various communication forms that have been used with deaf children during the past 200–300 years, and are still used today, can be classified under three major categories which represent two modes of communication, oral and manual, and two languages, English and American Sign Language. The major categories and subcategories are these.

Oral English
  Aural/oral
  Acoupedic (or unisensory) procedures
  Cued speech
Manually coded English
  General manually coded English
  Finger spelling
  Linguistics of visual English (LOVE)
  Seeing essential English (SEE I)
  Signing exact English (SEE II)
  Signed English
  Pidgin sign English
American Sign Language

The various communication modes and languages have been used singly or in combination to form teaching methods which have been widely used at various times. The *oral method*, which uses speech and speechreading as the primary means of communicating with and by deaf students, has its roots in the work of Ponce de Leon in Spain in the 16th century, of Samuel Heinicke, the founder of the German method in the 18th century, and of the Clarke School for the Deaf in the United States in the 19th century. This became the *aural/oral method* with the advent of electronic amplification (hearing aids) and the auditory training techniques developed by Urbantschitz in Austria and Goldstein at Central Institute for the Deaf in the United States in the early part of the 20th century. It is most commonly known as the auditory/visual/oral (AVO) method. The *acoupedic (or unisensory) method* is related to the *aural/oral method* but emphasizes amplification and auditory training and deemphasizes speechreading in the early stages of education.

The combination of speech and finger spelling is known as the *Rochester method* after the Rochester School for the Deaf where it was established by Zenos Westervelt in 1878. This method is directly related to the methods used by Juan Pablo Bonet, of Spain, who advocated the use of a combination of a one-handed manual alphabet and speech in his book published in 1620. This method had a resurgence in the Soviet Union in the 1950s under the name of *new-oralism* and in the United States in the 1960s.

Manually coded English, in some form, has been in use in programs for deaf students in the United States since the time of Gallaudet and Clerc. In the late 1960s and the 1970s, however, it achieved greatly increased popularity and usage through the development of several forms (SEE I, SEE II, Signed English) which have been defined and discussed. These systems use signs of ASL and invented signs in the structure of standard English. De l'Épée and Sicard in Paris in the late 18th century made similar attempts to conform the French language of signs to the structure of French. It is interesting to note that these efforts in France resulted in making the language of signs slower and more cumbersome to use, and the original French language of signs gradually reasserted itself (Moores, 1978). A similar occurrence seems to be taking place in the United States (Marmor & Pettito, 1979). The *simultaneous method* is the simultaneous use of oral and manual communication, usually with English structure. *Total communication* is a term for the philosophy or system which permits any and all methods of communication to be used with deaf children.

American Sign Language is probably not used systematically in any programs for deaf children in the United States, but it perhaps ought to be. This will be discussed in other chapters and in the final summation and synthesis of the book. Most of the information on the use and effects of ASL with deaf children comes from studies of deaf children of deaf parents and these, too, will be discussed later. It is possible that ASL will receive a great deal of attention and support during the next decade for use with deaf children in the home and in the school.

Language approaches

In this chapter, the various methods used in language development and instruction with deaf children have been classified under *natural approaches* and *structural approaches*. It is likely, however, that teachers are a great deal more eclectic than writers of textbooks and that elements of both approaches can be found in most programs. Schmitt (1966) listed a number of principles that seemed to represent the best practice in programs for deaf children at that time. Some of them are paraphrased here because they still seem current.

1. Multisensory channels (vision, audition, taction) should be used in language development and instruction.

2. The language that is developed and taught should be truly useful to the child.

3. Language should be taught in meaningful situations and contexts.

4.   Language should be considered a means to an end rather than an end in itself.

5.   Language learning must be begun as early in life as possible, preferably in infancy.

6.   Language is considered truly acquired when the child uses it spontaneously.

7.   Language acquisition is a continuous process and not simply a product of the classroom.

8.   The child's needs and interests should be the prime determiner of the content and sequence of language programs, although outlines and curricula may be useful as guides.

9.   The goal of language programs should be "automatic" language; formal devices and prompts should be considered temporary crutches and should be withdrawn as soon as possible.

These principles are in keeping with what have been defined here as the natural approaches to language. They also are consonant with the recent research on child language development. And they represent the major point of view of language development in this book.

A strong caution is in order. Although most hearing children acquire language in an easy interactive manner, and although procedures with deaf children should approach the model for hearing children as closely as possible, much structural knowledge about language is required on the part of the teacher to do this well. To use an analogy, the average person can be a skilled automobile driver with absolutely no knowledge of how an internal combustion engine works, just as the typical hearing person can use language fluently with no formal knowledge of its structure and function. But one cannot design, build, or repair that engine without a great deal of detailed knowledge about how it works. Similarly with the teacher of deaf children: That teacher must have detailed knowledge of many aspects of communication and language in order to design a language development program for deaf children and in order to use remedial techniques at older ages, if that becomes necessary.

Another caution is appropriate. A good case can be made that about every communication system and language method that could be applied to deaf children has been applied at one time or another and usually with limited success in the case of the *average* child. For example, the natural, interactive procedures emphasized in language development with deaf children today are strikingly similar to those advocated by Groht (1958) in the mid-1950s, by Greenberger (1879) in the latter half of the 19th century, and by Hill in the mid-1800s. Yet those procedures, in the past and in the present, have met with limited success and teachers find it necessary to use more structural approaches as the child grows older. This is pointed out to stress another viewpoint of the present book—the teacher of deaf children should know as much about language and communication content, development, and instructional methods as the teacher of any subject needs to know about that subject. This means being knowledgeable about, and proficient in, oral English, manually coded English, and American Sign Language; the various natural and structural approaches to language development and instruction and the content and skill areas in normal language and communication that underly these; and in methods of bilingualism and the learning of English as a second language.

chapter 2

Cognition and language

Two questions have engaged the interest of researchers in the areas of cognition (thinking) and language, and resolution of these questions has practical significance for teachers, clinicians, and other practitioners with deaf children and adults. First, there is theoretical and practical significance to knowing whether quantitative or qualitative differences exist between deaf and hearing people on various aspects of cognitive functioning such as memory, perception, creativity, and so forth. If certain differences do exist, they might indicate limitations on deaf persons' abilities to acquire particular cognitively based skills that are acquired readily by hearing people (such as reading), or they might dictate that in order to acquire those skills different developmental and teaching approaches need to be used with deaf children than are used with hearing children. Second, study of the cognitive and language functioning of deaf individuals might shed light on the persistent philosophic and scientific question of whether there is a relation between language and thought and if there is, what is the nature of it. Is language dependent on thought; is thought dependent on language; are the two mutually dependent; or are they mutually independent? This question, too, has practical significance. For example, if language is dependent on thought (cognition), then any differences or deficits in cognitive development will likely affect language acquisition.

Pintner and a group of colleagues, starting in the 1910s, were among the first to study these questions (and the psychology of deafness) in a systematic way with deaf people, and their resulting research conclusions led to the first of three positions that have been taken on the first question. This was that deaf people were intellectually inferior to hearing people and showed definite deficits in various aspects of cognitive functioning (Pintner & Reamer, 1920; Pintner, Eisenson, & Stanton, 1941). It is important to note that most of the tests used by these investigators were paper-and-pencil tests which often required verbal manipulation and verbal responses in the English language. Much of the historical development in the study of cognitive functioning of deaf people is a history of increasingly successful attempts by investigators to devise truly nonverbal tests of cognition. The goal is to assess the deaf person's performance on cognitive tasks, such as sequential memory, without the involvement of language. This is extremely difficult because of the pervasive influence of language in most of human behavior, but as attempts to accomplish it have been increasingly successful, differences between deaf and hearing persons in various cognitive abilities have tended to decrease and often to disappear.

The theoretical position of Pintner and his colleagues was dominant until the 1940s when it was challenged by the formulations proposed by Myklebust (1960). Myklebust interpreted a series of studies by him and a number of his students as showing that there are quantitative similarities but qualitative differences between deaf and hearing individuals when verbal factors in cognitive and intellectual tasks are controlled. The types of differences found by Myklebust and his students led him to conclude that on global measures (e.g., total score on IQ tests such as the WISC) deaf individuals equaled hearing individuals, but that the profiles of deaf and hearing individuals on specific abilities differed. That is, deaf and hearing persons performed differently on the various subtests of such tests as the WISC. Similar findings were revealed on tests of a variety of cognitive functions such as memory and creativity. The findings led Myklebust to conclude that deaf individuals were more concrete and less abstract cognitively than hearing individuals. He further concluded that the basic experiences of deaf people are altered as a direct consequence of hearing impairment and that all subsequently developed behaviors are also altered thus making the deaf person inherently different from the hearing person in many ways. Myklebust proposed the "organismic shift hypothesis" to explain these alleged inherent differences of deaf people.

The third stage of this historical perspective is the one that seems to prevail today—that deaf people are intellectually and cognitively similar to hearing people in all important abilities. Rosenstein (1961), Furth (1966b) and Vernon (1967) have taken the position that few if any differences exist between deaf and hearing individuals in cognitive functioning. This position is based on a substantial body of research conducted by numerous individuals (mostly in the 1960s and 1970s), some of which is discussed in this chapter. It is now generally accepted by researchers that any differences that do exist between deaf and hearing individuals on cognitive abilities are the result of environmental or task influences rather than being inherent in deafness. Quigley and Kretschmer (1982, p. 51) categorized these task influences as: "1) the inability of the researcher to properly convey the task demands because of language differences or deficits on the part of the subjects, 2) implicit bias within the solution of the task, or 3) general experiential deficits (including verbal language and communication in general) on the part of the subjects."

The second question posed, concerning the relationship between cognition and language, has also had various answers at different historical stages. The early position (known as the language dominant position) was that language was primary and that thinking (beyond early and primitive stages) took place in language. This position is exemplified by the linguist Sapir (1958) who states that

> It is quite an illusion to imagine that one adjusts to reality without the use of language and that language is merely an incidental means of solving specific problems of communication or reflection... we see and hear and otherwise experience as we do because the language habits of our community predispose certain choices of interpretation. (p. 162)

In this view, the child's linguistic development is determined largely by experience with language, and language accounts for the acquisition of concepts that are expressed within it (Quigley & Kretschmer, 1982). The opposing (and the presently prevailing) view is the cognitive dominant hypothesis which proposes that basic perceptual and cognitive development precedes language and provides the basis or underpinning for linguistic development. Language, in this view, is a natural extension or subset of the previously developed cognitive processes.

The present evidence does not appear to support the language dominant hypothesis (also known as the Whorfian hypothesis). Studies of hearing children by numerous investigators (notably Piaget and his followers) and of deaf children (notably Furth and his colleagues) have shown that much perceptual and cognitive development takes place prior to language development and also concurrently but independently of early language development. In Piaget's view,

> A symbolic function exists which is broader than language and encompasses both the system of verbal signs and that of symbols in the strict sense...it is permissable to conclude that thought precedes language...language is not enough to explain thought, because the structures that characterize thought have their roots in action and in sensorimotor mechanisms that are deeper than linguistics. (1967, pp. 91–92)

Although the present weight of empirical evidence does not seem to support the language dominant (Whorfian) hypothesis, a number of recent investigators have presented a weaker version of this hypothesis (Cromer, 1976; Schlesinger, 1977; McNeill, 1978). This weak form of the Whorfian hypothesis suggests that although language does not dictate thought, it can and does influence thought. The evidence for this position comes primarily from linguistic intuitions rather than from direct studies of cognitive and linguistic development. It has been pointed out, for example, that there are certain distinctions made in languages, such as gender and verb transitivity, that are language specific, and do not have real world correlates or referents.

It is not the purpose of this chapter to analyze in depth the enduring question of the relationship between thought (cognition) and language. The present weight of evidence in favor of the cognitive dominant hypothesis is accepted. Interest in the issue and in the comparative cognitive functioning of deaf and of hearing individuals is concerned with how it, and more importantly the data collected in pursuing it, can illuminate the problem of language development in deaf individuals. This interest is centered in two questions. First, how does the cognitive development of deaf individuals compare with the cognitive development of hearing individuals? Second, what are the internal symbolic mediators of thought in deaf people?

Both questions have direct implications for educational practice with deaf children and youth. As stated earlier, it follows from the cognitive dominant hypothesis that problems (differences or deficits) in cognitive development will be reflected in problems in language development. In relation to the second question, hearing people are known to use their initial phonologically based language as an internal mediator (internal speech) in various thinking tasks and to a certain extent in reading. It is important to developing language and reading in deaf children to know what internal codes they use (visual imagery, internal speech, signs, manual alphabet, etc.) as symbolic mediators. In pursuing answers to these questions, some definitions and background information are presented. Then research in three areas is examined: (1) research on how deaf persons perform on certain cognitive tasks in comparison to hearing people; (2) research on the coding and mediating processes that deaf people use to perform certain cognitive tasks as compared to those used by hearing people; and (3) the language systems deaf persons use as mediators of thought. Finally, some conclusions are presented to show the implications for language development practices with deaf children.

DEFINITIONS AND BACKGROUND INFORMATION

Slobin (1979) has defined *cognition* as the processes and structures of knowing, and the branch of psychology which studies knowing, including the study of perception, attention, memory, problem solving, thinking, and language. It can be seen that this is a cognitive dominant point of view which includes language as an extension or subset of cognition. *Language* has been defined as "a code whereby ideas about the world are represented through a conventional system of signals for communication" (Bloom & Lahey, 1978, p. 4). This definition is broad enough to include any conventionalized symbol system such as American Sign Language (ASL) as well as the more typical spoken languages.

Much of the cognitive research with deaf individuals has been influenced by the work of the Swiss psychologist, Jean Piaget. Piaget (1955) portrays the child as progressing through four stages to the development of mature thinking. The first stage is the period of *sensorimotor* intelligence and typically occupies the first 2 years of life. During this period, the child perceives and reacts to sensory data as related to basic needs and begins to organize and integrate these data into schemas. He/she goes through a process of establishing an equilibrium between adapting to the environment (accomodation) and acting upon the environment (assimilation). Interactions between accomodation and assimilation further develop schemas as the child's representations of experience. According to Yussen and Santrock (1978) these schemas are the units necessary for an organized pattern of sensorimotor functioning. The child, for example, will organize the schema for face as an integrated pattern of eyes, nose, and mouth in a spatial relationship to each other. Schema theory has become a highly developed area of cognitive psychology and has been incorporated into modern theories of reading as will be discussed in chapter 4.

Piaget's second stage is known as the *preoperational* stage of cognitive development and extends from about 2 to about 7 years of age. This represents a period of establishing relationships between experience and action. The child's symbol system is expanding during this period and language use and perceptual abilities continue to develop well beyond the child's capabilities at the end of Stage 1 (Yussen & Santrock, 1978). In this stage, egocentrism prevents the child from separating his perspective from that of others and is manifested in the child's social interactions. In this stage, also, the child is limited in his cognitive processes by inability to understand such basic Piagetian concepts as conservation and reversibility. The classic Piagetian example of conservation and reversibility is the ball of clay which when changed into another shape still retains the same mass and can be restored to its original shape. Another example is the volume of water remaining the same when poured from a short wide glass into a tall narrow one. Again the process can be reversed. Such concepts are difficult for children to grasp until they reach what Piaget calls the *concrete operations* stage.

The *concrete operations* stage is the third of Piaget's four stages of cognitive development and extends from about 7 to about 11 years of age. The child is now capable of distinguishing himself from others (egocentrism and relativism), and begins to understand such concepts as conservation and reversibility (Yussen & Santrock, 1978). The final stage is *formal operational thought* which begins at about 11 years of age. This stage is characterized primarily by abstract thinking and a shift from the need for concrete objects and experiences.

Piaget divides the development of children's language into two stages. The first stage includes egocentric speech which emerges from noncommunicative thought. This involves monologues and language play where the child repeats simply for the pleasure of talking. The second stage involves socialized speech which develops to include eventually all the forms required for social communication such as information, criticism, commands, requests, questions, and so forth. Piaget does not specifically attach importance to language as a major influence on cognitive development.

Various psychological investigators have used deaf children and adults as controls in examining the existence of these Piagetian stages of development. The assumption has been that deaf children lack formal symbolic language and thus cognitive development can be examined in the absence of language influence, something which is difficult to do with hearing children where language is so pervasive that it is difficult to devise cognitive tasks that are symbol free. One of the foremost investigators was Hans Furth whose book, *Thinking without Language* (1966b), presents much of the early Piagetian research with deaf children.

Several cautions should be observed in interpreting the work of Furth and others in this area who have assumed that deaf children used as subjects in these investigations have been truly nonverbal. First, as is unfortunately true with much other research using deaf individuals, hearing threshold levels are not given in some cases and in others subjects had thresholds as low as 60 dB (probably ASA standards). At least some of those subjects must have had internal auditory based language which could have contaminated experimental results. Also, Conrad (1973) has shown that even some deaf (90+ dB, ISO) children use internal speech as a mediating code. Finally, it cannot be assumed that because deaf children are deficient in standard oral English that they are deficient in language abilities in general. As will be shown in this chapter, many deaf individuals might be using internal language-mediating coding systems other than speech codes.

PERFORMANCE ON COGNITIVE TASKS

Furth (1966b) perceived his research as confirming that cognitive operations exist largely independent of language and that language is of minor concern in investigating cognition. His research can also be interpreted, however, as being supportive of the view that language and its acquisition are a natural outgrowth and direct result of basic cognitive processes and operations. According to this orientation, it is the dominance (but not independence) of cognition over language that explains why deaf individuals are able to function adequately in most situations even though they have not acquired fluent command of the core culture's language. Furth's investigations were characterized by the construction of ingenious tasks for assessing various thinking processes and by their comprehensive coverage of the various stages in Piaget's theory of cognitive development. The research of Furth and other investigators discussed here is only a sampling of a large literature. The research is organized in several sections. The first attempts to present an overview of the research based directly on Piagetian theory. Other sections deal with the more specific processes of memory, abstract thinking, and creativity all of which relate importantly to language acquisition.

Piagetian tasks

As stated earlier, one of the greatest difficulties in assessing nonverbal cognitive development is to devise tasks which are truly nonverbal or symbol free. This includes performance of the task itself and the directions given to the subject. Numerous studies have been designed specifically for studying nonverbal cognitive development in deaf persons and Quigley and Kretschmer (1982) have categorized them as follows:

> Studies into 1) the abilities of deaf children to learn or discover various pre-determined concepts or principles (rules), 2) the ability to transfer knowledge of a concept or principle (rule) to novel exemplars, 3) the ability to associate stimuli, 4) the ability to multiply, sort, or categorize objects requiring flexibility, 5) the ability to solve Piagetian and practical problems, and 6) the ability to demonstrate complex logical thinking and symbol manipulation. (p. 57)

Extensive summaries of these studies are provided by Furth (1970) and Ottem (1980). Only a few examples are discussed here.

Russell (1964) required subjects to discover or learn a concept and to engage in a reversal shift in categorization. Groups of deaf subjects and groups of hearing subjects were shown a number of metal tumblers that differed from each other only in height and color—the tumblers were either black or white and tall or short. One group of hearing and one group of deaf subjects were taught to respond to color (black and white) and to ignore height. Black was the correct response for half of these subjects and white the correct response for the other half. Another group of hearing subjects and one of deaf subjects were taught to respond to the height dimension, half to tallness and half to shortness, and to ignore color. Then half of each group and subgroup were required to unlearn their initial categorization scheme in favor of its alternative. The results showed that the deaf subjects were able to learn the categorization schemes and to make the categorization shifts or reversals as well as the hearing subjects. It can be concluded that the deaf subjects were as capable in concept learning and as flexible in concept shifting as the hearing subjects as measured by this task.

Furth and Youniss (1971) provide an example of a study of logical thinking and symbol manipulation. Forty deaf students, 14 years of age and older, were matched on age with 40 hearing students. Half of each group had above average and half had below average scholastic achievement. All subjects were presented three formal operational tasks. Task 1 was a symbolic logic task, Task 2 a probability exercise, and Task 3 required the subjects to generate all possible combinations of several numbers. As an example of the tasks, Task 1 required the subjects to verify certain logical statements using a symbol–picture task. If presented with the logical statement $\dot{H} + \dot{B}$, meaning something that is both not a house and not blue, the subject had to decide if a yellow tree was appropriate. The mode of response involved choosing between an arrow, ⟶ (true), or negated arrow ⟶̸ (not true) which were placed between the logical statement and the picture. A number of similar statements were presented. Results were that the hearing subjects performed better than the deaf subjects on all three tasks. There were, however, marked similarities in the problem solving strategies of the two groups. In spite of the differences found in the study, the investigators argued that there were no differences in formal operations between the deaf and hearing groups and that logical functioning at the Piagetian stage of formal operations does not require a spoken symbol system.

Furth (1973) attempted to demonstrate the importance of clearly controlling the nature of the task, the directions, and subject response in a comparative study using the classical Piagetian tasks involving the conservation of liquid. He found that responses of the subjects became more appropriate as the directions were adapted to the needs of the subjects. This was interpreted as another indication that cognitive differences between deaf and hearing individuals are the result of verbal influences in directions and responses rather than inherent consequences of deafness.

This issue was further explored by Rittenhouse (1977) with reference to the conservation of matter. He hypothesized that the performance of hearing as well as deaf children might be influenced on such tasks by the verbal instructions and by the subjects' perceptions of the experimenter's expectations of performance. Comparisons were made between the standard instructions of four conservation tasks and parallel sets of instructions designed to focus on the task attributes. It was found that the modified instructions improved the performance of both the deaf and the hearing subjects, but the deaf children still had an average 2- to 3-year delay in performance.

This pattern of improving performance of deaf children on nonverbal cognitive tasks as instructions and responses are designed to eliminate verbal influences has been demonstrated by other investigators also. As a consequence, Furth and others have argued that if directions and responses for such tasks could be made completely nonverbal then differences on the tasks between deaf and hearing individuals would disappear. This has yet to be demonstrated. Although appropriate modifications of directions and responses decrease these differences (Furth, 1973; Rittenhouse, 1977), differences still remain. It is also extremely difficult to construct cognitive tasks that are completely nonverbal. Hearing subjects can almost always verbalize the tasks for internal, silent rehearsal.

In spite of a large amount of research during the 1960s and 1970s, it is not yet clear to what extent deaf children can successfully perform various Piagetian tasks. Deaf children have been observed to progress normally through the sensorimotor stage (Best & Roberts, 1976). Delays have been noted, however, in some aspects of the preoperational and concrete operational stages. Although essentially normal functioning has been demonstrated in seriation (the ability to rank order items), significant delays have been noted in the ability to conserve items (liquid and matter) and to engage in transitive thinking (Furth, 1964; Youniss & Furth, 1966; Rittenhouse, 1977). The ability to conserve involves recognizing that objects do not change weight or volume when they change shape, and transitive thinking involves understanding the following types of logical operation: $A > B$, $B > C$, therefore $A > C$.

There is even less certainty about comparable performance of deaf and hearing subjects at the formal operation stage of Piagetian theory. Furth and Youniss (1965) have shown that deaf adolescents and adults can be taught to use very complex logical operation principles, but they also found that their subjects had impaired ability to discover these principles spontaneously. Thus, it must be concluded that the performance of deaf individuals on Piagetian tasks show normal order of progression through the stages of development but delay in actual level of performance, particularly on the later stages of concrete operations and formal operational thought. The effects this delayed performance might have on language acquisition is a practical consideration for educational practitioners.

Memory tasks

Memory is a basic function which exerts an influence on all other cognitive abilities. It is usually considered as having three levels. The first of these is the sensory register which is rapid and describes memories that last for a second or less. The second level, short-term memory, is the working memory which lasts for a few seconds to a minute and provides temporary storage of approximately five to seven unrelated items. Presumably, there is a sensory information (register) storage system for each sensory modality which feeds directly into short-term (or working) memory. Long-term memory, which lasts from a minute to weeks or years, is the third level.

Certain processes of memory allow information to be transferred from short-term (or working) memory to long-term memory. One such process is *rehearsal* which is simply the repeating of a response. A second process is *elaboration* in which new information is associated with already familiar information to facilitate retention. A third is *organization* whereby new information is incorporated into meaningful units with already familiar information to improve retention. Chunking information is one form of organization which has found application in the development of special reading materials (Quigley & King, 1982).

A distinction in type of memory that is important in studies with deaf individuals is that of spatial (or simultaneous) and sequential memory. This distinction is also related to the way in which different senses process information. Hearing processes input in a temporal sequential manner whereas vision can process spatially (simultaneously) as well as sequentially, although it might be a less efficient sequential processor than hearing. The spatial/sequential distinction might be important for the processing of speech as compared to the processing of signs and print. The several studies reported here are concerned largely with this spatial/sequential distinction.

Blair (1957) examined deaf and hearing children on three simultaneous (or spatial) memory tests (Knox Cube, Memory-for-Design, and Object Location) and four sequential memory span tests (Digit Span Forward, Digit Span

Reversed, Picture Span, and Domino Span). The results showed that the deaf children were equal or superior on the simultaneous (or spatial) memory tests whereas the hearing children were able to retain spans of greater length in the sequential memory tests.

Withrow (1968) tested 14 hearing children, 14 orally educated deaf children, 14 fluent manual deaf children, and 14 special deaf children (probably learning disabled). Familiar silhouettes, familiar geometric forms, and random geometric forms were presented first simultaneously, then sequentially. It was found that the deaf group performed the same as the normally hearing group for immediate recall when stimuli were presented simultaneously, but the normally hearing group was significantly superior in its recall of all levels of meaningfulness of stimuli presented sequentially. An interesting analog to this is the study by Stuckless and Pollard (1977) in which 19 deaf students were tested on their ability to process words in print as compared to words finger spelled. It was found that the printed letters were processed more readily than those finger spelled. The difficulty of finger spelling was attributed to its temporal–sequential characteristics. White and Stevenson (1975) have reported similar findings in favor of print as compared to signs.

Belmont, Karchmer, and Pilkonis (1976) tested seven college bound deaf students and seven normally hearing young adults on a short-term memory sequential recall task. Each subject paced himself through a list of consonant letters and then was asked to specify where in the list a particular letter had appeared. Left to their own strategies the deaf subjects performed more poorly than the hearing group. When the deaf subjects were instructed in finger spelling mnemonics involving primary and secondary memory components two things happened. 1. The mnemonic strategy brought the performance of the deaf subjects up to the level of that of the hearing subjects for the number of correct responses. 2. The response time for sequences with strategies directed toward primary (echo) memory was the same for both groups; however, the response time of sequences directed toward secondary (rehearsed) memory was significantly slower for the deaf subjects. Even when the deaf subjects were well rehearsed and recalling accurately, their secondary memory retrieval functions revealed slower access to the stored content. The authors state that

> The instruction strategy led the deaf subjects to such striking immediate increase in recall accuracy...that their original gross deficiencies in these measures must in large part be reflecting a simple ignorance of or disinclination to use effective information-processing strategies. (p. 46)

However, they declined to support a suggestion by Conrad and Rush (1965) that "the intellectual deficiencies of the deaf result because 'they lack practice in the exercise of those communication modes that are most efficient for them' " (p. 342).

It can be seen from these studies that deaf individuals seem to perform more poorly than hearing individuals in memory abilities primarily on tests involving sequential memory. Since auditory language is processed sequentially, and since some visual language inputs (such as print, signs, and finger spelling) can be considered to have sequential components also, this difference has implications for both primary and secondary (reading and writing) language acquisition. Recent research with hearing individuals indicates that this form of memory and information processing might be particularly important in the reading of connected prose.

Abstract thinking

Pettifor (1968) tested hearing-impaired children and normally hearing children on the Pettifor Picture Sorting Test designed to measure levels of conceptual thinking in a manner which did not require expressive speech on the part of the subjects. Instructions were given orally with gestures and repetitions to both groups. There were six acceptable ways of sorting the pictures: large–small; border–no border; figure on right–figure on left; male–female; adult–child; summer–winter. The first three are intended to be visual–perceptual–concrete; the last three, verbal–ideational–abstract. The results were that the normally hearing children were superior to the hearing-impaired children on both kinds of conceptual thinking. The superiority of the normally hearing children on the abstract thinking tasks was significantly greater than on the concrete tasks. Visual and verbal scores increased with age in both groups.

Rosenstein (1960) compared orally trained deaf children with normally hearing children on tasks of perceptual discrimination, multiple classification, and concept attainment and usage. Perceptual discrimination meant choosing the dissimilar object in a group based on some physical aspect. Multiple classification required some abstracting of certain perceptual categories as being the unifying quality. Concept attainment and usage was tested by observing the child's ability to apply a nonperceptive attribute to a group of words. Instructions were given verbally and in mimed gestures that were considered equivalent to verbal explanation. The results indicated that the two groups perceived, classified, and conceptualized equally well. The author believed the result to be due to the fact that the language involved was within the capacity of the deaf children and that in other studies where conceptual deficits were reported, there might have been tasks involving linguistic abilities beyond those of the deaf children tested. As was true in the studies of Piagetian tasks, it is important to be sure that language ability does not influence the ability being tested.

Creativity

Laughton (1979) conducted a study of deaf and hearing students in which the figural form of the Torrence Tests of Creative Thinking was administered in conjunction with the Peabody Language Development Kit in order to ascertain to what extent nonverbal creative processes of fluency, flexibility, originality, and elaboration might have counterparts in linguistic components. All directions were given in written, signed, and spoken form until the children appeared to understand the tasks. Transcription of language samples was done by recorders experienced in receptive sign language and in listening to speech of severely hearing impaired children. Phrase-structure-transformational grammar was used to analyze the language samples of the children.

The four linguistic components that were compared to the creative processes were: phrase structure, single words, transformations, and morphology. The canonical correlation between the nonlinguistic creative processes and the linguistic components was .58 (p < .000). Significant (p < .05) correlations between predictor variables as well as with personal data are as follows:

	r	R^2	
Phrase structure	.46	.21	Originality
Phrase structure	.53	.29	IQ
Phrase structure	.58	.34	Sex
Single words	.38	.14	Sex
Single words	.52	.27	Originality
Morphology	.44	.20	Originality
Morphology	.51	.26	Sex
Morphology	.56	.32	Elaboration
Transformations	.29	.08	Originality

Since 30 of the children had been trained in an auditory/visual/oral (AVO) environment and 47 had been trained in a simultaneous environment the two groups were compared statistically and it was found that the AVO children were superior to the simultaneous method children in both nonlinguistic creative abilities and linguistic abilities. The authors believed that because a significant relationship existed between the predictor variables (although they account for a relatively small amount of the variance as per low R^2s) there must be an interrelation between cognitive and linguistic systems.

Summary

Only a limited number of areas of cognition have been considered here and within each of those areas only a small number of studies have been presented, but they are representative of the body of findings on the cognitive abilities of deaf individuals. Several major conclusions can be drawn from the literature presented.

First, there are enough inconsistencies in the findings in the literature on the cognitive development of deaf individuals to warrant caution in making any definitive conclusions. Although better understanding of the various factors influencing cognitive studies, and increasing experimental control over those factors, has led to findings of smaller and smaller differences between deaf and hearing individuals in cognitive performance, certain differences still exist in various areas. Even when extreme care has been taken to control possible sources of error, differences still have been found in favor of hearing individuals on various Piagetian tasks, memory performance, abstract thinking, creativity, and other cognitive areas.

Second, even though some such differences still are found, there is disagreement as to how they should be interpreted. It can be concluded that the differences are real and represent a true cognitive penalty of deafness. This would be supportive of the Myklebust "organismic shift hypothesis" that deafness imposes a different view of the world through the remaining senses, resulting in qualitative differences between deaf and hearing people. This could result in similarity on overall quantitative cognitive performance but differences on specific aspects of cognition, with deaf people being superior in some areas and hearing people being superior in others.

It can also be concluded, however, that the remaining differences in cognitive performance are due to a remaining lack of experimental control over verbal and other factors that influence performance on tasks that are believed to be nonverbal. It is extremely difficult to construct nonverbal tasks, because hearing individuals can usually verbalize almost any task internally which would aid in performing the task. In addition to the pervasiveness of language, it can also be argued that lack of the language of the core society deprives the deaf individual of the interaction with his/her environment, including people in it, that is necessary for exposure to certain experiences that contribute to cognitive growth. The important point about blaming language and experiential differences for the differences in cognitive performance is that they are remediable. From this point of view, it should be possible to provide an early environment in which the deaf child can be exposed to appropriate experiences through some appropriate language and communication forms that will permit appropriate cognitive development.

The third conclusion that can be drawn from the studies of cognition is that cognitive development is not critically dependent on language in many instances. But although language might not be enough to explain thought, as Piaget claims, some of the studies cited indicate that it becomes so intertwined with cognition after language has developed, that the differential effects of language and cognition are almost inseparable for practical purposes. Perhaps what is most important from all this for the teacher, the clinician, and other practitioners, is summarized by Quigley and Kretschmer (1982).

> Most researchers and most educators of deaf children presently accept that any differences that do exist in intellectual and cognitive functioning between deaf and hearing persons are not significant for adequate functioning in society,

and that educational, occupational, and other deficiencies in deaf people are the result of our present inability to fully help deaf people develop and use their abilities rather than the result of any inherent deficiencies in those abilities. (p. 63)

SYMBOLIC MEDIATION

The second question of major interest in this chapter concerns what internal symbolic mediators of thought deaf people use. This question is of particular interest and importance in studying the development of primary language and of reading with deaf children. Since most people learn to listen and speak before they learn to read and write, it is assumed that a person's lexicon must be coded internally for speech; that is, initially one needs a speechlike representation of a word to access its meaning. This has led to the formulation of the speechrecoding hypothesis that readers must convert a printed word to its speech (phonological) equivalent in some internal way to understand its meaning. As will be shown in chapter 4 on reading, evidence now indicates that words in reading can be accessed directly through internal visual representation as well as indirectly through phonological mediation. But phonological (speech) mediation retains importance in reading, and a question of interest is what do deaf people use as symbolic mediators if they do not have phonological representations of words. Do they use visual imagery, partial or full, of the direct referents of words? Or do they use visual representation in the forms of signs, manual alphabet letters, or what? A considerable number of studies of this matter have been conducted. A limited number of studies are discussed here to illustrate the issue, its importance, and some present thinking concerning it.

Sign coding

At about the same period that Furth and his colleagues were studying cognitive processes in deaf people, a number of investigators were considering the internal coding and mediation processes of language in deaf persons. Odom, Blanton, and McIntyre (1970) tested deaf students and hearing students on their ability to remember words with sign equivalents and words without sign equivalents. The groups were matched on reading ability. It was found that deaf students had little difficulty memorizing words in signs but greater difficulty memorizing words that did not have sign equivalents. Other studies by these investigators found that deaf subjects could understand connected prose better when the syntax of printed messages had been changed to the syntactical order of American Sign Language. Bellugi, Klima, and Siple (1974) reported that deaf children could remember in signs without recoding into printed or acoustic words.

Moulton and Beasley (1975) tested hearing-impaired students who were fluent signers with a paired-associate verbal learning task to determine perceptual coding strategies. Four lists of word pairs were devised in which the word pairs in each list were characterized as sharing:

Similar sign	Similar meaning	e.g., mad–angry
Dissimilar sign	Similar meaning	e.g., cold–freeze
Similar sign	Dissimilar meaning	e.g., black–summer
Dissimilar sign	Dissimilar meaning	e.g., doctor–green

Hearing-impaired subjects were required to replace a word missing from the word pairs. The results showed that, while the subjects were able to code the verbal material on both a sign basis and a semantic basis, the semantic coding strategy appeared to be more efficient than the sign coding strategy for long-term memory. The study indicates that at least two coding strategies might be used by hearing impaired individuals and it is possible that they are capable of switching codes depending upon the communication situation.

In order to determine whether signs could be stored in memory in terms of their semantic characteristics, Siple, Fischer, and Bellugi (1977) conducted a long-term memory experiment using hearing-impaired college students and normally hearing college students. Specially prepared lists of items were presented to the subjects—printed and signed to the hearing-impaired subjects; printed and spoken to the normally hearing subjects. One significant result was that subjects in the printed/signed condition group did not falsely recognize items on the basis of their physical sign similarity. In a second experiment, subjects ignorant of sign language were presented lists of signed and printed words. Signs were meant to be meaningless visual stimuli in this second test. This resulted in formationally similar signs being falsely recognized 38% of the time. The authors concluded that if the hearing-impaired subjects had experienced intrusion errors of a visual nature as the normally hearing group did in experiment two, they would have been encoding items according to their visual characteristics; however, since this was not the case, it was concluded that signs were stored in long-term memory on the basis of semantic organization in the same way that spoken or written language is stored for normally hearing people.

Another study, by Tweeney, Hoeman, and Andrews (1975), sought to learn how words were organized semantically in deaf adolescents. A list of concrete nouns, a list of pictures, and a list of words representing sounds—for instance, meow, toot, hiss, crash—were presented to severely/profoundly hearing impaired persons and to hearing persons. Subjects were asked to sort each set into categories of similar meanings. It was found that deaf and hearing subjects differed only in minor ways with the nouns and the pictures, but greatly for the words representing sounds. The sound words were apparently unfamiliar to the deaf subjects and they grouped them in ways not always based on semantic relations, some on visual similarity, for instance, *whine, whack*. The authors suggest that the deaf subjects resorted to such criteria for clustering only when they lacked adequate semantic grounds for classification.

In general, these studies indicate that deaf people store information in long-term memory in terms of semantic characteristics just as hearing people do. But important differences seem to exist in short-term memory coding and storage where many deaf people seem to code in terms of the visual characteristics of signs and manual alphabet letters whereas hearing people code phonologically. These differences are not clear-cut, however. Hearing people who are skilled readers can access meaning in long-term storage both directly by visual access and indirectly by phonological mediation (Vellutino, 1982). And, as the next group of studies shows, some deaf people also use phonological coding and mediation, as well as visual, in accessing meanings in long-term memory.

Speech coding

Probably the first clear evidence that many deaf persons code, store, and retrieve verbal information in short-term memory differently from the ways that hearing persons do came from experiments by Conrad and his collaborators (Conrad, 1964, 1970, 1971a, 1979; Conrad, Freeman, & Hull, 1965; Conrad & Rush, 1965). Conrad changed Furth's question "What do deaf people think in?" to "What do deaf people memorize in?" His substantive question became "Regardless of the sensory nature of the input. . . when the moment for recall comes, what form, state, code, image, etc., is the memory of the material stored or retained or held in?" Conrad presented clear evidence that many of his deaf subjects coded material according to visual characteristics, but that some even profoundly hearing-impaired (deaf) persons use phonological (speech) coding.

Speech coding of information in short-term memory is important because of the major role it has played in some theories of reading development and methods for teaching reading. These theories and methods have assumed that the internalized auditory language of the hearing child, besides providing a major cognitive tool for thinking, is the base on which reading and writing are developed. The lack of internalization of spoken language has been blamed as a cause of the deaf child's major problems with reading and writing. A number of studies have been interpreted as showing that speech mediation is important to reading.

Conrad, Freeman, and Hull (1965) tested 45 *hearing* subjects on their immediate recall of six-consonant sequences whose main factor contributing to ease of recall was acoustic confusability. Items that are acoustically similar (e.g., *d–t, hat–cat*) are more likely to be confused in recall than acoustically dissimilar items. Factors of acoustic familiarity and frequency of occurrence in the language were compared. It was found that the acoustic property of the letter was the dominant factor for short-term encoding.

Locke and Fehr (1970) tested 11 *hearing* adults in a sequential recall task using visually presented disyllabic words characterized by the presence or absence of letters representing labial phonemes. Analysis of electromyographic activity at a chin–lip site showed greater peak amplitudes for labial than for nonlabial words during presentation and rehearsal periods. The authors inferred from this that covert oral activity occurring during verbal learning and reading is most likely speech and is important in determining the nature of learning.

Conrad (1971b) tested *hearing* children ages 3–11 years in a sequential recalling task using matched pictures of common objects. Up to the age of 5 years it made no difference on the recalling whether the objects memorized had acoustically similar names or not. Beyond 5 years, there was systematic progressive advantage when the pictures had unlike sounding names. This change was taken to represent the onset of the use of verbal code as an aid to memorizing.

In another study, Liberman, Shankweiler, Liberman, Fowler, and Fischer (1977) tested 46 eight-year-old *hearing* children from three reading-skill groups—poor, marginal, superior—on phonetic recall skills to assess the effect of phonological coding on reading skills. They found that the superior readers were sharply distinguished from the inferior groups in their better recalling of nonconfusable items, but were nearly identical to the others in their recalling of confusable strings. The implication is that the superior readers felt greater effects of the phonetic confusability. One interpretation was that the superior readers relied on speech coding during reading.

These studies and others with hearing subjects (Hardyck & Petrinovich, 1970; Kavanagh & Mattingly, 1972) were supplemented by studies of deaf subjects on the assumption that lack of hearing would force the use of internal coding other than speech. To probe the nature of the imagery used by deaf children when memorizing verbal material, Conrad (1970) fashioned and presented a list of nine alphabet letters in sequences of five and six letters 1 sec. apart. Deaf subjects were to read the sequences aloud and silently before transcribing, hearing subjects read only aloud. Errors seemed to be based on articulatory confusions and possibly shape confusions. The hearing group and part of the deaf group made primarily articulatory errors, while the rest of the deaf subjects made primarily what seemed to be errors based on shape confusion. Compare on the chart:

Hearing subjects:	Articulatory errors	Significant
	Shape errors	Not sig.
21 Deaf subjects:	Articulatory errors	Significant
	Shape errors	Not sig.
15 Deaf subjects:	Articulatory errors	Not sig.
	Shape errors	Significant

From these results it was proposed that 21 of the deaf subjects were probably relying on speech cues (artic-group) and the other 15 were not (nonartic-group).

Speech ratings were obtained on the deaf students and these correlated significantly with the type of coding cues attributed to the subjects such that most members of the artic-group had speech ratings of above average; those of the nonartic-group were rated below average. It was also found that the nonartic-group experienced an increase in errors when members were requested to read aloud while members of the artic-group experienced no change after reading aloud, which is interesting, for hearing people usually experience fewer errors after reading aloud. Conrad suggested that forcing a nonartic-child to vocalize during an educational setting possibly imposes a hindrance on recall.

In another study, Conrad (1972) tested three groups for coding in short-term memory with six acoustically similar letters and six visually similar letters. Testees were 32 hearing subjects aged 10–11; 40 high-functioning deaf oral students aged 11–16; 56 normally functioning, deaf oral students aged 9–16. An *articulatory index* (AI) was computed as the proportion of acoustical/articulatory errors out of the total number of errors. A subject with a high AI would be one who found the acoustically similar letters difficult to recall. A high AI person is inferred to be using a speech (acoustic/articulatory) short-term memory code. The results of the experiment were that the hearing subjects had very high AI, the high-functioning deaf subjects had a middle-range AI, and the normally functioning deaf children had a low-range AI.

Conrad (1973) tested short-term memory coding of normally hearing women, and hearing-impaired college students with hearing impairment range of 47–115 dB (probably ISO), speech quality ratings from 2–5 (on 5-point scale), and speech hearing rating from 1–5 (on 5-point scale). Stimuli were a series of letters with high phonologic similarity and a series of letters with low phonologic similarity. Recall was measured against a speech coding index (SCI). SCI is the proportion of all errors that are phonologically based (same as AI in the preceding experiment except it is meant to imply the lack of focus on an acoustic component). SCI of hearing subjects ranged from 50 to 100 indicating a high level of speech coding; SCI of hearing-impaired subjects ranged from 0 to 96 with a median of 50. It was further found that there was no association between IQ and speech-coding index; however, there was a significant association between greater hearing loss and lower SCI, and between poor speech quality and lower SCI. Hearing-impaired subjects who had speech coding indexes in the same range of values as the hearing subjects used the same short-term memory code, namely one based on speech.

Additional studies by other investigators have confirmed the findings of Conrad that some deaf persons use speech as well as various forms of visual coding in storing and retrieving information in short-term memory. Chen (1976) tested 40 college students on acoustic factors in a visual detection task. Subjects were asked to cancel all the letters *e* in a passage from *Treasure Island*. Group A were congenitally deaf, HTL 80+ dB; Group B were adventitiously deaf, HTL 80+ dB; Group C were hard of hearing, HTL less than 80 dB; Group

D were hearing subjects. Results were that the hearing and the partially hearing subjects were more likely to miss silent *es* than pronounced *es* while there was no significant difference in which type of *e* was missed by the profoundly deaf subjects. The tentative conclusions drawn from the results were that for hearing and partially hearing individuals, acoustic image of a word is scanned with the written word, and so when an acoustic factor is lacking, the *e* is more likely to be missed; for deaf individuals, whether congenital or adventitious, acoustic image of a word is not easily available to them, and they rely on mainly visual information.

Locke (1978) conducted a test similar to that of Chen's using three target letters: *c, g, h*. Students were asked to cancel the target letters. Results were that hearing subjects were almost three times as likely to miss a nonphonemic use of the letters than they were to miss a phonemic use, whereas the deaf subjects showed no differences, suggesting the interpretation that deaf children, as a group, do not effectively mediate print with speech.

Locke and Locke (1971) tested three groups of adolescents on a grapheme recall test: 26 normally hearing subjects, 28 intelligible hearing-impaired subjects, and 28 unintelligible hearing-impaired subjects. Stimuli were three lists of letters paired either by (1) phonetic similarity, for example, *B–V*; (2) visual similarity, for example, *P–F*; or (3) dactylic similarity, for example, *K–P*. Analysis showed that the three groups recalled at essentially the same level, but confusion errors differentiated the groups. Overt coding was also observed.

	Hearing	Intel. deaf	Unintel. deaf
Phonetic errors	high	moderate	low
Visual errors	low	moderate	high
Dactylic errors	low	moderate	high
Phonetic coding (overt)	high	moderate	moderate
Dactylic coding (overt)	none	low	moderate

The researchers concluded that deaf children's communication capabilities and their apparent coding strategies in short-term memories seemed to agree closely.

Some of the studies discussed in this section indicate that many deaf people seem to store information in *long-term memory* in terms of semantic characteristics of signs just as hearing people do with spoken language. Other studies indicate that coding in *short-term (working) memory* is in different form for many deaf people than it is for hearing people. Although some deaf people seem to use speech coding as do hearing people, many others seem to code in short-term memory on the basis of visual characteristics of signs and manual alphabet letters.

Multiple coding

Probably the most extensive studies of the internal coding and recoding systems of deaf people have been conducted by Lichtenstein (1983). His research confirmed the findings of Conrad (1979) and Hanson (1982) that working memory capacity is related to the extent to which students can make efficient use of a speech-based recoding strategy in various language tasks and that this strategy is positively related to reading ability.

Lichtenstein reports extensively on the studies of working memory with hearing people to show that problems related to memory capacity and recoding processes are closely associated with difficulties hearing children have in learning to read, (e.g., Bakker, 1972; Shankweiler, Liberman, Mark, Fowler, & Fischer, 1979), even though those children already know the language they are attempting to read. He also cites evidence which indicates that reading a second or less familiar language places increased demand on working memory capacity (Sokolov, 1972). As Quigley and King (1982) have reported, deaf children confront the tasks of both learning a language (English) and learning to read at the same time, since few of them have adequate mastery of English in any form by the time reading instruction begins. Lichtenstein argues that this dual task must make large demands on the working memory and recoding processes of deaf children. Yet the evidence indicates that deaf children have quantitative and qualitative limitations in these processes as compared to hearing children.

Lichtenstein's (1983) extensive studies of the working memory processes of deaf individuals and their relations to language skills, particularly reading comprehension, involved students at the National Technical Institute for the Deaf (NTID), all of whom had reading abilities considerably above the average for prelingually deaf students. His subjects exhibited a considerable range of competence in English skills and came from a variety of educational and communication backgrounds. Lichtenstein's goal was to study their working memory processes with word and sentence memory tasks, obtain extensive self-reports through questionnaires of their conscious coding and recoding strategies, gather extensive descriptive and performance data on their auditory, intellectual, and linguistic abilities, and then analyze the relations among these data in the framework of a series of hypotheses connecting working memory to coding and recoding processes and to psycholinguistic functioning. His detailed investigations produced results and conclusions of critical importance to understanding the role of working memory in the development of primary and secondary (reading and writing) language in deaf children.

1. Lichtenstein found that individual deaf students usually used two or more codes rather than just one exclusively and that the various codes were used with varying degrees of effectiveness. The most commonly used codes were sign and speech.

2. There was clear evidence that working memory capacity is related to the extent to which students make use of a speech-based recoding strategy.

3. Lichtenstein used a model of working memory involving separate subsystems (Baddeley & Hitch, 1974). One subsystem, the *central processor* (CP), performs higher level or control functions but also has a limited amount of processing capacity which can be used for temporary storage of information. A second subsystem, the *articulatory loop* (AL), is a more peripheral system which maintains coded information by subvocal speech rehearsal. This model proved useful to Lichtenstein's research in suggesting why deaf persons generally have shorter memory spans than hearing persons for linguistically codable materials. He found that the more central cognitive components of working memory in deaf people appear to function as effectively as those of hearing individuals. He also found, as have other investigators (e.g., Conrad, 1979; Belmont & Karchmer, 1978; Hanson, 1982) that the more peripheral components of the deaf person's working memory system are not as capable as those of the hearing person's in maintaining English linguistic information in working memory.

Lichtenstein was also able to relate his experimental findings on the limited efficiency of the coding strategies available to his deaf subjects to the manner in which the codes are used during reading to represent English linguistic structure. Some of his findings have direct implications for the development of primary language and of reading in deaf children.

1. Although most of the students used speech, sign, visual information, and to a small degree finger spelling for recoding printed information during reading, the better readers relied very heavily on speech recoding. This confirms similar findings by Conrad (1979) and by Hirsh-Pasek and Treiman (1982).

2. Reliance on speech recoding was not confined to those deaf students who had intelligible speech. Just as Conrad (1979) had found for English and Welsh students, Lichtenstein found that many of his American students whose speech was not readily intelligible nonetheless were using internal speech of some form for recoding during reading.

3. Sign was rarely used consistently for recoding by the most highly skilled readers, although many of them used it selectively for specific memorial purposes.

4. The various codes used by students, particularly speech, sign, and visual, seemed to be selectively related to various aspects of English. Vocabulary test scores and semantic writing errors were not significantly related to working memory capacity or to recoding processes, especially when syntactic abilities were statistically removed from the relationships (partialed out). Research with hearing subjects has demonstrated that visual access to meaning is typical in reading without the need for recoding. This seems to be true also for deaf persons.

5. The primary relationships of working memory capacity and recoding processes seem to be with syntactic skills. Speech recoders tend to be better readers apparently because speech recoding can better represent the grammatical structure of English than sign or visual coding. This allows the short-term retention of enough information to decode grammatical structures

which often are not linear (e.g., medial relative clauses, passive voice). This finding of Lichtenstein's confirms similar findings reported by Lake (1980).

6. Lichtenstein found that skill in the use of bound morphology was most highly related to the self-reports of dependence on speech to represent English information in working memory and to the ability to retain visual word shape information in working memory.

From all of this, it would seem that speech recoding is important to reading development. Visual coding and sign coding might suffice for adequate vocabulary development, but faithful representation of English structure seems to be peculiarly sensitive to speech recoding. It does not necessarily follow from this that deaf children who do not develop speech recoding are doomed to be nonreaders. As is discussed in the chapter on reading, it might mean simply that new methods must be developed to teach reading to such children. It might also signify that means other than reading should be sought for imparting information to some types of deaf children. After having learned to read, children in school read primarily to learn, and other means than the printed word can likely be found to impart information.

MEDIATING LANGUAGE SYSTEMS

In addition to using some means for storing information in long-term memory (apparently semantic) and for coding information in short-term memory (apparently visual as well as phonological), deaf people must use some system of connected language (or grammar) for the manipulation of verbal thinking. Again, there is a question as to what form this connected language takes. And again, as with coding in short-term memory, the answer seems to be, various forms. Most hearing persons in the United States have spoken English as their primary language and printed and written English as their medium for reading and writing. The basic symbols (words) are connected in a common grammatical system, of which syntax is a primary component. Deaf people, however, may have any of several systems and a number of studies have revealed some of these.

Some deaf persons acquire sufficient fluency in spoken language that English becomes their primary internalized language system. A study by Ogden (1979) of 637 former students of three private oral schools for deaf children found them to be highly successful educationally and occupationally. Measures of their reading abilities and samples of their written language attested to the fact that English in some coded form was their internalized language and their medium for verbal thought. The former students themselves attributed their academic and occupational success largely to their development of oral English.

The low reading levels and inappropriate written language (see language samples in chapter 1) of most deaf children attest, however, that this situation is not typical. Many specific studies of written and spoken language samples of deaf persons confirm this (Brannon, 1968; Monsen, 1979;

Oller, Jensen, & Lafayette, 1978; Quigley, Power, & Steinkamp, 1977; Quigley, Smith, & Wilber, 1974; Wilbur, & Montanelli, 1974). If English structure is not the typical internalized language structure for deaf children, then what is? A number of studies indicate that the structure of American Sign Language is the functional structure for some deaf persons while some hybrid of ASL and English is for others. These studies explore both the linguistic characteristics of ASL and the emergence of semantic and syntactic relationships in deaf children exposed naturally to ASL, systems of manually coded English, and gestural systems. They demonstrate the adequacy of ASL and other manual systems as linguistic mediators of thought.

The following are a few of the studies that demonstrate and explicate the linguistic characteristics of sign language. Klima and Bellugi (1979) have shown how subtle modifications of movement of certain signs can impart a wide range of aspectual modifications to them (frequency, continuation, intensity, approximation, inception, result, etc.). Fischer and Gough (1978) showed how changing the spatial arrangement of a verb can incorporate both subject and object pronouns, location, reversibility, reciprocity, size, continuation, and manner into it. Bode (1974) videotaped 16 signers to study how communication of agent, object, and indirect object took place in signs. Ingram (1978) discusses how elements within a signing sequence are ordered to show different informational perspectives. Liddell (1975) discusses how facial expression is used as a syntactic marker to convey the equivalent of relative clauses in signs.

There also appear to be similarities between deaf children's acquisition of signing as their first linguistic medium and hearing children's acquisition of English. Newport and Ashbrook (1977) found the emergence of eight semantic relationships in the expressions of five deaf children learning sign language to be in the same order as they were for four hearing children in a study by Bloom, Lightbown, and Hood (1975). Other systems in sign language that do not have exact parallels in English nevertheless seem to evolve in a developmental way in deaf children. Hoffmeister (1978) traced the development of a pronominal referential system until it was completely learned by a 6-year-old girl. Ellenberger and Staeyert (1978) report that a deaf child they studied learned the directional modification of verbs and the structuring of space by age 5. Collins-Ahlgren (1975) found a facilitative and simultaneous effect of sign language with English. Two deaf girls she observed produced complex grammatical functions in simple signs first and then gradually moved into standard English form using function morphemes.

In an educational setting Higgins (1973) found sign language effective for communicating factual information. Bellugi and Fischer (1972) found that although signs were communicated slower in their study, the rates for producing propositions were similar in both signs and English. They agreed that signs could compact linguistic information in ways not available to English. Jordan (1975) compared the communicative speed and abilities of deaf signers with hearing speakers and found that both groups communicated with the same degree of accuracy, but that the deaf signers included more information per unit of time than the hearing people did. Dalgleish (1975) studied reports from educational institutions in the United States, Holland, and England and reported that sign language was the preferred mode of communication by deaf children.

Studies by Babb (1979) and Brasel and Quigley (1977) suggested that signs might be a valuable medium of early linguistic input contributing to later academic improvement. Max (1935) used a biofeedback approach to test whether deaf subjects might be dreaming in sign language. Electrodes were fastened to the fingers and hands of deaf and hearing subjects. Electromyelograms were obtained during undisturbed sleep and during dream sleep. The onset of dreams caused a current response in the arm and finger muscles of the deaf subjects but not in the hearing subjects. Other studies by Hawes and Danhauer (1978), Crittenden (1975), and Lane, Boyes-Braem, and Bellugi (1976) have supported the concept of distinctive perceptual features for the hand configurations and movements of sign language.

These studies demonstrate a growing belief among psychologists and linguists that a gestural form of language, such as ASL, is probably as efficient a thought mediating system for deaf persons as English and other spoken languages are for hearing persons.

SUMMARY AND CONCLUSIONS

Present resolution of the enduring question of the relationship between language and cognition (thought) seems to favor the primacy of basic cognitive processes with language being dependent on them. Perception, attention, memory, and other abilities need to develop appropriately to ensure the adequate development of the abstract thinking processes and language on which educational development is largely based. Deficits or problems in the development of basic cognitive processes will be reflected in problems of language development and ultimately in most academic educational areas. This is why the work of psychologists such as Piaget and others with hearing children and Furth and others with deaf children have major implications for teachers and clinicians.

While the language/cognition question seems at this stage to have been resolved in favor of the primacy of cognition, the question of how deaf individuals compare with hearing individuals on cognitive tasks seems to have been resolved in favor of equality of performance; however, this should be treated with caution. It has long been obvious from the successful social and occupational functioning of deaf individuals that the Pintner position of deficits in the general cognitive and intellectual functioning of deaf people is untenable. As greater control has been exerted over the variables that influence studies of cognitive abilities, especially verbal language, differences between deaf and hearing individuals have decreased, and in some cases disappeared. They have not disappeared in all areas, however. Some differences continue to be found on various Piagetian tasks and in areas such as sequential memory which are important to language and educational development. There is a tendency to assume that even greater experimental control will eventually eliminate those differences also. But the possibility that they are true differences should also be entertained. This is particularly true of linguistically codable materials where studies have consistently shown deaf people to have shorter memory spans than hearing people (Lichtenstein, 1983).

It does not follow from the acceptance of true differences between deaf and hearing individuals in some cognitive areas, that *inferiority* in cognitive, linguistic, and educational development will inevitably follow. Knowing the nature and effects of any true differences allows developmental and educational programs to be shaped to capitalize on the differences. For example, if deaf people do perform as well as, or better than, hearing people on tests of spatial memory, but less well on tests of sequential memory, and if these are true differences, there are several implications for educational practice. First, since hearing is an efficient processor of temporal–sequential input (such as auditory language), while vision is more efficient at processing spatial information, ASL might have some advantages over spoken language as the initial linguistic input for at least some deaf children. ASL makes use of motion and position in space to convey some concepts that depend on temporal–sequential transmission in spoken language. This might be particularly true in connected discourse where certain syntactic constructions might be heavily dependent on temporal–sequential storage in short-term memory. According to the work of Lichtenstein, this type of processing of information is important in comprehending embedded or interrupted syntactic constituents such as sentences with medial relative clauses (e.g., The boy who kissed the girl ran away) which require integration of information from the beginning and end of a sentence for proper understanding. Deaf persons have great difficulty in understanding the spoken and written forms of such syntactic constructions (Quigley, Smith, & Wilbur, 1974), yet it is possible that the constructions can be readily understood through ASL where they are conveyed in terms of space, movement, and facial expressions. ASL might be uniquely adapted to capitalize on the cognitive differences between deaf and hearing individuals by using space and motion where spoken language uses time for the same purpose.

A second implication in the same area is that manually coded English systems might have some advantage over spoken language in that, like ASL, they make the individual units of language (words) more visible than does speech, but they might have the same disadvantage as speech in connected discourse in that they rely on time rather than space as an important element in syntactic transmission. A third in this chain of implications derived from possible differences between deaf and hearing individuals in spatial and temporal–sequential memory is that teachers and clinicians, in order to teach deaf children the language of the core society, need to know some of the basic ideas of cognition and the comparative performances of deaf and hearing children in various cognitive abilities. They need also to know ASL and perhaps the various manually coded English systems as well, but particularly ASL.

At first glance, the findings on the importance of speech recoding in the reading process, particularly with regard to grammatical structure, appear to present a dilemma for the teaching of reading to deaf children. Most deaf children presently do not learn to read English well; and if this is due in any considerable part to the lack of a speech coding system, then those deaf children who are unable to acquire this coding system might simply be unable ever to learn to read well or even adequately. At second glance, the findings on speech recoding do not present as bleak a prospect. There are at least three potential solutions to the problem.

1. Speech could be developed far better with far more deaf children than is presently the case. Ling (1976), Ling and Ling (1978), and others have shown that this is possible. And there is no strong evidence that this requires the abandonment or prohibition of ASL or whatever other manual means of communication deaf children prefer naturally.

2. Other means of teaching reading could perhaps be developed that are not dependent on speech coding or recoding. If reading, as we presently conceive it, is not possible without a speech code, then using ASL as the first and basic language of young deaf children might preclude the learning of reading. This *is* a dilemma. Proponents of developing ASL as the first language of the deaf child with English being developed later as a second language seem to overlook that not only a new language must be learned but also a new code (speech vs. sign) and a new modality (auditory/kinesthetic vs. visual). This might be a much more difficult task than the learning of a second spoken language by a hearing person who already has a first spoken language and a well developed cognitive and experiential base. In this case the modalities (auditory) and the codes (speech) are the same for both languages. As is discussed in chapter 4, ASL-using deaf children of deaf parents often read better than other deaf children, so perhaps a speech code is not indispensable. Conrad (1979) and Lichtenstein (1983) have shown, however, that many of those deaf children might be using internal speech coding even though their speech is unintelligible or rarely used.

3. One basic purpose for reading is to acquire information. But it should be possible to find other means than the printed word to accomplish this purpose. Talking books for blind people are one means by which this is done. Translation of the printed or written word to signed videotapes in ASL for deaf people is another possible means.

chapter 3

Primary language development

In a spoken or verbal language, it is axiomatic that speech is primary and that written language is a secondary component derived from the primary one. In other words, *sound* is the medium in which a spoken language is embodied and the written language results from the transference of speech to a secondary, visual medium (Kavanagh & Cutting, 1975). Thus, primary language development refers to the development of speech within the conceptual framework of the various established components of a spoken or verbal language (i.e., phonology, syntax, semantics, and pragmatics). For most hearing children, the comprehension and production of spoken language present little difficulty; the hearing child's ability to understand the spoken message is limited primarily by the extent of his/her linguistic and cognitive development (Dale, 1976; de Villiers & de Villiers, 1978). Still, controversies do exist in child language research and these can be grouped into three major areas for discussion: (1) methodologies for gathering data, (2) interpretation or categorization of data within the various linguistic components (e.g., phonology, semantics), and (3) the construction of grammars or theories that achieve explanatory adequacy or that best fit the data (Chomsky, 1965; Howe, 1981; Schlesinger, 1982).

Describing the primary language development of deaf children is a more complicated matter. Such description can include a spoken and/or signed language or some other communication form (e.g., finger spelling, cued speech). Signed languages, in general, are visual–gestural in nature and differ from spoken languages in the modes of perception and production. It is only recently that signed languages have come within the purview of linguistics and psycholinguistics, and that at least one signed language, American Sign Language, has been generally accepted as a bona fide language (Lane & Grosjean, 1980; Liddell, 1980). In addition, within the United States, there has been a proliferation of contrived sign systems (e.g., SEE II, signed English) which have generally borrowed and altered signs from the lexicon of ASL and have also created additional sign markers (see Stokoe, 1975 and Wilbur, 1979 for a discussion of the complex notion of "borrowing" signs from ASL). The three groups of controversies previously mentioned in language research with hearing children also apply to research on the primary language acquisition of deaf children. There are, however, some additional concerns uniquely attributed to this population. For example, one of the major issues in the education of deaf children can be stated as a question: How do deaf children acquire language? This question has been discussed in depth by King (1981) who suggested that it has two parts: (1) *How well do* deaf children acquire language and *how do* deaf children acquire language? This *how do* aspect of the major question can be rephrased and further differentiated for the purposes of this chapter. For instance, one could inquire about the nature and process of the primary language development of deaf children. More specifically, is this development similar to or different from the primary language development of hearing children? In what ways is it similar? In what ways is it different? Is the primary language development of a signed language similar to or different from a spoken language? Do the contrived sign systems or other esoteric communication forms possess the same functions and purpose as a spoken or signed language? Is the primary language development of these systems similar to or different from either a spoken or a signed language?

Because of these special considerations of type of communication and language input and usage with deaf children, their language development must be considered in relation to the particular type of input to which they are exposed in infancy and early childhood. This can be an unfortunately large variety, but for the purposes of this book three categories have been proposed which include most of the varieties: oral English (OE), which includes supplemental cueing; manually coded English (MCE), including pidgin sign English (PSE); and American Sign Language (ASL). As stated in the Preface, an attempt is made to trace the development of language in deaf children in each of these categories. The attempt is admittedly only partially successful due to the lack of data in the categories. Descriptions of the three approaches and the various specific varieties within them, such as signed English, is possible, but evaluation of the effectiveness of each approach in developing language lacks an adequate data base. This will become evident as the research is presented in each of the categories following presentation of theoretical considerations and some basic data on the language development of hearing children.

THEORETICAL PERSPECTIVES

A theory of the nature of a language can be closely related to a theory of the acquisition and use of a language. This notion, however, has been established only in recent years. Historically, the study of language has been undertaken by philosophers, linguists, and psychologists (Blumenthal, 1970). Linguists have generally concerned themselves with description of the overt structure (in particular, phonology and syntax), whereas psychologists have been concerned with the observable function (i.e., the speaking and listening behaviors). In the past, neither group was interested in studying the acquisition of meaning (or the structure of the mind), although some linguists, notably Bloomfield (1933), acknowledged that such an entity could exist but probably could not be studied. Thus, until Chomsky appeared on the scene, the researchers in linguistics and in psychology were primarily concerned with descriptions of the surface features or output of a language (i.e., speaking, writing). Consequently, most language theories were developed to explain the acquisition of these surface features. Chomsky, however, attempted to understand the relationship between linguistic structure and the processes of speaking and listening. Consequently, his notion of innate structures in the mind and his distinction between the competence (underlying knowledge) and performance (observable speaking behavior) of a native speaker started a revolution in linguistics and, in time, spawned a number of subdisciplines investigating the acquisition of language (e.g., psycholinguistics, developmental psycholinguistics, educational psycholinguistics, sociolinguistics).

Subsequently, in recent years, a theory of a language has been defined to be a grammar of that language. Like any other scientific theory, it is an attempt to explain some domain or range of natural phenomena (de Villiers & de Villiers, 1978; Howe, 1981; Schlesinger, 1982). This "domain of natural phenomena," however, is dependent upon one's theoretical perspective. Some investigators focus on describing the knowledge that is possessed by every native speaker of the language (Chafe, 1970; Chomsky, 1968; Fillmore, 1968). Others investigate what speakers say in different social situations or contexts (Bates, 1976a, 1976b; Labov, 1972; Snow, 1977). Thus, some researchers still focus on the surface structure of linguistic strings as the primary correlate of human verbal behavior while others are more concerned with an abstract linguistic analysis of underlying representation. Most investigators agree that a linguistic grammar or theory should be able to explain how native speakers of a language proceed from the sounds (or some other observable output such as signs) to the corresponding meanings.

Theories of language have been grouped into several categories. Different researchers have employed a variety of terms to label these categories; a close inspection of these terms reveals more similarities than differences. Several researchers (e.g., Cruttenden, 1979; Slobin, 1979) employed terminology similar to Menyuk's (1977): (1) behavioral, (2) biological, (3) cognitive, and (4) sociocultural. Cruttenden (1979) employed (a) innatist instead of (2) biological, and (b) sociological instead of (4) sociocultural. Cruttenden (1979) argued that the term, innatist, is the general notion which is associated with Chomsky (1965) whereas maturation (biological) is part of this theory which was contributed by Lenneberg (1967). Bloom and Lahey (1978) argued that only three groups of linguistic theories have been most influential in the study of child language and language development: (1) generative transformational grammar (similar to biological and innatist); (2) the semantic theories; and

(3) variation theory (combination of 1 and 2). They claimed that *behaviorism*, at the present time, has exerted very little influence on language theory. Other researchers, however, have argued that *neobehaviorism* can explain some of the linguistic data, and that the theory of behaviorism, itself, has been misinterpreted (Salzinger, 1979; Schlesinger, 1982). It should be noted that the semantic theories were a reaction against Chomsky's view of syntax as depicting the structure of the mind. More specifically, the issue of semantics became a dominant concern in generative grammar after some researchers argued that syntax was inseparable from underlying meaning (Chafe, 1970; Fillmore, 1968; McCawley, 1968). The variation theory described by Bloom and Lahey (1978) combines aspects of generative transformational grammar and the semantic theories. The proponents of this theory argue that a linguistic analysis must proceed beyond the sentence level into the level of discourse where a different set of rules applies (Bates, 1976a, 1976b; Halliday, 1975; Lindberg, 1979; Snow & Ferguson, 1977). In this respect, this theory is similar to the category *sociocultural*. For the purposes of this chapter, the terminologies suggested by Menyuk (1977) (except for biological theories) are employed in the brief, ensuing discussions of the current, major theories of child language and language acquisition. In addition, the reaction against innatist theories (i.e., that syntax depicts the structure of the mind) is discussed under the heading, *Transformational Generative Grammar*.

Behaviorism

Most recent studies in child language have not been conducted within the behavioristic framework, however, an understanding of current theorizing, as well as of Chomsky's revolutionary notions, requires a brief discussion of how the behavior theorists attempted to explain the acquisition of language. The major argument against behaviorism is that it fails to take the notion of meaning into account. It is further argued that the theory of behaviorism cannot account for the productivity of language; that is, native speakers can produce an infinite number of sentences, many of which they have never heard previously.

A theory of behaviorism emphasizes the influence of the environment in the learning of language. Behaviorism has been labeled stimulus–response (S–R) psychology (Slobin, 1979) in which behaviors are described as connections between stimuli and responses. In general, a stimulus is said to elicit a response, and then, this response becomes a stimulus for the following or next response. Within this framework, the behaviorists either deny that the child possesses innate abilities to aid in learning language or assert that such abilities cannot adequately be described (Cruttenden, 1979). This assertion is explicitly a noncognitive approach. In addition, this approach places a great deal of emphasis on such notions as *imitation, reinforcement,* and the role of parental and social *approval*. More recently, behavior theorists have reacted against transformational generative grammar by asserting that it has little or no psychological reality, and at best is only a metaphor (Miller & Johnson-Laird, 1976; Salzinger, 1979). These theorists have focused on studying the psychological concept of meaning which others have interpreted as a return to the consideration of the environment in which language behavior is emitted. This new approach has been labeled neobehaviorism, radical behaviorism, and ecolinguistic (Salzinger, 1979; Skinner, 1974).

Recently, it has generally been accepted that behavioral concepts such as approval, reinforcement, and imitation play very little role in the child's acquisition of language (Bloom & Lahey, 1978; Cruttenden, 1979). For example, parental pressure for correct syntax is generally not very successful (Brown, Cazden, & Bellugi, 1973). It should be born in mind, however, that a more general approval of successful communication of meaning may actually have a role in language acquisition; for example, parental approval in the development of the first words from babbling (Moerk, 1977). The major objection to the aspect of approval in the theory is that it offers no explanation for how such interaction takes place. Likewise, imitation has a limited role for it fails to account for such statements of children as "I goed" and "all gone cookie."

It was previously mentioned that behavioristic theories fail to account for the productivity of language. This argument, however, does not invalidate all S–R theories of language learning, some of which are productive. An S–R theory does not require that each sentence a child produces or comprehends be learned in its entirety. Staats (1971) has shown that a relatively small number of S–R links may account for a larger number of sentences. Consider the following examples. Suppose the child has learned to associate the word *the* with *boat, table,* and *bicycle.* Then the child could produce *the boat, the table,* and *the bicycle.* Now suppose the child has learned that certain words could precede *the;* words such as *see* and *made.* It is then possible for the child to produce six strings of phrases without ever having heard all of them. An even more productive model has been proposed by Braine (1963a, 1963b) in his notion of contextual generalization. In general, this theory, called a pivot grammar, asserted that certain morphemes and phrases are followed by other words and phrases. Several objections have been levied against these proposals. One is that the grammars are too productive; that is, they do not *exclude* linguistic strings not permitted by the grammar. Other objections were put forward by Bever, Fodor, and Weksel (1965a, 1965b) and Van der Geest (1974). These investigators argued that this and all theories of behaviorism (including the more recent ones) cannot answer the following barrage of questions: (1) How does the child learn to segment utterances into morphemes and phrases? (2) How does the child deal with statements and questions with different word orders? and (3) How does the child deal with ambiguity; for example, sentences like *Visiting linguists can be dangerous?* The crux of these objections is that behaviorism, in any form, takes no account of meaning, which must be considered in any theory of language.

Transformational generative grammar

In the history of psycholinguistics, certain linguistic grammars or theories were compatible with (and influenced by) behaviorist theories; these theories were labeled structuralist or constructivist. They developed phrase structure grammars which parse sentences into constituent elements (phrases). There was a degree of productivity in phrase structure grammars; however, they required only the relatively simple cognitive capacity of forming and arranging categories. In essence, these grammars only dealt with surface features and had the same difficulty as behaviorism with the previous sentence, *Visiting linguists can be dangerous* (Slobin, 1979). These surface structure grammars or theories set the stage for Chomsky.

Chomsky (1957, 1965), deviating from the then prevalent emphasis on phonology, based his early work almost exclusively on syntax. He claimed that sentences are the basic units of communication in language. He further argued that regardless of a person's understanding of the meanings of words or morphemes or pronunciation, understanding of sentences could still be completely inadequate. This, of course, has been indicated by the earlier sentence, *Visiting linguists can be dangerous.* In particular, transformational grammar, as proposed by Chomsky, is concerned not only with the surface arrangements of words, but also with abstract structures that underlie the sentences. According to Chomsky, not everything the native speaker knows about a sentence is revealed in the words which are spoken. This distinction between underlying (or deep) structures and surface structures is one of the major contributions of transformational grammar. Consequently, the basic position of Chomsky's theory (1968) is that children possess an innate predisposition to language. This notion has reintroduced the issue of rationalism and empiricism into psychology and philosophy. Chomsky further argued that these innate structures are syntactic in nature; that is, the syntactic forms depict the structure of the mind.

The notion of innate structures is argued for on three counts: (1) the existence of linguistic universals; (2) the structure or form of the linguistic input to children; and (3) the speed of the acquisition of language. In spite of unobservable structure and an inadequate sample of sentences, children acquire a language in all its complexity within a brief time span. It appears that children must possess some innate predisposition which influences them to observe or search for certain linguistic features and these must be common to all languages. Consequently, Chomsky has argued that humans are unique, rational animals since they are the only species to have evolved language. This has led to the notion that the human capacity for language is different from other animals' capacity for communication. Finally, a corollary to the theory is Chomsky's distinction between *competence* and *performance*. *Competence* refers to the native speaker's underlying knowledge of the rules of a grammar; this knowledge exists on an unconscious level. *Performance* refers to the actual utterances of the native speaker. The performance of native speakers is fraught with errors due to psychological factors such as distractions, memory lapses, fatigue, and other factors. Thus, performance only approximates a native speaker's knowledge of a language since under ideal conditions (i.e., no errors), performance reflects competence. This ideal condition cannot exist, thus, transformational generative grammar is actually a theory of the competence of a native speaker not a theory of performance which Chomsky (1975) argued can never reach explanatory adequacy.

Because transformationalist theories of language emerged as a reaction to S–R accounts, it was expected that more attention might be paid to semantics by these theories. Chomsky's (1965) model of grammar did include a semantic component and this model attempted to show the manner in which the child expresses meaning through sentence structure. This new model, however, was still not acceptable to those theorists who felt that semantics was more basic than syntax (Chafe, 1970; Fillmore, 1968). Most recent researchers argue that semantic information is important for language learning; however, they disagree on the appropriate formalism for representing the underlying semantic structures. One of the earliest attempts to represent additional dimensions of meaning within transformational grammar was Charles Fillmore's (1968) case grammar. Fillmore argued that the deep structure of sentences contained consistent meaning relations which can not be revealed by transformational grammar. A good description of case grammar can be found in Slobin (1979). Bloom and Lahey (1978) have argued that, of all the semantic theories, case grammar appears to be the most promising for analyzing child language. But a number of linguistic models have attempted to generate sentences from more complex underlying semantic structures than those of case grammar. A good discussion of these can be found in Parisi and Antinucci (1976). Case grammar has been expounded by Fillmore (1968) and Bowerman (1973), generative semantics by McCawley (1968), and Chafe's (1970) theory of semantic structures by Nelson (1975).

In sum, Chomsky's revolution contributed two major notions which have affected all aspects of components of linguistic study: (1) the distinction between competence and performance; and (2) the notion that language is generative, that is, a finite number of rules can generate an infinite number of sentences. These notions have led to the development of generative phonology and generative semantics.

Cognitive theories

As previously mentioned, the neglect (or rather the low status) of semantics in the transformationalist theories gave rise to a countermovement—the semantic view. Essentially, the semantic theorists argue that syntax is not separable from semantics and that, in fact, semantics or meaning is more basic in language than syntax. A similar kind of argument was presented in another countermovement, that of the cognitive theorists. The relationship between semantics and cognition can be seen in the fact that semantic theorists lean toward a cognitive interpretation of linguistic structure and principles (Fillmore, 1968; Lucas, 1980; McCawley, 1968; Moerk, 1977). In essence, the cognitive theorists oppose the notion that language is independent of other cognitive functions, and argue that language is a mapping out of existing cognitive skills. These theorists have taken as axiomatic that cognitive development is a prerequisite for grammatical and lexical development in the same way that perceptual and motor development are said to be a prerequisite for phonological development (Cruttenden, 1979; Menyuk, 1977; Schlesinger, 1982). It can be seen that both the semantic approach and the cognitive approach were reactions to the claim of an innate component of specific linguistic knowledge.

The groundwork for researchers interested in demonstrating that language learning is based on general cognitive development was laid by Jean Piaget. A comprehensive and lucid overview of Piaget's work can be found in Gruber and Vonéche (1977). The sensorimotor period of early child language has been discussed by Sinclair-de Zwart (1973) and Brown (1973). Other studies based upon Piaget's work are in Morehead and Morehead (1974), and Greenfield and Smith (1976). Excellent critical reviews may be found in Cromer (1974) and Bowerman (1976). A review of the relationship between cognition and language in the literature on deafness can be found in chapter 2 of this book.

Questions that still remain to be answered in cognitive theories of language are (1) what is the nature of this cognitive ability, (2) how can it be studied, (3) how does it develop, and (4) do language and cognition interact in any way? It has been argued that most studies of cognitive development are useless for comparison with language development because cognition is studied through language (Cruttenden, 1979). The one framework of cognitive growth researched in part independently of language is, of course, that of Piaget (Piaget, 1954, 1971). The recent trend in cognition is to acknowledge or show that there are cognitive underpinnings but that after a short period of time (sensorimotor period), cognition and language exert some influence on each other. The nature of these influences (or the interaction approach) is still being explored (Schlesinger, 1982).

Sociocultural theories

In recent years a number of special disciplines have developed within the social sciences with the purpose of including the study of language in its sociocultural context within the purview of linguistic inquiry (Cruttenden, 1979; Ervin-Tripp & Mitchell-Kernan, 1977; Mey, 1979; Moerk, 1977). It is interesting to note that sociocultural theorists, like semantic and cognitive theorists, also reject Chomsky's hypothesis of language (in particular, grammar) as an autonomous system whose acquisition depends on innate linguistic structures. These theorists, however, differ from both semantic and cognitive theorists by emphasizing that the development of language is due to a child's interaction with other members of society. Such thoughts have engendered the development of the ethnography of communication (Gumperz & Hymes, 1972), sociolinguistics (Labov, 1972), and conversational analysis (Turner, 1974). *Pragmatics*, as a component of linguistics, has also emerged from this movement (Bates, 1976a, 1976b; Moerk, 1977).

In general, sociocultural research shared several notions: (1) Natural conversation is a bona fide source of data; (2) sentences are not the highest level of analysis; (3) social context is relevant to linguistic rules; (4) variability is a component of linguistic rules; and (5) language functions are diverse in nature (Ervin-Tripp & Mitchell-Kernan, 1977; Lucas, 1980; Mey, 1979). The main problem is to discover systematic rules in each of these areas.

It has been argued that natural conversation might be the most profitable and the basic source of linguistic data (Lindberg, 1979). Hitherto, transformational theorists have argued that knowledge (linguistic competence) can be assessed by judgments of sentence grammaticality, acceptability, presuppositions, or invariance of meaning (Chomsky, 1975; Slobin, 1979). These tactics are termed introspection; however, this method is impractical for the study of child language, informal styles, and vernaculars (Brown, 1973; Ervin-Tripp & Mitchell-Kernan, 1977; Labov, 1972). Introspection is even less adaptable for the study of semantics. For example, native speakers are not capable of reporting out of context a language aspect which varies according to social or situational context (Hymes, 1974). The use of natural conversation as a data source, however, raises problems which need to be resolved: (1) What kinds of activities, or groups should be investigated? and (2) How large should a sample of these be?

One of the most controversial tenets of sociocultural analysis is: Sentences are not the highest level of analysis (Lindberg, 1979). Most of the previous linguistic analyses and explanations of grammatical rules have employed sentences as the unit of analysis. Recent work in discourse structure has suggested different levels for analysis: moves, turns, exchanges, stories, conversations, and speech events. The boundaries of these units for study can be indicated by such factors as code switches, paralinguistic cues, and lexical markers. Consequently, the current trend in pragmalinguistics is to identify those linguistic features which are systematic and interpretable.

There is increasing support that social context is relevant to linguistic rules (Bloom & Lahey, 1978; Ervin-Tripp, 1976; Mey, 1979; Moerk, 1977). The major function of context is to provide an interpretation for the rules and substance of conversations. Bloom and Lahey (1978) and de Villiers and de Villiers (1978) argue that child language cannot be studied without reference to context. In fact, it is argued that the interpretation of the data is primarily dependent upon context or situation cues since a child's language does not possess the same level of sophistication as that of adults, and furthermore, it is not open to introspection (Brown, 1973). The limits and problems of contextual interpretation have been discussed elsewhere (Bloom & Lahey, 1978; Howe, 1981; Schlesinger, 1982). In spite of these concerns, most theorists agree that context is of primary importance in sociocultural research.

Variability is a systematic part of both phonology and grammar. Previously, it has been shown to be due to linguistic context (Robins, 1980). For example, when spoken in conversation, the sentence *I want to go to the store* may be heard as *I wanna go to da store.* As another example, some native speakers might omit the final consonant in *next* but not in *mixed.* Variability of this type is not only related to linguistic context but also to social features such as gender, age and setting (Hymes, 1974; Labov, 1972). Thus, it has been argued that variability must be considered as an aspect of linguistic rules.

The last notion of sociocultural theroists for discussion here is the diversity of language functions. This notion of diversity in function is revealed by natural conversations. Some theorists believe that some language functions are universal; however, the social emphasis on the different language functions appears to vary culturally and developmentally (Ervin-Tripp & Mitchell-Kernan, 1977; Mey, 1979). In the area of language acquisition, Halliday (1975) has proposed that shifts in functions produce a change in the structures of language. Thus, as children acquire language they spontaneously change forms in order to meet new functions. This spontaneous structural change has also been observed in mature speakers as society alters the functions of language.

COMPONENTS OF LANGUAGE

Currently, a flurry of activity exists in the field of language acquisition and development. New findings are constantly being published, and the interests of researchers seem to proceed from one problem area to another. The various components of language have been the primary focus of investigators at one time or another. The movement has gone from phonology to syntax to semantics and, currently, to pragmatics. One of the recent primary issues is the argument over which of these components is fundamental: syntax, semantics, or pragmatics (Schlesinger, 1982; Slobin, 1979). The grammar of a language is intended to be a complete description of the language as it is actually spoken. Thus, there are grammatical rules that deal with each of the four (as of now) major components of language. Taken together, these rules should form a complex system that describes and explains all aspects of linguistic structure and function. These linguistic components are briefly described in the ensuing paragraphs. More detailed descriptions can be found elsewhere (Bloom & Lahey, 1978; Kretschmer & Kretschmer, 1978; Schlesinger, 1982).

Phonology is the study of sounds and their structures. It is agreed by most researchers that phonology is dependent upon the requirements of the other linguistic components; however, there is disagreement concerning the entity or reality of the other components (Aaronson & Rieber, 1979; Moerk, 1977). In general, the most important concepts associated with phonology are segmental aspects, that is, phonologic distinctions, and suprasegmental aspects like intonation and stress (Cruttenden, 1979). This component has also felt the influence of transformational grammar and the new term that emerged is generative phonology (Chomsky & Halle, 1968). Recently, it has been argued that child language, in particular child phonology, should act as a potential source of constraint on the construction of linguistic theory (Menn, 1982). Menn discusses two current theoretical approaches which attempt to constrain generative phonology. One approach attempts to minimize the distance between Chomsky's notions of underlying or deep structure and surface structure representation. The other approach is concerned with the psychological reality of the derivation rules. These issues have been discussed extensively (Diver, 1979; Fromkin & Rodman, 1978), yet they still remain to be resolved.

The syntactic component is concerned with the way words are combined to form sentences. As previously discussed, syntax is/was the primary concern of tranformational grammarians. Chomsky, the main proponent, also argued that syntactic structures reflect the structures of the mind. On a sentence level, there are three major aspects of syntax: phrase structure rules, lexical insertion rules, and transformational operations. Discussion of these terms may be found in Russell, Quigley, and Power (1976) and Kretschmer and Kretschmer (1978). In the literature on deafness, the syntactic component has been researched most extensively in secondary language development (Quigley, Wilbur, Power, Montanelli, & Steinkamp, 1976). It should be clear, by now, that a syntactic description should be an adjunct to semantic and pragmatic descriptions of language.

The study of meaning or semantics is said to exist on two levels: the sentence level and word level. As previously mentioned, the theoretical model that currently is deemed most applicable to the study of child language is that of case grammar (Fillmore, 1968). Good discussions of this theory and of generative semantics can be found in Kretschmer and Kretschmer (1978), Slobin (1979), and Schlesinger (1982). In essence, the study of semantics may be concerned with such issues as the nature of propositions, case relations, relational categories, and semantic features or componential analyses.

The fourth linguistic component that has been delineated is pragmatics. Pragmatics has been defined as the study of linguistic structures and the contexts in which they are used (Mey, 1979; Moerk, 1977). This component deals with such topics as logical and pragmatic presuppositions, the analyses of propositions, and the structure and functions of speech acts. On a higher level, the study of pragmatics is concerned with communicative competence, in particular, the organization of discourse, that is, the manner in which conversations are opened, sustained, and terminated. Further discussions of the component can be found in Lucas (1980).

METHODOLOGIES FOR STUDYING CHILD LANGUAGE

There are two major approaches for obtaining data for the description of children's language. One is to observe and describe children's verbal and nonverbal behaviors in natural interactions or situations. The second is to experimentally manipulate an aspect in one of the components of language discussed previously and record the behaviors (Bloom & Lahey, 1978; Dale, 1976; Lindfors, 1980; Slobin, 1979). In general, both approaches entail (1) gathering data, (2) interpreting or categorizing the data, and (3) formulating a hypothesis to explain the data.

Data collection

Observations can be cross-sectional or longitudinal. In cross-sectional analyses, a number of children are observed at different ages. In a longitudinal research design, a child or a group of children is observed for a long period of time. This type of design is useful for observing developmental changes. In general, most experimental studies are cross-sectional and evaluate the comprehension capacity of children (Bloom & Lahey, 1978; Clark & Clark, 1977; Dale, 1976). The research is designed in a manner that requires children to respond in some way, for example, manipulating objects and toys. Sometimes, the researcher attempts to manipulate or elicit the speech of children. This design may require children to describe an event, complete a sentence, or imitate the speech of the investigator (Bloom & Lahey, 1978; Kretschmer & Kretschmer, 1978). Naturalistic observations are generally longitudinal in nature. In the past, the researcher followed the child and wrote down each utterance and the surrounding context. More recent studies employ tape recorders and video tape systems either to supplement or supplant the paper-and-pencil method. In essence, the children are typically recorded for set periods of time in the home environment while additional notes are written on the surrounding context. This method has been used to describe the developmental progress of deaf children exposed to ASL or a signed system (Hoffmeister & Wilbur, 1980; Schlesinger & Meadow, 1972).

In sum, in the literature on language acquisition, experiments have been used mainly to study children's comprehension; that is, to find out how much they really understand and to what degree they rely on contextual cues. A few experiments have concentrated on production and have used various techniques to elicit speech from children. It should be remembered that the younger the children, the more difficult it is to collect experimental data (Brown, 1973; de Villiers & de Villiers, 1978). A discussion of additional problems related specifically to deaf children can be found in Kretschmer and Kretschmer (1978).

Data interpretation

The next step is interpretation of the data; that is, to discover or uncover the patterns of regularity in children's utterances. Interpretation can be based on consistencies among the words (or signs), structures, lengths, or other surface features of children's utterances (Bloom & Lahey, 1978; Dale, 1976; Slobin, 1979). For example, the examiner can group or list children's utterances according to the number of words—one-word, two-word, or three-word utterances. Additional groupings can be based on consistencies of word order; for example, the number of times a word appears in a particular order (Braine, 1971). Still another analysis can be performed employing the terminologies of semantic theorists; for example, the relational categories or the propositions of case grammar. Finally, pragmatic analyses can be performed; for example, describing the specific characteristics or rules associated with turn-taking and speech acts.

Hypotheses formulation

The final step is for the researcher to formalize the information about the observed behaviors. This is a difficult task, and is fraught with controversies. In essence, the researcher hypothesizes about the rules or rule systems that appear to underlie the observed behaviors. While the behaviors can be observed and categorized, the rules can only be inferred and hypothesized. There are discovery procedures for detecting regularities in observations of behavior but there are no discovery procedures for formulating rules of grammar (Chomsky, 1965). The task becomes even more complicated with respect to the close intimate relationship between theoretical perspectives and the nature of the data obtained (Slobin, 1979). The most critical issues in the study of child language are the interpretation of data and the formulation of hypotheses (Bloom & Lahey, 1978; Howe, 1981; Schlesinger, 1982). For example, it can be argued that both transformational grammar and case grammar can provide an adequate explanation of child language. Neither model, developed for adult language, however, provides a complete grammar of child language. Part of the problem in describing child language is due to the production of verbless sentences (Bowerman, 1973). In sum, one of the major goals of linguists and psycholinguists is to create a grammar suitable for both adult and child language.

HEARING CHILDREN

With little difficulty, most hearing children learn the language(s) of their society, that is, the one(s) to which they are exposed. Upon a first inspection, this process appears effortless and relatively simple; however, an in-depth analysis reveals its complex and intricate nature. Despite voluminous research, the exact nature of this language learning process is still open to question. Even the manner in which child language development should be studied abounds with controversies. It seems obvious that descriptions of the primary language development of hearing children should be based on analyses of their spoken utterances, that is, their performance. A number of linguists have argued, however, that such analyses do not and cannot yield an adequate linguistic grammar (Chomsky, 1968; McNeill, 1970). These linguists maintain that any description of primary language development must be based on the competence of the native speaker, not the performance (see the earlier discussion under *Transformational Generative Grammar*). There are others who argue for an opposing view (Bloom & Lahey, 1978; Brown, 1973; Labov, 1972). These investigators are more interested in collecting data on the performance of children than in uncovering innate language acquisition devices. They support this approach by arguing that the methods for analyzing a native-speaking adult's competence (i.e., introspection) are not useful for analyzing children's grammar (Brown, 1973; de Villiers & de Villiers, 1978).

Analyses of the spoken utterances of children are also not devoid of problems. It is extremely difficult to interpret the performance of children, especially in the early stages of development. A major controversy is the extent to which nonlinguistic data (e.g., context cues) should be used as an adjunct to linguistic data in descriptions of language development. Another area of difficulty is the relationship between comprehension and production (de Villiers & de Villiers, 1978; Schlesinger, 1982). These controversies have placed in question the psychological reality of the various linguistic terminologies (e.g., the semantic relation categories) used in describing child language development (Howe, 1981; Schlesinger, 1982). Despite these controversies, it is possible to provide a general description of child language development within a conceptual framework of two time periods, prelinguistic and linguistic, and within the four components of language previously discussed.

Prelinguistic development

Jakobson (1968) remarked that the prelinguistic period, that is, the period prior to the emergence of a child's first words has only recently attracted the attention of linguists. More recently, this period has come within the purview of developmental psychologists and developmental psycholinguists (Lindfors, 1980; Lucas, 1980; Menyuk, 1977). In the past, most researchers viewed this era as uninteresting albeit important to the later linguistic development of the child. Several factors contributed to a renewed, intense interest in this area: (1) the emergence of new apparatus for data collection; (2) the notion that later development is dependent upon early linguistic and cognitive precursors; and (3) the recent focus on the functional aspects of language (e.g., pragmatics) as opposed to the structural aspects (de Villiers & de Villiers, 1978; Menyuk, 1977). In addition to the increasing emphasis on the communicative intent of the utterances, there are a few studies regarding the infant's discrimination of speech sound categories. In essence, the major focus of research in the prelinguistic period is on the descriptions of linguistic and cognitive precursors and their importance to the later mature development of both language and cognition.

Precursors of phonology

Phonologic precursors can be discussed with respect to two aspects of speech: segmental and suprasegmental (Cruttenden, 1979). The segmental aspect refers to the sounds of speech (i.e., vowels and consonants), while the suprasegmental aspect refers to such factors as intonation, stress, and rhythm. These aspects of speech can be examined with respect to the findings on speech production and perception capabilities of infants during this period.

Segmental aspect: Production. Kaplan and Kaplan (1971) delineated four major stages of prelinguistic development. Stage 1 contains crying behaviors, Stage 2 has other vocalization and cooing behaviors, Stage 3 is the babbling period, and Stage 4 is the transitional period between babbling and the emergence of the first words. It should be kept in mind that these stages are not distinct or mutually exclusive, but rather are continuous. In addition, not all children proceed through them in a similar manner or at the same time. Nevertheless, it is possible to present a few salient findings of Stages 3 and 4.

It is generally agreed that the beginning of the babbling stage occurs around the 3rd or 4th month (Cruttenden, 1970; Wolff, 1969). This stage is characterized by two salient events: (1) the emergence of pulmonic–lingual sounds, and (2) the infant's pleasure in producing such sounds (Brown, 1958; Cruttenden, 1970; Wolff, 1969). Pulmonic–lingual sounds refer to those produced as air is interrupted when passing through the tongue along with vowel-like or vocalic sounds. Few generalizations can be made concerning the pattern of development of these sounds for most children (see the reviews in de Villiers & de Villiers, 1978; Menyuk, 1977). It is safe to conclude, however, that the production of consonants moves from the back of the mouth to the front. Another observed pattern concerns the structure of the babbling syllables. In general, vocalic sounds occur initially followed by consonant-vowel (C-V) combinations. Next to occur are the V-C-V combinations, then the V-C combinations, and finally the reduplication of C-V combinations (Cruttenden, 1979; Dale, 1976; Menyuk, 1977). Also, during this period, the child realizes that producing sounds is pleasurable (Wolff, 1969). In fact, this activity may occur with or without the presence of an adult/caretaker. In sum, in producing the segmental aspect of speech, the child is beginning to coordinate his/her tongue, lips and teeth.

Segmental aspect: Perception. Studies of the infant's discrimination of speech sound categories are few in number (see the reviews in de Villiers & de Villiers, 1978; and Menyuk, 1977). It should be born in mind that discrimination is not similar to recognition or comprehension. This issue is discussed in detail in Bruner and Bruner (1968). The studies of Eimas, Siqueland, Jusczyk, and Vigorito (1971) and Morse (1974) have shown that infants as young as 1 month are responsive to speech stimuli and are able to perceive differences between voiceless /p/ and voiced /b/ phonemes produced by an adult. In addition, infants between the ages of 2 and 7 months inclusive have been observed to possess crude localization abilities for sound as evidenced by these infants turning their heads in the direction of a particular sound. It has also been shown that infants, by the age of 3 months, respond differently to their mother's voice as compared to those of other adult females. In general, the infant's ability to discriminate between speech contrasts is superior to his/her ability to discriminate between nonspeech contrasts. This finding implies that sensitivity to speech or speechlike sounds may be unique to human infants during this period.

Suprasegmental aspect: Production and perception. While suprasegmental precursors of pitch, stress, and rhythm have been observed during the prelinguistic period, very little is known regarding the production and perception of this aspect (see the reviews in de Villiers & de Villiers, 1978; Lindfors, 1980; and Menyuk, 1977). Intonation patterns have been observed to emerge during Stage 2 and by Stage 3 (babbling) these patterns begin to resemble those of adults. Halliday (1975) has reported that a contrast between rising and falling intonation is produced by the 10th or 11th month. He stated, however, that this contrast is not present in adult speech; it is, rather, an idiosyncratic system unique to the child. After analyzing several studies, Bloom and Lahey (1978) concluded that the rise–fall contour of infant vocalization may be a more important precursor to the later production of words rather than for the later production of sentence types, that is, statements, questions, and explanations. Other researchers have suggested that early intonation patterns are precursors of the later process of determining old information from new information (pragmatic function) and to interpreting direct and indirect speech acts (Lucas, 1980; Searle, 1969). In sum, a number of researchers have suggested that infants are sensitive to the suprasegmental aspect prior to the segmental aspect of speech (Eimas, 1974; Menyuk, 1974; Morse, 1974).

Relationship between perception and production. The relationship between speech perception and production during the early stages of the prelinguistic period and the later stages is not clearly understood (Cruttenden, 1979; de Villiers & de Villiers, 1978; Menyuk, 1977). One major problem is to explain the discrepancy in time between the perception and production of similar sounds. Another is to account for the differences in the structure of these early productions from the later ones. It has been previously reported, for example, that a child can perceive a distinction between the presence or absence of vocalic sounds by the age of 4 months. The child's production, however, does not reflect this distinction until sometime during the 2nd year of age. In general, the data on production during this period reveal sounds with unequal frequency distributions, and these data are not congruent with those on perception. In addition, the relationship between babbling and the emergence of intelligible speech is still not well understood. Menyuk (1977) has delineated three issues which still need to be resolved by investigators: (1) the uniqueness of speech to the human infant during the prelinguistic period; (2) the existence of a universal developmental sequence in perception and/or production of vocalization; and (3) the relationship of perception and production to each other and to the later development of speech.

Transitional stage. There is a transitional period between babbling and the emergence of one-word utterances. During this stage (approximately 9 to 13 months), a change occurs in the child's repertoire of sounds, and this is known as the babbling drift (Brown, 1958). The child shifts from the production of four or more syllable utterances to those of one or two syllables. In particular, the structure of these utterances consists predominantly of plosives and nasal sounds (e.g., /b/, /d/, /g/, /m/, /n/) in conjunction with low vowels (Cruttenden, 1979). These syllables are of the C-V type described earlier. Several researchers have suggested that the early and late stages of babbling are vocalizations without reference to meaning. In other words, there is no intention to communicate and babbling merely reflects the feelings of the infant (Bloom & Lahey, 1978; de Villiers & de Villiers, 1978). In this view, the child seems to be playing with speech production by exercising the vocal organs in order to gain control over their movements. This development may also be influenced by the reactions from the caretakers. It should be pointed out, however, that precursors of meaning and communicative competence are also developing during this period.

Precursors of semantics–cognition

An overview of semantic–cognitive precursors necessary for the later development of referents is presented here. More detailed descriptions can be found in Bloom and Lahey (1978), Clark and Clark (1977), and Lucas (1980). In many ways, semantic development is isomorphic with cognitive development. Cognitive and semantic categories, however, are not exactly the same. A semantic category, such as a word, may be indicative of a non-linguistic conceptual category; however, it is not the same as a nonlinguistic conceptual category (i.e., schema). Nevertheless, it is safe to conclude the semantic development parallels observed patterns of behavior which correspond to different levels of cognitive development. Thus, prior to the emergence of the first words, semantic and cognitive precursors may be essentially the same.

The development of referents as well as communicative competence is dependent upon cognitive processes which emerge during one of Piaget's stages called sensorimotor (Piaget, 1951, 1971). Prior to learning about object concepts and relational concepts, a child must develop the ability to organize information. This process is inoperable without certain concepts such as object permanency; that is, a stable world replete with persons, objects, and events. Prior to the emergence of intentional and meaningful communication, a child explores the environment for about 1 year. With this exploration comes the realization that persons, objects, and events are separate from the self. By acting on these persons, objects, and events, the child discovers object and relational concepts, and realizes that s/he can have an effect on them. Further discussion of the importance of cognition to the development of language has been presented in chapter 2.

Precursors of pragmatics

Several investigators have suggested that the precursors of speech acts (Dore, 1974, 1975; Searle, 1969, 1975), the functions of speech acts (Halliday, 1975), and the overall communicative aspects of language (Bates, 1976a, 1976b; Bruner, 1974–1975) also emerge during a prelinguistic period. Bruner (1974–1975) states that a child learns about functions, rules, and referential concepts of language while engaging in joint activities with a caretaker. These concepts and rules are also part of the semantic development of the child. Rules of interactions, for example, are learned as the child and caretaker vocalize and respond to each other. The caretaker considers the child's vocalizations a response; this, in turn, prompts a return response from the caretaker. This interaction establishes the roles of speaker and listener which are important to the communicative process.

These intentional and purposive behaviors have been observed as early as 4 months in the motor patterns of the child (Bates, 1976a, 1976b). The child's endeavors to reach for objects while vocalizing simultaneously has been interpreted as a form of communication. In essence, these vocalizations apparently can perform certain functions without conforming to the linguistic structures of the native-speaking adult. In particular, Halliday (1975) delineated several functions in the early linguistic development of his son: (1) instrumental (*I want*); (2) regulatory (*do as I tell you*); (3) interactional (*me* and *you*); and (4) personal (*here I come*). The interactional function was observed to emerge at 9 months; however, it has been observed as early as 4 months (Bates, 1976a, 1976b). Also at nine months, the personal function emerged[1]. By 10½ months, the instrumental and regulatory functions emerged. It should be remembered that the primary forms of communication during this prelinguistic period are cries, smiles, eye-gazing, and vocalizations. All of this implies that the infant uses these behaviors to express his/her needs.

Linguistic development

Prelinguistic development does not simply culminate with the emergence of the first words. In fact, the development of the later stages of this period may parallel the beginning stages of linguistic development. Occasionally, the child may engage in behaviors which emerged earlier in both the prelinguistic and the linguistic periods. This should not be taken to mean that the child is regressing; rather, the child may be increasing understanding of—in Bloom and Lahey's words (1978)—the form, content, and use of language. The stages of linguistic development discussed here are (1) the one-word stage, (2) the two-word stage, and (3) linguistic maturity. An alternative way to view language development, particularly grammatical development, is to employ the stages of Brown (1973) based upon mean length of utterance. While this method is not adopted here, it is briefly discussed later to account for the development of inflectional morphemes. As with prelinguistic development, the development of the linguistic stages are continuous; the labels are used by investigators for the purpose of studying various parts of the stages.

The child's first words generally mark the beginning of linguistic development. Depending on the nature of the linguistic criteria established, different ages may be reported for the emergence of the first words. Dale (1976) cited three general requirements which have been reported in the literature: (1) The child must demonstrate an understanding of the word; (2) the child must use the word consistently and spontaneously with reference to an object or event; and (3) the word must be recognized as one from a native-speaking adult's lexicon. The age at which the first words emerge has been reported to be between 10 and 13 months (Bloom & Lahey, 1978; de Villiers & de Villiers, 1978; Schlesinger, 1982).

Analyses of the first words and later development are conducted within the conceptual framework of the four linguistic components. It has been argued that syntactical anaylses are not useful for determining the content of the first words (Bloom, 1973; Brown, 1958). More specifically, it is demonstrated that syntactic precursors do not appear until the end of the one-word stage (Bloom, 1973; Dore, Franklin, Miller, & Ramer, 1976). In addition, it is argued that syntax, as a linguistic component, does not emerge until sometime during the two-word stage (Bloom & Lahey, 1978; Cruttenden, 1979; Kretschmer & Kretschmer, 1978). Thus, descriptions of the child's first words are primarily phonologic, semantic, or pragmatic in nature.

Phonologic development: Second year and beyond

A review of the literature reveals three general conclusions regarding the description of the phonologic development of young children (Cruttenden, 1970; Eimas, 1974; Kaplan & Kaplan, 1971; Menn, 1982; Menyuk, 1974; Morse, 1974). The first, presented earlier, is that prior to the age of 2, the developmental data on perception and production are equivocal and inconclusive. The second is that there exist at least three units of phonologic analyses: phonemes, syllables, and words. The third is that, in general, there are two approaches to analyzing child phonology: (1) The developmental sequence of the child's sound system can be compared with that of the adult model; or (2) this development can be described with reference to the particular child's strategy, and this, in turn, can be compared with that of the adult.

Unit of analysis: Phonemes. Prior to the 1970s, most researchers employed the phoneme as the unit of anaylsis and their approach was to compare the child's development to that of the adult. Jakobson (1968) attempted to chart the order of phonemic acquisition by using his notion of distinctive feature analysis. He proposed several principles to delineate the order of acquisition; only two are presented here: (1) The description of phonologic development should parallel the mastery of distinctive features; and (2) the system of phonemic contrasts of the child may not always be similar to that of adults in distinguishing between words. It should be seen that the second principle is a move away from the dominant approach of this period. In essence, Jakobson argued that the pattern of phonologic development in all children is systematic and universal. The universal sequence proposed by Jakobson is as follows: (1) Children initially differentiate vowels from consonants; (2) then, they make a distinction between oral stop and nasal consonants; (3) next, they distinguish between labial (lip) and apical (tip of tongue) stops; and finally, (4) they differentiate the high vowels from the low vowels.

The difficulties in evaluating this theory are discussed in detail elsewhere (Fromkin & Rodman, 1978). Prior to the age of 2, the production and perception data are equivocal (Braine, 1971; Dale, 1976; Ferguson & Garnica, 1975). Some evidence for the theory, that is, for the reality of distinctive features, has been observed after the age of 2 (Menyuk, 1968). It seems that after children have mastered a particular phonemic contrast, they generalize this knowledge to other phonemes with similar distinctive features. In sum, there appears to be a wide variation in the early phonologic development of children. This development, however, may be systematic and probably should be analyzed with reference to the child's system of strategies (Menn, 1982).

Units of analyses: Syllables and words. More recent research has moved away from the phoneme as a unit of analysis to either syllables (Moskowitz, 1973) or whole words (Ferguson & Farwell, 1975). These investigators have argued that a child's phonological development does not proceed one sound at a time or by mastery of successive distinctive features. Instead, they proposed that development occurs according to certain strategies or rules. A good description of these general strategies can be found in Ingram (1976). In addition, de Villiers and de Villiers (1978) cite a major shortcoming of the earlier phonemic and distinctive feature analyses: the failure to consider error types and substitutions in the child's production. These researchers argued that such analyses are important for charting the phonological development of the child with reference to his/her own system. In addition, this approach sheds more light on the perception–production issue. While this is described in detail in de Villiers and de Villiers (1978) and Menyuk (1977), some major points are related here. In general, perception precedes production. Sometimes both processes, however, appear to be simultaneous, and occasionally production may precede perception. As discussed earlier, the sequence of phonemic development in perception may not be congruent with that of production. Finally, the contribution of additional unrelated factors (e.g., frequency of occurrence) to the process of phonological development needs to be studied.

Mastery of phonological rules. In general, most of the phonological rules are acquired by around 6 to 8 years of age (Moskowitz, 1973; Winitz, 1969). From age 3 onwards, the child attempts to acquire the rules associated with the various inflectional endings of nouns and verbs (Brown, 1973). The more general rules of phonology are acquired prior to the acquisition of the specific or less general rules. A description of some of these rules can be found in

Durkin (1978). The early stages of phonological development cannot be described with reference to phonemic contrasts or distinctive features. This development can be charted only after the acquisition of a certain number of words in the child's lexicon. The strategies the child develops may relate these words to each other or to an adult model. Finally, these strategies may be dependent upon the particular first words acquired by the child.

Syntactical development: The transitional and the two-word stages

Several investigators have identified syntactic precursors prior to the emergence of the two-word stage (Bloom, 1973; Dore et al., 1976). The notion of syntax, or that word order is meaningful, is marked by the production of successive utterances which do not, at this time, function as connected or cohesive linguistic units. Bloom (1973), for example, reported that a 16-month-old child consistently used one word (i.e., *wide*) with a certain phrase. She maintained that this lexical unit was not interpretable since it referred to *anything and everything*. Other notions of syntactic precursors are (1) the use of a nonsense syllable with a cetain lexical unit, (2) the reduplicated production of a single lexical unit successively, (3) the production of a single, phonetically, unstable unit prior to a lexical unit, and (4) the production of two words in combination consistently and restrictively (i.e., not with other word combinations).

The beginning of grammar, particularly syntax, commences with the combination of two or more words in sentences (Dale, 1976; de Villiers & de Villiers, 1978). The syntactic activity during this period prepares the child for the later acquisition of the major transformations of the language. An important question in the two-word stage is whether children possess knowledge of subject and predicate, and whether this knowledge is similar to that of adults. Several researchers have suggested that knowledge of the basic grammatical relation between subject and predicate is possessed by children (Bloom, Miller, & Hood, 1975; Smith, 1975a). Bloom and Lahey (1978), however, argue that such knowledge is not syntactic only, but rather semantic–syntactic in nature. They described two kinds of relationships: linear syntactical relationship and hierarchical syntactical relationship. In the former, relational words (e.g., *more, away*) are combined with other words, and the meaning of the relational word determines the meaning relation of the two-word combinations. In hierarchical syntactical relationship, these combinations involve the form classes of nouns and pronouns in relation to verbs. The meaning of these combinations (i.e., subject–predicate concepts), however, are not the same as the meaning of the individual words. In the latter combinations, the children must know both the category of word order relation between words and semantic relation between words. This position is also supported by Bowerman (1975). In addition, both syntactic and semantic complexity have been employed as adequate indices in accounting for the acquisition of the inflectional morphemes by Brown (1973). Essentially, Brown maintained that both components overlap making it difficult to distinguish their relative contributions. Other researchers agreed that knowledge of subject–predicate is present at this stage, but it is better explained by pragmatic terminology (Bates, 1976b; Greenfield & Smith, 1976). These investigators maintain that the use of word order by children is in accordance with a given–new concept. In the adult use of this concept, given or known information is presented first followed by new or unknown information. It has been reported that in children the order is reversed. Thus, the first word in the two-word stage is the comment about the topic which occurs as the second word. In sum, the notion of syntax is present in the two-word stage. This notion, however, may be inextricably related to those of semantics or pragmatics. While more research is needed in this area, it is safe to conclude that syntactical analyses alone are not adequate at the level of two words.

Semantic development: One-term and two-term relations

An important aspect in the language growth of a child is the development of semantic or meaningful referents (Lindfors, 1980; Lucas, 1980; Schlesinger, 1982). These referents reflect the organization of the child's knowledge concerning persons, objects, events, and relations (Bloom, 1970, 1973; Brown, 1973). The meanings of these one-term and two-term semantic relations have caused considerable controversy (Howe, 1981; Schlesinger, 1982). Essentially, it is argued that these early relations must be analyzed with respect to the surrounding context. de Villiers and de Villiers (1978) have cited several ways in which the meanings of the first words have been described in the literature: (1) categorization of objects and events; (2) categorization of relations between self and other persons, objects and/or events; (3) categorization of relations between others and objects and/or events. The psychological reality of semantic relations have been questioned due to the possibility of categorizing relations in an infinite number of ways (Bowerman, 1976; Howe, 1981; Schlesinger, 1982). In addition, the semantic attributes which contribute to the acquisition of the first words produced and comprehended by children are not agreed upon yet. These attributes have been termed functional (Nelson, 1973), perceptual (Bowerman, 1976; Clark, 1973), relational–categorical (Bloom, 1973), and relational (Greenfield & Smith, 1976). A detailed description can be found in Bloom and Lahey (1978), Dale (1976), and Menyuk (1977); a few salient findings are reported here.

Nelson (1973) investigated the nature of the first 50 words acquired by children. This investigator remarked that two-word combinations emerge after the acquisition of at least 50 words. Nelson reported her findings in six categories. The most common category was general nominals, for example, *milk, dog,* which consisted of 51% of the data. Next with 14% of the data each were specific nominals (e.g., *mommy*) and action words (e.g., *give*). Nelson concluded that the words that are learned initially are those which the child can manipulate; that is, these words are functional.

Clark (1973) reported on the phenomenon of overextension; that is, the use of a word to reflect a broader category than is appropriate. An example is the use of the word *daddy* to refer to all men encountered. Clark argued that overextensions may be based upon perceptual attributes which she classified into six categories: shape, sound, size, movement, taste, and texture. Her data revealed that the most common overextensions are concrete nouns occurring between the ages of 12 and 30 months.

Underextensions, as well as overextensions, were reported by Bowerman (1976). Underextension refers to a word representing a narrower category than is appropriate. This phenomenon is difficult to determine since the child is employing the label in a correct albeit restricted manner. Bowerman maintained that underextensions, like overextensions, are related to perceptual attributes of objects. It is suggested that underextensions occur prior to overextensions.

Bloom (1970, 1973) argued that the first words are relational–categorical. These relational words (e.g., *this, uh oh, no more*) reflect the behavior of objects and are predominant in the one-word or one-term utterances. Bloom labels the relation of object to itself as reflexive-object relation. This semantic category consists of four relations: existence, nonexistence, disappearance, and recurrence. At a later period, Bloom states that children produce words reflecting causality–locative relationships which focus on the various aspects of the communicative situation.

In many ways, the two-term stage is a continuation of those semantic relations identified in the one-term stage (Bloom, 1973; Brown, 1973; Greenfield & Smith, 1976). Greenfield and Smith (1976) argue that the semantic relation in this stage consists only of those expressed in the previous stage. In Bloom and Lahey's words (1978), children in this stage use old functions (i.e., relations) to gain mastery of new forms.

Semantic relations expressed in the two-word stage have been described extensively in the literature (Bloom, 1973; Bowerman, 1973; Brown, 1973; Cruttenden, 1979). Only the most common relations are discussed here. With little disagreement, these relations can be grouped into eight categories: nomination, attribution, recurrence, possession, notice or exclamation, negation, location, and action. Examples of the first five are: nomination—*that car*; attribution—*big car*; recurrence—*more car*; possession—*mommy car*; and notice or exclamation—*hi car.* The categories of negation, location, and action may be subdivided into further categories. For example, negation may reflect nonexistence (*no cookie*) or disappearance (*allgone cookie*). Location may reflect a noun plus noun category, *mommy car*; or verb plus verb, *walk car*; or noun plus prolocative, *car up there.* Action may reflect an agent–action category, *Daddy read*; or agent–object (noun plus noun), *mommy sock*; or agent–object (verb plus noun), *make cookie.* During this stage, the relations which initially occur in large quantities are possession, recurrence, negation, and location.

On the surface level, it appears that some two-term utterances (e.g., *mommy sock*) may be classified in any one of several relation categories. The interpretation of these semantic relations must be based upon the child's intent, and this intent is made clearer by the surrounding context. Bloom (1970) reported an example of one utterance (*mommy sock*) which could express two different semantic relationships with respect to two different contexts. In one context, this two-term relation referred to the concept of mommy putting on her own sock whereas, in the other, mommy was putting the child's sock on the child.

Pragmatic development: The functions of one- and two-word stages

In general, pragmatic development entails the acquisition of semantic rules which are necessary for engaging in purposive and intentional behaviors (Bates, 1976a, 1976b; Bruner, 1975; Lucas, 1980). The basic unit of analysis of pragmatics is the speech act (Searle, 1969, 1975). Speech acts have been investigated in very young children (see the reviews in Bloom & Lahey, 1978 and Lucas, 1980). For example, Dore (1974, 1975) attempted to describe the developmental stage of language acquisition by employing Searle's (1969) theory of speech acts. Several primitive speech acts (PSAs) were identified: labeling, repeating, answering, requesting an answer, requesting (action), calling, greeting, protesting, and practicing. Dore suggested that the one- and two-term semantic relations of children contain both a function and form and represent the content of the child's social interactions. Others disagree, however, that these early utterances have a form (Bloom & Lahey, 1978; Halliday, 1975). An interesting finding reported is that some of the PSAs of the child are different from the more mature adult's speech acts. These differences contribute to the difficulty of interpreting the intentions and purposes of the child. Dore maintained, however, that the development of clearer intentions and purposes parallels the acquisition of more advanced linguistic competency. Thus, the child eventually uses speech acts which are in accordance with those of the native-speaking adult.

The basic context for speech acts, or rather, communicative competence, is social interactions. During the prelinguistic period, the child expresses the beginnings of purposive and intentional behaviors in his/her motor patterns. Typical behaviors include crying, vocalizing, eye-gazing, smiling and various attempts to reach for objects in conjunction with some of these behaviors. By the 2nd year, due to an increase in mobility and cognitive structures, the communicative gestures consist of showing, giving, and pointing (Bates, 1976a). This phase commences with the child showing an object to an adult. Then, the child engages in such behaviors as giving objects and pointing out objects (deixis). The major function of these acts is to direct the adult's attention to the object. The attention and acceptance of the adult/caretaker is important for the child. The emergence of the first words coincides with these early communicative behaviors of showing, giving, and pointing (deixis). A more detailed description of the substance and function of interaction/deixis may be found in Kretschmer and Kretschmer (1978), Lindfors (1980) and Lucas (1980).

The functions of speech acts have also been reported by Halliday (1975). Phase I, described earlier, contained four functions. Halliday maintains that during Phase II the child continues to master the functions of language by using utterances which resemble those used by adults. In addition, Halliday reported that a fifth function, heuristic, emerges during this phase around the 13th or 14th month. This function entails the use of vocalization in exploring and learning about the environment. In the earlier heuristic period, a child demands the names of objects, and later on, this behavior evolves into questioning behaviors. Halliday maintains that it is possible to make a distinction between the *mathetic* and pragmatic functions of language. The mathetic function is the use of language to learn about persons, objects, and events in the environment. The precursors of this function are the personal and heuristic functions. The pragmatic function refers to the regulation of others' behaviors and attempts to satisfy personal needs. The precursors of this function are the instrumental and regulatory functions. The interaction function contributes to the development of both the mathetic and pragmatic functions. In sum, Halliday argues that the functions of language are expressed in isolation prior to the age of 2. During the 2nd year, however, a child's utterance contains both mathetic and pragmatic functions.

Comprehension–production

Central to the analyses of the first words is the comprehension–production issue. This issue was discussed earlier with respect to the sounds of speech; it is presented here with respect to the nature of the first words. This relationship has not been investigated extensively. The productions of children have received more attention than the corresponding comprehensions of words. The paucity of research is not due to a lack of interest, but rather to the difficulty of measuring the comprehension of children. A more detailed description of these difficulties can be found in Bloom and Lahey (1978). This issue has not been resolved; however, a few tentative findings are presented here.

It is suggested that the one-word utterances of children are analogous to the sentences of adults (Antinucci & Parisi, 1973; McNeill, 1970). This phenomena is termed holophrastic speech, implying that children understand more than they say. While the word-or-sentence hypothesis has been discussed extensively (Antinucci & Parisi, 1973; Bloom, 1973; McNeill, 1970), most of the evidence seems to support Bloom's (1973) argument that the extent of children's early knowledge is restricted to lexical meanings, not grammatical meaning, that is, syntax or relations between words. The question of whether comprehension precedes production or vice versa has been investigated by Huttenlocher (1974) with four 1-year-old children. Huttenlocher devised procedures to assess comprehension by minimizing the influence of contextual cuing. A list of words with precise meanings, that is, those understood by the subjects, was obtained. This is contrary to Clark's (1973) and Bowerman's (1976) contentions that obtaining precise meaning is extremely difficult at this stage. The results of this study also supported Bloom's (1973) arguments. In sum, Huttenlocher concluded that at the one-word stage (1) the comprehension of children is dependent upon contextual cues rather than on verbal comprehension, and (2) there are no instances of overextensions; thus, comprehension of lexical items precedes production.

Shipley, Smith, and Gleitman (1969) investigated the comprehension issue in two groups of children: One group used single-word utterances and the other used telegraphic two- and three-word sentences. Commands were presented to these children in (1) single words, (2) telegraphic speech, or (3) well-formed sentences. Conflicting results were reported. The single-word group responded best to commands of first words, thus substantiating the claim that comprehension precedes production at this stage. The telegraphic group, however, reponded best to well-formed commands. This latter result cannot be interpreted in the same way as the former.

In sum, Bloom and Lahey (1978) suggested that different kinds of questions should be asked concerning comprehension and production. Instead of investigating which one precedes the other or the relationship between the two, they suggest studying the processes that underlie each and the relationship of the two processes to linguistic and cognitive development. They suggested that "the developmental gap between comprehension and speaking probably varies among different children and at different times, and that the gap may be more apparent than real" (p. 238).

Linguistic maturity

As the child proceeds through the three-word stage and beyond, it still is difficult to assess the relative contributions of each linguistic component *in isolation* to this development. For example, it was mentioned earlier that Brown (1973) reported on the developmental sequence of the first inflectional morphemes. While syntactic and semantic complexity were adjudged to be good indices of development, it is difficult to isolate the relative contributions. Kretschmer and Kretschmer (1978), however, contend that an analysis of Brown's data reveals that semantic complexity precedes syntactic complexity and is predominant. After some kind of order (semantic) is established, syntactic complexity comes into operation. This view is not shared by others (de Villiers & de Villiers, 1978). Nevertheless, most of the contributions to the development of language have been attributed to syntax and semantics; however, the effects of pragmatics is beginning to be noticed (Ervin-Tripp & Mitchell-Kernan, 1977; Lucas, 1980). The importance of pragmatics is not questioned; rather, the precise nature of the effects of this component on language development still needs to be determined (Bloom & Lahey, 1978).

Beyond the three-word stage, the child begins to produce and comprehend linguistic forms and functions of a more complex nature. Now the child is learning the general, adult rules which govern the application of rules for the various linguistic components. The child plays an active role by discovering regularities and formulating hypotheses regarding the application of the rules (Berko, 1958; Bloom & Lahey, 1978; de Villiers & de Villiers, 1978; Menyuk,

1977). Through the joint social interactions or deixes (pragmatic), the child acquires semantic referents and functions for persons, objects, and events, in his/her environment. The form of the referents entails the combinations of the arbitrarily defined symbols from phonology, morphology, and syntax. The application of linguistic form, content, and function correspond to a rule system (Bloom & Lahey, 1978; Lindfors, 1980; Lucas, 1980).

The mature linguistic forms are acquired through the processes of modulation and refinement. The basis of these processes is the acquisition of morphemes which alters meaning and form (Brown, 1973). The early syntactic–semantic utterances are modulated and subsequently expanded (or refined) into structures similar to those used by adults. Initially, two operations are in effect: embedding and conjoining (Brown, 1973). An example of embedding is: *no cookie* and *make cookie* becomes *make no cookie*. *No cookie*, which expresses a functional relation, is inserted or embedded into *make cookie* to form a grammatical relation. An example of conjoining is: *Mommy make* and *make cookie* becomes *Mommy make cookie*. In conjoining, two grammatical relations sharing a common term are conjoined with the redundant term deleted. In sum, an increase in semantic information parallels the increase in structure complexity, and this phenomenon is reflected in the complex utterance produced (Lucas, 1980).

In general, beyond the three-word stage, the syntactic development of the child consists of learning the major transformations of the language (Dale, 1976; de Villiers & de Villiers, 1978). Initially, the child adheres to a noun–verb–noun or a subject–verb–object word order which present problems in some transformations, notably passivization (de Villiers & de Villiers, 1978). Nevertheless, the major transformations, for example, question formation, relativization, are acquired in a systematic manner. For example, in question formation, yes/no questions precede Wh-questions, which in turn are acquired prior to tag questions. In addition, there are smaller acquisition steps within each group. Discussions of these terms and the acquisition process can be found in Dale (1976) and Russell et al. (1976). In general, most children have internalized much of the grammar of the language by the age of 4 or 5 years and have mastered nearly all of the grammar by age 9 or 10.

As stated earlier, semantic development (and probably pragmatic development) is isomorphic to cognitive development (Lucas, 1980). Pragmatics consists of utilizing the rules of semantics. Semantic referents can be categorized as objective and agentive, action, dimensional, and spatial and temporal. The beginning of social interaction or deixis is characterized by the identification of referents with corresponding labels (Bruner, 1974–1975). This process helps the child organize knowledge about persons, objects, and events. The growth in vocabulary and other linguistic variables is hypothesized to be influenced by these interactions (Lucas, 1980). In essence, most of the semantic referents are acquired by the second stage of cognition as delineated by Piaget (1971). This is nearly congruent with syntactical development. By the age of 10, 11, or 12 years, the child has reached linguistic maturity; that is, s/he has mastered most, if not all, of the finite set of the native-speaking adult *rules* regarding the form, content, and function of language.

DEAF CHILDREN

As previously discussed, describing the primary language development of deaf children is much more complicated than describing the primary language development of hearing children. Quigley and Kretschmer (1982) have stated that descriptions of the language development of deaf children must consider two important issues: (1) the nature of the language input, that is, English or American Sign Language, and (2) the nature of the communication mode used, that is, manual or oral. In addition, these languages and communication modes may be employed in various combinations and may emphasize one or other of the primary sense modalities, that is, audition or vision. With this in mind, the language development of deaf children may be charted in each of three categories: oral English (OE), manually coded English (MCE), and American Sign Language (ASL). These three categories probably are representative of most of the language input to deaf children in infancy and early childhood. As much as possible, research findings are reported here within each of these categories with reference to the various components of language described previously (cherological [phonologic], morphological, syntactic, semantic, and pragmatic). It should be remembered that there is a paucity of data on the primary language development of deaf children in each of these approaches and a variety of research designs were used in gathering the data. Some of the research involved retrospective studies employing secondary language assessments, that is, the read and written modes, in evaluating the efficiency of these approaches for developing primary language. There are a few studies, however, which are developmental; that is, these studies attempted to chart some aspect of primary language development.

Language and communication categories

Prior to delineating the most commonly used approaches in each category, several remarks should be made concerning the general nature of the categories themselves. It has been claimed that deaf children exposed to the OE and MCE approaches are, in fact, exposed to some representation of standard English (King, 1981). The relationship of this visual linguistic input to that of the primary aural–oral linguistic input of hearing children is not well understood. The developmental rate and extent of English for some deaf children, however, has been reported to be similar to that of hearing children (Ogden, 1979). The main purpose of the pedagogical approaches associated with OE and MCE is to teach standard English as a first language. In this respect, most deaf children are exposed to some form of English in infancy and early childhood (King, 1981; Luetke-Stahlman, 1982; Rawlings & Jensema, 1977).

American Sign Language, on the other hand, is a language with a grammar different from that of English (Lane & Grosjean, 1980; Liddell, 1980). It is important to remember that ASL is a *signed language* whereas the various approaches of MCE are contrived *signed codes,* designed to represent the grammar of English. Thus, description of grammatical development in ASL is different from that of English, in the same manner that Chinese is different from English. There is, however, another important difference, ASL is a *signed* language (i.e., visual–gestural) whereas both Chinese and English are *spoken* languages (i.e., aural–oral). In essence, ASL differs from English in both grammar and modality. The nature and importance of these differences, or more specifically, the relationship between signed languages and spoken languages, is currently being debated (Siple, 1982). It is possible that the primary language development of deaf children exposed to ASL parallels that of hearing children exposed to an aural–oral language (Lane & Grosjean, 1980; Siple, 1982). Another question, however, concerns the manner in which English must be taught to these children, if it is to be taught at all. As discussed in the chapter on bilingualism, it is possible that English should be taught as a second language to ASL-oriented deaf children.

Definitions of the major communication and language categories (OE, MCE, and ASL) and specific approaches used within some of the categories (e.g., signed English, cued speech) have been provided in the first chapter and are discussed again in the chapter on bilingualism and English as a second language (ESL). It is important to emphasize repeatedly that the definitions and categories are idealized versions of what usually occurs in practice. For example, Marmor and Pettito (1979) and Reich and Bick (1977) have shown that MCE approaches in actual practice tend to resemble pidgin sign English (PSE) more than they do standard English. One imperative of this is that future studies of the primary language development of deaf children should describe specifically the form of language input to which the children were consistently exposed.

It is helpful in remembering the somewhat arbitrary and idealized nature of the definitions and categories to consider the various language and communication approaches as a continuum ranging from least representative to most representative of the grammar of standard English (Baker & Cokely, 1980; Wilbur, 1979). The relationships of the various approaches to standard English are depicted in Figure 1. ASL is a *signed language* with a grammar different from that of English (and other *spoken languages*) and least resembles English in vocabulary and structure. It therefore anchors one end of the continuum. The various MCE approaches are *signed codes* which are invented and contrived means of representing the vocabulary and structure of standard English. The manner in which each of the signed codes represents a written English word determines its placement on the continuum in Figure 1. For example, the English word *Beautifully* can be represented by (a) one manual

Figure 1: Relation of Approaches to English Grammar

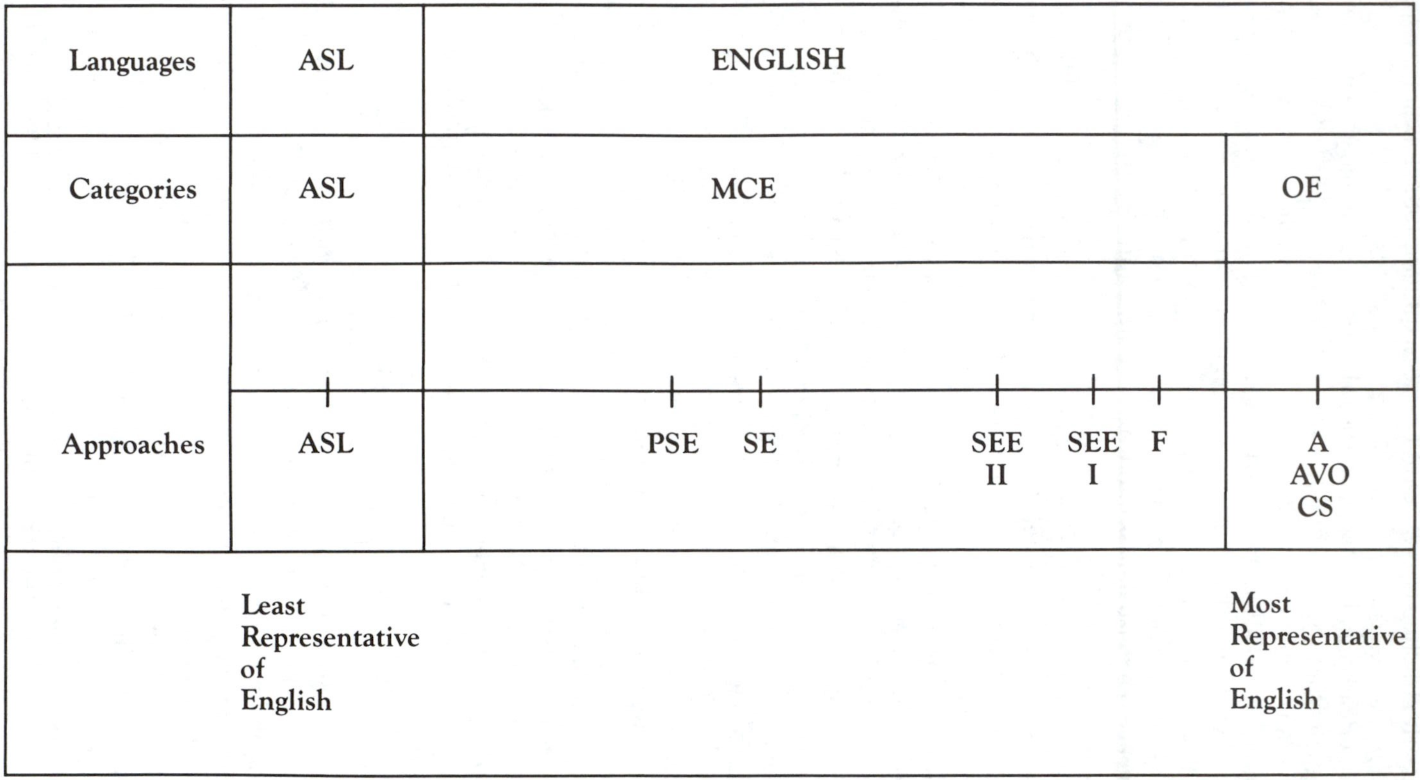

	Least Representative of English				Most Representative of English
Languages	ASL	ENGLISH			
Categories	ASL	MCE			OE
Approaches	ASL	PSE SE	SEE II	SEE I SEE F	CS AVO A

marker (sign) for the whole word as in PSE (Wilbur, 1979; Woodward, 1973); (b) two manual markers, one for *Beautiful* and one for *-ly* as in SEE II (Gustason, Pfetzing, & Zawolkow, 1975); or (c) one manual marker for each letter as in finger spelling (Scouten, 1967; Quigley, 1969). From this (a) is considered to be least representative of English and (c) most representative (Bornstein, 1973; Wilbur, 1979). In this line of reasoning, finger spelling is considered to be most representative of the vocabulary and structure of English. Next is SEE I, then SEE II, signed English, and PSE. Since all OE approaches, including those supplemented by cued speech, use standard English, these anchor the other end of the continuum in Figure 1. This concept of a continuum allows for the various gradations in the communication and language approaches that are likely to occur in actual practice.

The relative merits of the various communication approaches used in developing language in deaf children are shrouded in controversy. Most of the arguments, however, are polemic rather than data based. The extensive historical backgrounds of the various approaches have been described in chapter 1. The crux of the matter is that these approaches are not new. The controversy which still exists after more than 200 years of practice is indicative of the notion that none of these approaches has proven adequate for *all* deaf children. In fact, it is possible that a universal approach does not exist (Moores, 1978; Quigley & Kretschmer, 1982). Obviously, the controversies cannot be resolved by polemics. It is possible, however, that they may not yield even to scientific study. Nevertheless, a scientific, research approach is much more likely to produce shared, objective knowledge for assessing these approaches both as instructional methods and as means for developing primary language. Systematic research has been conducted only in the last 20 years, so, as stated earlier, the contributions of research have not yet been substantial.

OE and language development

Research on OE approaches are presented in two major categories: cued speech (CS) and the traditional oral English approaches. It is shown that the data on OE approaches are extremely limited. In addition, favorable data on OE approaches appear to be restricted to select groups of deaf children. These data, however, do seem to indicate that these deaf individuals are successful both educationally and vocationally.

Cued speech (CS)

Very little empirical data exist on the pedagogical use of this approach. A few studies have attempted to assess primarily the reception of CS by deaf children (Clarke & Ling, 1976; Ling & Clarke, 1975; Nicholls, 1979) with one of them also investigating corresponding expressive, that is, speech and language, development. Speech reception scores were obtained under different experimental conditions involving various combinations of audition, lip reading, and cuing. Superior scores resulted from the lip reading plus cues condition in two studies (Clarke & Ling, 1976; Ling & Clarke, 1975); whereas, in a longer study conducted in Australia, superior scores resulted from lip reading plus cues plus audition (Nicholls, 1979). No corresponding development was reported for expressive speech and language.

A more recent study attempted to assess the effects of cued speech on the language development of deaf children as well as to compare those effects with those of an oral program previously attempted (Mohay, 1983). In this study, language development was operationally defined as (1) the production of cues, (2) the frequency of communication, that is, the total number of noncued gestures and words, (3) the range and depth of lexical development, and (4) the length and structure of spoken utterances. Three deaf children served as subjects, one of whom did not meet the criteria for deafness as defined in this book (i.e., HTL was 72 dB). All three subjects were transferred to a cued speech (CS) program from an oral program. Of the four areas listed above, the most positive effects of CS were reported in Category 4. In essence, all subjects began to produce word combinations after the introduction to CS. Mohay suggested, however, that other factors may have played a role; namely, increased maturity, vocabulary growth, cognitive development, or a combination of these. It was concluded that the effects of CS on this, and other aspects of language development, need further investigation.

Oral English

To adequately evaluate studies of this approach, several cautions should be born in mind: (1) The children in these studies should be deaf as defined earlier; (2) the studies should contain deaf children who have been exposed *primarily* to an oral approach; and (3) the studies should contain deaf children from highly structured, comprehensive oral programs, for example, Central Institute for the Deaf (CID), or from those integrated into regular education programs. These considerations have been discussed in detail elsewhere (Quigley & Kretschmer, 1982). In essence, the studies reported here are limited as much as possible to the above considerations. Several of these studies indicated that the mean performances of these deaf children were inferior to those of comparable hearing children. It should be remembered that most of these deaf children still attain an achievement superior to most of those educated in the other approaches. It is difficult, however, to generalize from the findings; this issue is discussed in the summary.

Phonologic and syntactical development of oral deaf students

Mavilya and Mignone (1977) investigated the oral development of three deaf children from birth to 5 years of age at the Lexington School for the Deaf. A comprehensive list of speech stages was reported. Typically, the children began the babbling stage at 6 months. This finding is almost 2 to 3 months later than that observed for hearing children (Cruttenden, 1979). Similar to hearing children, however, these deaf children were producing one and two words at 24 months. By the age of 30 months, these children began to use their voices with other deaf children. In addition, the 3- to 4-words stage emerged around age 3. Finally, the children's speech began to approximate that of an adult around age 5.

This study seems to indicate that at least some deaf children can master aspects of speech and language at rates comparable to that of hearing children. This has been confirmed in another study using the syllable as a unit of analysis (Ling, Leckie, Pollack, Simser, & Smith, 1981). It has been argued, further, that most educational programs do not have adequate provisions for developing speech communication skills (Ling, 1976). Thus, adequate oral language development is not as commonly achieved with deaf children as it ought to be.

Dodd (1976) conducted a two-part study on the speech of deaf children to determine if their phonological systems were rule governed. In the first part, the speech of 10 deaf children, age 11 years, was analyzed. The results indicated that each subject produced more than half of all the 42 phones of English. Additionally, it was concluded that the phonologic systems of these children are, in part, rule governed, and used by hearing children at an earlier stage. It was hypothesized that the systems are only partially rule governed due to the incomplete information provided by the residual hearing and speech reading abilities of these deaf children. The second part of the study was conducted to ascertain the existence of nine phonologic rules derived from the findings on the first part. Significant predictive values were obtained for six of the nine rules under a lip reading experimental condition.

Presnell (1973) investigated the syntactic ability of both deaf and hearing children, aged 5 to 13 years, by analyzing spontaneous language samples and the results of the Northwestern Syntax Screening Test (NSST; Lee, 1969). Some deaf children in this study had hearing threshold levels of less than 90 dB; however, all were prelingually hearing impaired. The findings depict a profile which is reported later in the studies in the section on MCE approaches. In essence, the rate of syntactic development in deaf children was slower than that of comparable hearing children. It was noted that the older deaf children outperformed the younger ones. In addition, it was found that the most rapid rate of language development occurred between the ages of 5 and 9. Analyses of the spontaneous language samples revealed no significant improvement associated with age. Finally, Presnell reported that deaf children acquire some verb constructions in a different order than that reported for hearing children. It was hypothesized that this difference was due to the unnatural order of teaching verbs by the instructors of hearing-impaired students.

A more recent study (Geers & Moog, 1978) assessed the spontaneous language and imitated language of deaf children, ages 4 to 15. Several of these subjects also had hearing threshold levels of less than 90 dB. The subjects were administered the Developmental Sentence Analysis (DSS; Lee, 1974) and the Carrow Elicited Language Inventory (CELI; Carrow, 1974). Similar to Presnell's findings, the most rapid language development occurred between the ages of 4 and 9. On the DSS, the scores of more than half of the subjects were inferior to the scores of the average 3-year-old hearing child. Similarly, on the CELI, more than half of the deaf subjects produced more errors than the average 3-year-old hearing child. Qualitatively, the deaf subjects produced more structurally complex sentences, albeit with a greater number of grammatical errors, than the hearing children. This difference, however, may be due to a difference in age; that is, the deaf children ranged from 4 to 15 years of age whereas the hearing children ranged from 2 to 6 years of age.

Semantic and pragmatic development of oral deaf children

A few studies have explored the development of semantics and pragmatics in oral deaf children. As with the other components, it is concluded that the development of deaf children is similar to—albeit, slower than— that of comparable hearing children. Skarakis and Prutting (1977) studied the early linguistic behaviors of four deaf children, ages 2 years 1 month to 4 years 3 months, at the John Tracy clinic. These behaviors were categorized into 13 semantic functions and 8 communicative intent (pragmatic) functions. These functions are similar to those observed in hearing children at 9 to 18 months of age (Halliday, 1975; Lucas, 1980). Some of the semantic functions reported in the literature on hearing children, however, were not present in the data on deaf children. It was interesting to note that the verbal data indicated that the number of semantic functions exceeded that of pragmatic functions whereas the nonverbal data demonstrated that pragmatic exceeded semantic. In essence, similar to Halliday's contention for hearing children, it was suggested that both types of functions may not be differentiated in the early linguistic stages of deaf children.

This similar—but slower—rate of development has been reported also by Jarvella and Lubinsky (1975), studying the development of temporal semantic functions. It should be remembered that these semantic functions are difficult even for hearing children, most of whom achieve mastery around 8, 9, or 10 years of age (Lucas, 1980). Twenty deaf children, age 8 to 11 years, and twenty hearing children, age 8 to 9 years, served as subjects. The deaf children were enrolled in a day school in Cleveland, Ohio. Several tasks were administered; however, only the oral listening tasks are pertinent here. Both groups of children were required to listen to sentences spoken by the experimenter, and then to arrange pictures in a sequence. In general, deaf children performed similarly to hearing children when the temporal order in the sentences was preserved, that is, *after* clause first or *before* clause second. The performance of deaf children, however, was inferior to the hearing children and only at chance level when the temporal order was reversed.

Oral deaf children in regular classes

It has been hypothesized that oral deaf children with adequate language skills are likely to be integrated into regular classrooms with hearing children.

Some evidence has been found to support this notion (Doehring, Bonnycastle, & Ling, 1978; Geers & Moog, 1978). Geers and Moog retested 14 oral deaf students, some of whom had been integrated into regular classrooms, on the DSS and the CELI. Mixed results were reported. The integrated students outperformed the special oral deaf students (i.e., those at CID), on spontaneous language (DDS). The special oral deaf students, on the other hand, produced significantly fewer errors than the integrated students on the CELI. No other information is provided to determine whether the performance of the integrated students was on grade level appropriate for their age.

Doehring et al. (1978) also assessed reading and language skills of integrated students. In general, the results indicated that those students who were profoundly hearing impaired performed at or above normal grade level on reading related tests. These subjects, however, were below normal grade level on four of the five language related measures. In sum, it was observed that the language scores correlated somewhat with the reading scores.

MCE and language development

Much of the educational and research activity during the past two decades has been conducted on the MCE approaches. Despite this, it has been argued that the usefulness of these approaches in helping deaf children acquire competence in English has not been demonstrated (Baker & Cokely, 1980; Bockmiller, 1981; Erting, 1981; Wilbur, 1979). The few studies reported here are those which adhered as closely as possible to the principles of the particular approach investigated. It should be pointed out that the consistency with which these approaches are used is open to question (Marmor & Pettito, 1979; Reich & Bick, 1977; Schlesinger & Meadow, 1972). This issue is discussed further in the summary.

Pidgin sign English (PSE)

PSE appears to be analogous to two hearing speakers who speak a pidgin for communicating when they do not know each other's language. Cokely (1983), however, has questioned the use of this term to describe the contact between ASL signers and English-speaking signers. He argued that the present situation may best be described as *moving toward pidginization*. Thus, Cokely maintains that the use of terms from bilingualism, for example, fossilization, recommend themselves as the better descriptions of this process (see chapter 6 on bilingualism). In spite of this, it is still safe to conclude that PSE represents a method of signing which combines some of the grammatical aspects of ASL and some of the contrived sign systems and uses these in a *predominantly* English word order (Bragg, 1973; Wilbur, 1979; Woodward, 1973). Within this framework, it is synonymous with several other terms, for example, Siglish, Ameslish, manual English, and even *total communication* (Marmor & Pettito, 1979; Reich & Bick, 1977). The studies discussed in this category are those which either (1) made no mention of a specific manually coded system, or (2) used ASL like signs and some inflection—markers from another contrived system, or (3) use total communication.

The first study examined is one which described the communication approach used in school and at home as total communication. Griswold and Cummings (1974) investigated the expressive vocabulary of 19 preschool deaf children, aged 2 to approximately 5 years. Results indicated that a composite vocabulary list of 493 words and expressions were used by two or more students; however, the size of the vocabulary was smaller than that reported for hearing children of comparable ages. In spite of this, the composition of the vocabulary of the deaf children was similar to that of hearing children regarding (1) the proportion of nouns and verbs, (2) the number and usage of specific prepositions, (3) the usage of numbers (words), and (4) the usage of specific question words. The deaf children, however, differed from the hearing children in that they rarely used connectives, articles, and auxiliary/modal verbs. These investigators concluded that a correlation existed between the size of the vocabulary and two other variables: the length of time spent in a preschool program and the amount of exposure to total communication in the home environment.

The developmental order of manual English morphemes was investigated by Crandall (1978). The communication approach was manual English which entailed signs from an ASL lexicon and sign markers representing morphemes, demonstratives, and articles from SEE II (Gustason et al., 1975) and from a basic text on manual communication (O'Rourke, 1973). Twenty pairs of hearing mothers and their young deaf children served as subjects. In particular, Crandall was interested in ascertaining whether the developmental order of the morphemes used by the deaf children was (1) related to age, (2) similar to that of hearing children of comparable age, and (3) related to their mother's use.

In general, all three hypotheses were supported. Mixed results, however, were obtained for the first hypothesis. It was reported that the deaf children's production of the inflectional morphemes did not increase significantly with age. The mean number of morphemes per utterance, however, did show an increase with age. With respect to development order, it was found that the first six morphemes used by the deaf children were similar to those reported for hearing children (Brown, 1973). This finding is consistent with those obtained in other studies (Raffin, 1976; Raffin, Davis, & Gilman, 1978; Schlesinger & Meadow, 1972). Finally, it was reported that the mother's use of the morphemes influenced the child's use of these same morphemes. This last finding is typical of others in that it reveals the importance of the home environment.

The emergence of semantic relations within a PSE environment was observed by Layton, Holmes, and Bradley (1979). Three deaf children, aged 5½, 6½, and 7 years 7 months, served as subjects. They had been exposed to sign language 9 to 15 months prior to the inception of the study. Sign language is taken to mean a total communication system in which speech is simultaneously combined with manual signs, predominantly selected from an ASL lexicon. The signs needed for inflections and articles (determiners) were selected from SEE II (Gustason et al., 1975). The subjects were exposed to signed/spoken utterances that were one-word/one-sign in advance of their productions. For example, a subject at the one-word/one-sign stage was exposed to two-word/two-sign sequences. The findings indicated that the semantic–syntactic categories of the deaf subjects were proportionately different from those reported for younger hearing children at less developed and equivalent linguistic levels (Bloom et al., 1975). For example, hearing children produced more recurrence utterances (more,), whereas the deaf subjects produced more state, negation, and attribution utterances. It was noted that these latter types of utterances did not emerge until a later stage of hearing children's development. These investigators attempted to account for these differences by suggesting that (1) deaf children were exposed to advanced categories prior to their understanding of the basic concepts, and (2) the differences may be due to a difference in age, that is, the older deaf subjects processed at a more sophisticated cognitive level than that of the younger hearing subjects in the study by Bloom et al. (1975). As in the study on OE by Presnell (1973), it was suggested that instructors of hearing impaired children should be aware of the normal developmental patterns of hearing children.

The studies presented thus far seem to indicate that the use of PSE is effective for primary language development if (1) it is used in the home and (2) its practitioners use structures that follow the developmental patterns of hearing children. The effect of this approach on the later educational performance of deaf children has been studied (Brasel & Quigley, 1977). The research design permitted the investigation of the effects of type of communication (oral and manual), type of language (ASL and English), and intensity of early language input. Eighteen deaf students between 10 and 19 years of age were located in each of four language groups: manual English (PSE), ASL, intensive oral, and average oral. The intensive oral group represented those students who received intensive oral training involving both the school and the parents. The parents of the average oral group left the education of their children to the schools.

The results indicated that the manual English group significantly outperformed both oral groups in five of the six major syntactic structures as measured by the Test of Syntactic Abilities (Quigley et al., 1978). In addition, the manual English group significantly outperformed all other groups on all subtests of the Stanford Achievement Test (SAT). On the Paragraph Meaning subtest, the manual English group's mean score was 7.24 years which was nearly 2 years better than the nearest group, intensive oral. The overall mean score of the manual English group on the SAT was 5.25 years. In sum, the findings were interpreted as indicating that both type of communication and type of language input are essential variables in the language development of deaf children and that manual English (PSE) might be a superior system for teaching deaf students.

Signed English (SE)

The effects of SE on the language development of deaf children has been investigated by Bornstein and his associates (Bornstein, 1982; Bornstein & Saulnier, 1981; Bornstein, Saulnier, & Hamilton, 1980). Certain aspects of vocabulary and syntactical, in particular, morphological, growth were studied. It was found that the growth was similar to that of hearing children but at a slower rate.

Bornstein, Saulnier, and Hamilton (1980) conducted a 4-year longitudinal study on twenty 4-year-old prelingually deaf children. Each subject was evaluated annually with the Peabody Picture Vocabulary Test, the Northwestern Syntax Screening Test, and a morphology test designed to measure skill on the 14 SE inflectional markers. The results indicated that the vocabulary level of these deaf children was similar to those reported for other deaf children who were 3 years older. In addition, the rate of growth of receptive vocabulary was reported to be 43% of that observed in hearing children of comparable age. Finally, the most impressive finding was that the rate of growth in the reception of the inflectional markers was *similar to* that of hearing children.

The similar rate of growth of the inflectional markers was not maintained by these deaf students in a follow-up study (Bornstein & Saulnier, 1981). Two rating scales, devised by these researchers, were administered to each subject's instructor. The instructors rated each subject's continual used of the sign markers and changes in the overall use of the entire marker system. Only a slight improvement in the overall use of the markers was observed. In general, the most frequently used markers were the *regular plural* and the *possessive* followed by the *-ing* and the *regular past* markers. The remaining 10 markers were rarely used. In sum, a large gap existed in the developmental sequence of inflections when compared with hearing children since the deaf subjects were using only *half* of the 14 markers by 9.5 years of age.

Signing exact English (SEE II)

It has been reported that SEE II is the most widely used educational approach with deaf children (Jordan, Gustason, & Rosen, 1976, 1979). In spite of this, a perusal of the literature revealed only one study assessing the effects of this approach on the language development of deaf students (Babb, 1979). Babb studied 36 deaf children who had been exposed to SEE II for at least 10 years. The research design was similar to that used by Brasel and Quigley (1977). Half of the subjects were exposed to SEE II only in school and the other half were exposed to it both in school and in the home. These groups were compared with each other, with a hearing comparison group, with the groups in the Brasel and Quigley study, and with normative data for hearing-impaired students on the Stanford Achievement Test for Hearing Impaired Students. The school-only group performed no better than the average oral group in the Brasel and Quigley study and no better than the norms for the general population of deaf students on the SAT. The group exposed to SEE II in the home as well as school performed significantly better than the school-only group and the general school population on all educational measures. In addition, this group performed almost as well as the manual English group in the Brasel and Quigley study. This study demonstrates the importance of family influence on the language development of deaf students at school.

Seeing essential English (SEE I)

Schlesinger and Meadow (1972) described the primary language acquisition of four deaf children. Three of their subjects were exposed to at least some SEE I signs. The beginning of these subjects' exposure to SEE I ranged from 15 months to 3 years of age. Fairly substantial development was observed in both syntax and vocabulary, and some support was found for Bloom's two-word syntactic–semantic relations (1970). The data on one subject were analyzed with respect to the pivot-grammar proposed by Braine (1963a, 1963b), the counterfindings on pivot-grammar argued by Brown (1973), and the relations proposed by Bloom (1970). It was reported that the bulk of the data supported Brown's arguments against pivot-grammar. In addition, the use of two-word/sign utterances by this subject seemed to support Bloom's contention that such utterances tend to expose a variety of structural meanings in relation to the surrounding context cues. For example, this subject signed/spoke: *Daddy shoe*. This is an example of the agent–object relation (see the discussion on hearing children) in which the subject is attempting to tell her father to remove his shoes and get into the sandbox with her. The data on another subject focuses on the acquisition of some English morphological rules. It was found that this subject, exposed to SEE I markers at age 3, began to use the markers by age 4. In sum, on the basis of spontaneous language samples and tests of grammatical competence (Menyuk, 1963), it was concluded that these deaf children were acquiring grammatical competence in the same sequence as hearing children; however, the rate of development was slower.

This same trend has been observed in more recent investigations of the morphologically based SEE I approach (Gilman, Davis, & Raffin, 1980; Raffin, 1976; Raffin et al, 1978). In general, those studies were concerned with the effects of the system on the acquisition of eight commonly used morphemes. Raffin (1976) developed the evaluative instrument used in these studies. The test material consisted of sentences, spoken and signed simultaneously, which represented both correct and incorrect usage of the morphemes. Forty-eight items were presented, six items for each of the following morphemes: past tense /-ed/, third person singular present indicative /-s/, present progressive /-ing/, present perfect /-en/, plural /-s/ on nouns, possessive /'-s/, comparative /-er/, and superlative /-est/. Two of the six items used the morphemes correctly while the other four used them incorrectly. The numbers of years the subjects were exposed to SEE I ranged from 2 to 6. Results indicated that the developmental sequences of these English morphemes were generally similar to those reported for hearing children (Brown, 1973). These findings support those of Schlesinger and Meadow (1972) in that the use of SEE I may aid in the acquisition of English morphemes. Despite these results, however, there was still a 2- to 6-year delay in the acquisition when compared with hearing children.

Finger spelling

Two early studies designed to assess the effectiveness of finger spelling as an educational tool were conducted between 1963 and 1968 (Quigley, 1969). One was a longitudinal survey of the use of finger spelling in conjunction with speech (Rochester method), and the other was an experimental comparison of the Rochester method (RM) and the oral method (i.e., OE) with preschool aged deaf children in two residential schools. In general, in both studies, the deaf children exposed to RM performed better than the comparison groups on most measures of language and educational assessments. Quigley concluded that the use of RM with young deaf children is a useful educational tool, but is not a panacea.

More recently the effectiveness of using finger spelling (i.e., RM) to teach certain morphological structures of English has been studied (Looney & Rose, 1979). Twenty-four prelingually deaf students, age 8 to 15 years, were assessed on their ability to acquire past tense inflectional suffixes. After demonstrating the ability to express through writing and finger spelling a few basic English kernel patterns, these subjects were randomly assigned to three groups. Group 1 was exposed to the Rochester method, Group 2 to print, and Group 3 was the control group. The two treatment groups were exposed to a systematic, 4-week instruction of selected morphological rules, that is, those involving past tense inflectional suffixes. These groups were administered pre- and posttests to assess their ability to recognize, select, determine grammaticality, and to produce the appropriate past tense morphemes. The results indicated that both treatment groups made significant gains whereas the control group failed to demonstrate such a trend. In addition, no significant differences were reported between the two treatment groups. This led the researchers to conclude that finger spelling, as well as print, is useful in representing inflectional suffixes when taught in a systematic manner.

ASL and language development

Traditionally, the study of spoken languages has contributed to much of the prevailing linguistic thinking. The study of signed languages, however, has only recently attracted the attention of linguists and psycholinguists. Most researchers agree that one signed language, ASL, is a bona fide language (Lane & Grosjean, 1980; Liddell, 1980; Siple, 1982; Wilbur, 1979). Recent research focuses on comparing the processing of signed languages with that of spoken languages (Siple, 1982). In addition, researchers may find it useful to study the manner in which skills can be transferred from a signed language to a spoken language. This last issue is of importance for teaching deaf children whose first language is ASL to read and write standard English (see chapter 6 on bilingualism). In sum, there are two areas in which research on ASL can be conducted: (1) charting the developmental sequence of ASL within the four components of language, and (2) describing the effects of ASL on the later development of English.

Primary development of ASL

As stated previously, it is only recently that some aspects of a grammar of ASL have been delineated (Lane & Grosjean, 1980; Kantor, 1980, 1982). Descriptions of ASL grammar abound in controversy similarly to any other new field of scientific inquiry (e.g., attempting to establish new terminology or directions for research). This situation, in turn, makes it extremely difficult to describe the acquisition of ASL grammar by deaf children. For example, the feasibility of applying spoken language analyses (e.g., mean length of utterance, one-word stage) to a signed language has been questioned (Siple, 1978; Wilbur, 1980). The meaning of a sign probably should not be described without considering its accompanying nonmanual cues. Such description, however, is only in the beginning stages (Baker & Cokely, 1980; Liddell, 1980; Wilbur, 1979). In spite of that problem, it is still possible to state that deaf children learning ASL may be comparable to their hearing peers at the early stages of language acquisition (Bellugi & Klima, 1972; Schlesinger & Meadow, 1972).

Cherological development. Research on the structure of ASL signs commenced with Stokoe (1960). He studied the formation of signs, called *cherology,* and treated it as analogous to the phonology system of spoken languages. Just as spoken words can be divided into phonemic elements, signs can be divided into *cheremic* (hand) elements. Stokoe described three elements of a sign: (1) the handshape, (2) the location of the hand with reference to the body, and (3) the movement of the hand. These he labeled *dez, tab,* and *sig.* Battison (1974) argued for a fourth element, called orientation, which refers to the orientation of the palm (e.g., to differentiate between the sign for *SHORT* and that for *TRAIN*). The distinctive features in spoken language are combined from vowels and consonants. In a similar manner, the four elements described here are combined to produce a sign.

It has been reported in the literature that the first words of hearing children emerge between the ages of 10 to 13 months (Dale, 1976; de Villiers & de Villiers, 1978). The literature on the emergence of the first signs in deaf children contains conflicting reports. A similar age period to hearing children's first words has been reported (Schlesinger, 1978; Schlesinger & Meadow, 1972). Other accounts indicate that the first signs emerge 2 to 3 months earlier (Hoffmeister & Wilbur, 1979, 1980). It is hypothesized that the earlier emergence of signs is due to earlier control of the musculature of the hand as compared to the speech articulators (e.g., lips, tongue, teeth).

The study of phonologic acquisition in ASL has focused thus far on the acquisition of handshape (Hoffmeister & Wilbur, 1980). In general, similar to hearing children, deaf children acquire easier (unmarked) elements prior to more difficult (marked) elements. McIntire (1977) studied the acquisition of handshapes in one deaf child at ages 13, 15 18, and 21 months. It was reported that pointing and grasping handshapes were acquired initially (e.g., A, S, L, 5, C, and "baby O"). The acquisition of more complex handshapes (e.g., H, W, 8, X) occurred with the increasing maturity of cognitive and physical abilities. In addition, substitutions produced by the subject involved similar cheremic elements, for example, using the 5 handshape instead of the F handshape to sign *cat*. This phenomenon parallels substitution of phonemic elements in hearing children. Thus, the cherological development of deaf children appears to be similar to the phonologic development of hearing children. That is, both proceed from easier, less marked elements to more difficult, more marked elements and both substitute easier, similar elements for more difficult ones.

Syntactic development. Siple (1978) remarked: "It is easy to say that the grammar of ASL is uniquely its own; but it is more difficult to identify and describe the actual syntactic devices used" (p. 10). Consequently, researchers are attempting to discover syntactic devices which are not present in spoken languages, for example, reduplication, verb directionality, and systematic nonmanual cues (see the discussion of these terms in Kantor, 1980 and Wilbur, 1979). The study of these devices is important for a description of word order in ASL which is still shrouded in controversy (Fischer, 1975; Friedman, 1976; Liddell, 1980; Padden, 1981). In addition, nonmanual cues, a relatively unexplored area, are deemed to be of importance for the production of some major linguistic structures, for example, negation, question formation, and relativization (Liddell, 1980).

Studies of syntactic development, like those on cherological development, are few in number. Those concerned with three major linguistic structures are briefly described here: negation, the pronominal reference system, and classifiers. Data on negation and the pronominal reference system are taken from Hoffmeister and Wilbur (1980), and those on classifiers are from Kantor (1980).

Hoffmeister and Wilbur (1980) reviewed a number of studies investigating the beginning stages of the acquisition of negation. In general, in the earlier stage the use of the sign for *no* is present as well as the more frequent negative headshake. The later stage is characterized by the emergence of two signs *not* and *can't*. Similar to hearing children learning a spoken language, the notion of *can't* is acquired prior to that of *can*. In sum, it was concluded that these developmental stages appear to parallel those reported for hearing children learning English (Brown, 1973).

Hoffmeister and Wilbur (1980, citing Hoffmeister, 1978) described a study on the acquisition of the pronominal reference system of ASL. A deaf child of deaf parents served as a subject. Results are presented in five stages. In Stage 1, for example, it was reported that pointing behaviors refer to objects that are visible in the immediate environment; for example, the signer, objects. The subject indicated a possessor–possessed relationship by initially pointing to an object and then pointing to the self. Analogously, Nelson (1973) and

Bates (1976a, 1976b) also found similar deictic (pointing) gestures which preceded the spoken language development in young hearing children. These pointing behaviors of the deaf child also were the precursors to other pronominal concepts, for example, plurality, the use of *that* and *all,* which are later executed by formal adult signs. By Stage 3, the previously learned operations began to refer to events and objects not in the immediate environment. By Stage 4 (age 4 years 2 months), reflexivization emerged as a set. Finally, it was concluded that this deaf subject had mastered the ASL referential system by Stage 5 (4 years 5 months of age).

Kantor (1980) studied the acquisition of ASL classifiers by deaf children. Similar to classifiers in spoken languages, ASL classifiers appear as part of syntactic forms (e.g., the verb or the noun) and reflect certain semantic properties of their noun referents. Nine deaf children, age 3 to 11 years, of deaf parents served as subjects. Similar to other studies on acquisition of ASL, these findings indicated a developmental sequence similar to those that have been identified for hearing children learning a spoken language (Menyuk, 1977). In particular, it was reported that classifiers emerged around age 3 and were mastered by 8 or 9 years of age. It was concluded that classifiers are not acquired as lexical items, but rather as a complex syntactic process. In sum, this study, and others, suggested that rule acquisition in both ASL and spoken languages is affected by similar phonological and syntactical environments.

Semantic–pragmatic development. A few studies have investigated the development of semantics and/or pragmatics in deaf children (Kantor, 1982; Newport & Ashbrook, 1977). Again, development was noted to be similar to that of hearing children.

Newport and Ashbrook (1977) conducted a study to compare the emergence of semantic relations in deaf children learning ASL as a first language to that of hearing children learning English as a first language (Bloom et al., 1975). Five young deaf children served as subjects. In general, the findings indicated that the *existence* relation emerged prior to *action* relations which preceded *state* relations. In addition, *nonlocatives* emerged prior to *locatives.* A detailed description of these relations can be found in Bloom and Lahey (1978) and Lucas (1980). It was concluded that the sequence of the acquisition of semantic relations by deaf children was similar to that reported for hearing children despite the differences in modality and syntax.

Kantor (1982) conducted phonologic, syntactical, semantic, and pragmatic analyses on data obtained from interactions of two deaf mothers with their deaf children. This researcher was interested in (1) describing the modifications of deaf mothers in communicating with their children, and (2) describing the developmental sequence of deictic (pointing) behaviors and modulated verbs in deaf children exposed to ASL. In general, it was reported that the deaf mothers, similar to hearing–speaking mothers, modified their language to fit the child's, that is, they used more simple and direct structures. The developmental sequences of the pointing behavior and verb modulations were essentially similar to those reported early in this section by Hoffmeister and

Wilbur (1980). In addition, it was suggested that pointing, in the early stage, indicated a few semantic relations, for example, the use of demonstratives. Additional semantic and pragmatic functions emerged at a later stage with the occurrence of locatives, pronominals, and indexing referents present in the context.

ASL and later development of English

There is ongoing research on the development of ASL in some deaf children; however, the effects of having learned ASL in early childhood on the subsequent learning of English in a formal educational program has not been assessed in detail. Most of the studies employed the paradigm of comparing deaf children of deaf parents to matched deaf children of hearing parents. Previously, it was assumed that deaf parents of deaf children use ASL with no accompanying speech (Charrow & Fletcher, 1974; Meadow, 1968). These assumptions, however, have been questioned since (1) some deaf parents may use ASL signs with accompanying speech (Collins-Ahlgren, 1974; Schlesinger & Meadow, 1972), and (2) others may not use any form of manual communication (Corson, 1973). With these caveats in mind, it is still reasonable to assume that many deaf children of deaf parents are reared in an environment where ASL is the dominant language used by the parents and children. At any rate, this assumption is implicit in the studies cited here.

Most of the earlier studies reported similar results; namely, that deaf children of deaf parents (DCDP) scored higher than deaf children of hearing parents (DCHP) on certain educational and psychological tests (Meadow, 1968; Quigley & Frisina, 1961; Stuckless & Birch, 1966). Quigley and Frisina, for example, reported the DCDP significantly outperformed DCHP in vocabulary, finger spelling, and educational achievement. Meadow (1968) reported higher self-image and academic achievement for DCDP. In addition, she reported the DCDP were at a reading level more than 2 years higher than DCHP. These early findings were interpreted to mean that early exposure to manual communication (probably in the form of ASL) was beneficial to English language development in deaf children. This assumption has since been questioned (Brasel & Quigley, 1977; Corson, 1973). Quigley and Kretschmer (1982) discussed this issue in detail and concluded that such factors as the type of manual communication and parental acceptance of the deaf child must also be considered.

SUMMARY AND CONCLUSIONS

Oral English

Due to the paucity of studies on cued speech, it is not possible to state even tentative conclusions. The study by Mohay (1983), however, did indicate some favorable effects of cued speech on language development. In essence, cued speech is in need of further research.

The studies cited in OE approaches involved those deaf students in indisputably oral programs or those integrated into the regular classroom. In general, it was found that the primary language development of these students was similar in sequence but slower in rate to that of hearing children. Also, a good number of these deaf students performed on grade level with their hearing peers. It is difficult to generalize these results to other deaf students on two counts: (1) An active, comprehensive oral approach to language development may be present only in a few educational programs; and (2) deaf children in these programs often are more select in IQ, socioeconomic status, and highly educated and motivated parents than deaf children in the general school population. Despite the select nature, these studies indicate that deaf children in incontestably oral programs or those select few integrated into regular classrooms develop superior language and academic skills compared to those in the general school population. In essence, the success of these students is attributed mainly to their development of oral English.

Manually coded English

Most of the MCE approaches cited in this chapter have been in use for 15 years or longer, yet, very little research has been conducted and very little educational success has been reported. Almost all the studies indicate that certain aspects of English grammar, for example, morphology, can be taught through a particular approach. The studies demonstrating the most success (e.g., Babb, 1979; Brasel & Quigley, 1977), however, indicate that certain conditions are necessary for this level of achievement: (1) active involvement in the home and school, and (2) instruction which adheres to the developmental patterns of hearing children. Other additive factors are high socioeconomic status and high IQ. As with OE, the primary language development of deaf children is similar to—albeit slower than—that of hearing children. Studies showing an early, rapid morphological and syntactical development (e.g., those of signed English and SEE I) indicate that this development slows in the later years. In addition, it may be difficult to evaluate the usefulness of approaches most representative of English (e.g., SEE II, SEE I, and Finger spelling) since it has been reported that many practitioners do not adhere strictly to English structure in the manual component of these systems (Marmor & Pettito, 1979; Reich & Bick, 1977; Schlesinger & Meadow, 1972). Thus, these systems may evolve into some form of PSE.

American sign language

The discussion of ASL is presented in two areas: (1) the developmental sequence of deaf children acquiring ASL, and (2) the effects of such acquisition on the later development of English. More research is available in the former area; however, even this research is limited. Research on the structure of ASL began with Stokoe (1960) delineating the elements of a sign. Since that time, it has been demonstrated that ASL is a bona fide language with a grammar different from that of English (Lane & Grosjean, 1980; Wilbur, 1979). Psycholinguistic research indicated that the acquisition of ASL may be similar to and parallel to that of spoken language acquisition (Hoffmeister & Wilbur, 1980; McIntire, 1977). For example, such strategies as over-generalization have been observed in both ASL and English (Hoffmeister & Wilbur, 1980). Another example is that certain semantic relations (Newport & Ashbrook, 1977) and pragmatic functions (Kantor, 1982) observed in hearing children have also been reported in the early acquisition stages of deaf children. Linguistic description of ASL, however, is far from complete. Certain areas of syntactical development need further investigation; for example, word order (Liddell, 1980) and nonmanual cues (Baker & Cokely, 1980). In sum, more data is needed since most of the findings are based upon research with very few deaf children.

The effects of early exposure to ASL on later development of English have not been extensively studied. Care must be taken when interpreting studies employing the paradigm of comparing DCDP with DCHP. It cannot be assumed that DCDP are exposed only to ASL as defined by researchers (Brasel & Quigley, 1977; Corson, 1973; Schlesinger & Meadow, 1972). In addition, it is concluded that issues other than type of language input must be considered (Brasel & Quigley, 1977; Corson, 1973) in evaluating the performance of these children. The major issue in this area is for researchers to discover whether or not certain skills can be transferred from a signed language, for example, ASL, to a spoken language, for example, English (Siple, 1982). This issue is of utmost importance if the ability to read and write English is a desirable goal in the education of deaf children.

chapter 4

Reading

Tens of thousands of children in American schools do not read well. . . Many of these poor readers have difficulty because they cannot decode unfamiliar words. . . [Our] research suggests that poor readers and immature readers do not make inferences that integrate information across sentences, do not link what they are reading with what they already know, do not successfully monitor their own comprehension, seldom engage in mental review and self-questioning, and do not make effective use of the structure in a story or text to organize learning and remembering. (Anderson, 1981, pp. 8)

This statement illustrates the extent of reading problems in the United States and lists a number of elements of the reading process in which problems can arise. Although the decoding process is clearly acknowledged as one source of difficulty, problems in higher order mental processes are assigned roles at least as prominent in problems of reading comprehension. The statement emphasizes the importance in reading of (1) prior knowledge of a topic, (2) the ability to relate text data to prior knowledge through inferential processes, (3) the ability to integrate information at various levels of the text (words, phrases, sentences, paragraphs, whole texts), and (4) the ability to use the metacognitive processes of monitoring, mental review, self-questioning, and knowledge of text structure to organize learning and remembering from printed material. Reading is thus seen as being driven, or controlled, by higher order mental processes and not simply as a matter of decoding letters or words. It involves the construction of meaning from written material and the interpretation of that meaning in terms of the general experiential, cognitive, and linguistic store of meaning in the reader's possession.

A vast amount of theoretically based and empirical research information has been accumulated on reading since the classic book by Huey (1908). Most of the issues raised in Huey's work, however, remain unresolved: the extent to which word recognition involves serial versus parallel or holistic processing of component letters, direct versus phonologically mediated lexical access; and bottom-up (sequential/heirarchical) versus top-down (context driven), and/or interactive processing of printed information (Vellutino, in Rosenberg, 1982, p. 33). Research information on the reading process in hearing individuals presented here includes: (1) requisites for reading; (2) the three types of current theories (bottom-up, top-down, and interactive); (3) a selected sampling of research on various aspects and problems of the reading process organized under the categories of the text, the reader, and socioeconomic and cultural factors; and a summary of what seems to be the present state of knowledge. Research information available on the reading process and problems in deaf individuals is then presented. A final section attempts to relate what is known about the reading of deaf individuals and of hearing individuals and makes some comments about present practice and future research.

REQUISITES FOR READING

Skilled reading involves, in addition to decoding printed words, the use of higher order mental processes in constructing meaning from text. If normal early development has taken place, the necessary higher order processes will have developed at least partially by the time the child begins to read. If the child has been exposed in the early environment to a wealth of stimulating and relevant learning experiences that were made meaningful for the child through interaction with the parents and other people by means of a fluent and intelligible communication system, then a cognitive base for language will have been established, a structured symbol system will have been internalized, and the child will have stored in structured form a variety of experiences and the learning strategies to manipulate and expand the experiences and the symbol system (Quigley & Kretschmer, 1982). For most of the population, the symbol system is, of course, oral language. But this is not true for most deaf children, and it is likely that much of the difficulty deaf children have with reading text is a result of experiential and linguistic deficits incurred in infancy and early childhood.

Besides bringing to the reading task a rich background of experiential, cognitive, and linguistic experiences, the prereading normally hearing child also has the strategies to link textual information to these experiences. In particular, such a child has developed inferential and figurative language abilities that enable him or her to understand textual information by relating it to experience and information which he or she already has acquired. Inferential processes are ubiquitous in reading comprehension. While much of the special materials prepared for beginning readers is literal or text explicit in that all the information required for comprehension is stated explicitly in the text, most reading materials beyond the third grade rely heavily on inference for full comprehension. A simple example from a study by Wilson (1979) of inferencing in deaf children illustrates this process.

The shirt is dirty.
The shirt is under the bed.

The cat is on the shirt.
The cat is white.

It can be inferred readily from this that the cat is under the bed, even though this is not explicitly stated in the text. Inferencing is a process essential to reading text which seems to create major problems for deaf children (Wilson, 1979) and is considered later in more detail.

Just as considerable use of inference has been demonstrated in prereading children by recent research (Gelman, 1978; Trabasso, 1980), so also has figurative language usage. Reynolds and Ortony (1980) and Winner, Engel, and Gardner (1980), among others, have shown that even very young hearing children have some figurative language comprehension. Like inferencing, figurative language seems to present major obstacles to the reading of standard English for deaf students (Payne, 1982; Giorcelli, 1982). The importance of this is emphasized by the findings of a detailed examination by Dixon, Pearson, and Ortony (1980) of reading series (Grades K through 6) published by Houghton-Mifflin, Ginn, and Scott, Foresman. The investigators found that, with the exception of the Scott, Foresman series, the materials use an abundance of figurative language (especially metaphors and similies) at all levels.

All of the abilities and mental processes which have been briefly discussed are important to the reading process and most of them, as part of the larger domain of cognitive development, have developed at least to some extent prior to the usual age for beginning reading. The practical needs and developing interests of the child in early life shape his/her experiences and cognitive and linguistic development. These practical considerations are also reflected in the developing area of pragmatics. They have led to the consideration of written discourse as a form of pragmatic speech acts—the view that speakers or writers (just as children and parents) use words to *do* things or to get a hearer or reader to believe or do something (Searle, 1969; Morgan & Sellner, 1980). In this view, larger units of text, or discourse, become the unit of study rather than words and sentences. The prereading child uses spoken discourse in this same practical way—as a means to satisfy needs and curiosities—and does not consciously perceive the stream of speech as being segmented into sentences, phrases, words, and phones. This metacognitive knowledge is acquired later—often in connection with learning to read.

Of the various abilities and mental processes discussed thus far in connection with beginning reading—early experience, cognitive development, linguistic development, the use of inferencing and figurative language, communication acts as pragmatic acts expressed in discourse units, decoding, and metacognitive processes—only decoding is unique to reading and only decoding and metacognitive processes are probably acquired at or after beginning reading. It would seem then that "the only knowledge that is unique to reading is that which is specifically related to the printed medium" (Anderson, 1981, p. 57). This perhaps explains why difficulties at the level of letter and word processing have been found consistently to be the single best class of discriminators between good and poor readers (e.g., Biemiller, 1977, 1978; Graesser, Hoffman, & Clark, 1980). These processes are the ones that are unique to the printed medium and uniquely foreign to the beginning reader (Anderson, 1981, p. 57).

THEORIES OF READING

Three types of theories (bottom-up, top-down, and interactive) are examined in some detail and selected evidence is presented in support of each. It is concluded that interactive theories provide better explanations for more of the established empirical data than do bottom-up or top-down theories. It is further concluded that the class of interactive theories known as schema theories seem most promising at present. Schema theories incorporate the idea of schemata (or plans) as organizing frameworks for knowledge based on recent research in memory and cognition (Bobrow & Norman, 1975).

Bottom-up theories

Bottom-up theories place initial emphasis in reading on word recognition, either as a whole unit (whole word or look–say approach) or as strings of letters, or letter clusters, which are related to spoken equivalents (phonics approach). Reading at the phonics level is seen as putting together small units (letters, letter clusters) to form words; words are then combined into the larger units of phrases and sentences to arrive at textual meaning. Beyond the level of decoding, reading comprehension also is seen as an hierarchy of subskills, such as locating details, recognizing main ideas, and so forth, which combine into larger units to provide the meaning of a text (Mason, Osborn, & Rosenshine, 1977).

The issue of the place and form of decoding in beginning reading in bottom-up theories has been at the heart of a long-standing controversy in reading instruction (Chall, 1967; Flesch, 1955) as to whether emphasis should be placed on the whole-word approach or spelling–sound correspondences (phonics). It has also been an issue in the psychological study of the unit of perception involved in word recognition as summed in the question posed by Vellutino (1982), How does a skilled reader recognize a word? Vellutino uses this question as the basis for an exhaustive analysis of an impressive body of literature on the topic extending back to the work of Cattell in 1886. In the course of his analysis, he presents much of the significant research literature, and the bottom-up reading theories related to the research.

Vellutino's extensive analysis of almost a century of research concludes that the unit of perception in word recognition is relative, that it involves the basic perceptual recognition and interpretation of graphemic details, that it is heavily influenced by contextual clues in the text being read, and that it is also heavily influenced by prior knowledge and skills of the reader (in particular, the linguistic and nonlinguistic knowledge and information processing strategies the reader brings to the task).

Top-down theories

Top-down theories are best exemplified in the writings of Goodman (1967, 1976) and Smith (1975b, 1978). Both reject what they term the emphasis on reading as a precise process which involves exact, detailed, sequential perception and identification of letters, words, spelling patterns, and larger units. According to Goodman (1976), phonic centered approaches are concerned with precise letter identification. In word centered approaches, the focus is on word identification. In place of this, Goodman sees reading as a "psycholinguistic guessing game" involving an interaction between thought and language. Skill in reading is seen not as involving greater precision but more accurate guesses at the unfolding meaning of a text based on better techniques for sampling the text, greater control over language structure, broadened experiences and increased conceptual development. Increasing skill and speed in reading are accompanied by decreasing use of graphic cues.

Smith's views (1978) are similar to Goodman's with some differences in terminology. Smith refers to the primary role of "prediction" in reading rather than "hypothesis testing" or "psychological guessing" (Goodman's terms). The concepts, however, are similar. Smith presents four main arguments for the primary role of prior knowledge, context, and prediction in reading and against the precise sequential/hierarchical view of the reading process. (1) Individual words are often polysemous (have multiple meanings) and their intended meanings can only be obtained from context aided by prior knowledge. (2) According to Venezky (1976), there are more than 300 "spelling-to-sound correspondences rules" of English and there is no precise way of knowing when any of the rules must apply or when an exception to the rules is being encountered. In brief, the rules of phonics are very complex. (3) The amount of visual information from print that the brain can process at any given moment in reading is limited to four or five letters or other units, according to a substantial body of research. (4) Short-term memory (or working memory) is limited; only a small number of items can be stored at any time and increased input leads to displacement of items already in storage.

Referring to data from information theory, Smith (1978) points out that there are sequential dependencies in English among letters, words, and larger units which aid in comprehension. A large body of research data attests to this: Individual letters are recognized more readily when embedded in groups (Wheeler, 1970); even more readily when the letter groups form pseudowords, such as *gorp* (Adams, 1979); and more readily still when in real words (Adams, 1979). The same situation applies to words in the context of meaningful phrases and sentences and phrases and other syntactic units in the context of sentences and larger units. Meaningfulness apparently allows the reader, or listener, to group the material in larger and larger chunks in working memory and aids in comprehension. As Smith (1975b) states:

> The limited capacity of short-term memory is overcome by filling it always with units as large and as meaningful as possible. Instead of being crammed uselessly with half-a-dozen unrelated letters, short-term memory can contain the same number of words, or better still, the meaning of one or more sentences. (p. 309)

Two basic conditions that Smith states must be met for children to use prediction for learning to read are: (1) The material which children are expected to learn to read must be potentially meaningful to them; and (2) the children must feel free to predict even though this will result initially in errors rather than precise reading.

The importance of context and prior knowledge in reading is now generally accepted (Anderson, 1981). But there is less acceptance of the lack of importance of textual detail to the reading process. Top-down theories, such as espoused by Goodman and by Smith, assert that textual detail (letters and words) need only be sampled from the text. The remainder of the text presumably can be "guessed at" or "predicted." This concept of sampling of text is not supported by the data on skilled reading.

Recent developments in computer techniques make it possible to control the text displayed on a screen (a cathode-ray tube) contingent upon eye movements and to make various changes in the text during the reading process. For example, it is possible to change a particular letter or word in the text from one eye fixation to the next. It then can be determined from the reader's reports of what he saw and from the analysis of eye movements whether the reader perceived the change. It is also possible to place errors in the text for a single eye fixation and to physically shift the text on the screen during a saccadic eye movement and thus change where the eyes come to rest.

Data from the use of these and other recently developed techniques (McConkie, 1982) to study mental processes involved in reading through analyzing eye movements contradict the top-down theorists contention that skilled readers only sample words and letters from text. A substantial body of data now attests that the skilled reader responds to letters as units and that words are not identified strictly on the basis of more global stimulus patterns. Rayner, McConkie, and Zola (1980) and Zola (1981) confirm that specific letters are being used during one fixation and used to facilitate perception of the word on the next fixation. Zola (1981) demonstrated that even replacing a single letter in the center of a highly constrained (predictable from context) word with its most visually similar letter resulted in some disruption of the reading process compared to a no-error control situation, thus indicating that even minimal visual distortion in a word was evident to skilled readers. These, and many other studies, attest that, contradictory to top-down theorists' contentions, skilled readers fixate virtually every content word in a text and use individual letters and other graphemic knowledge and skills extensively in the course of reading (Just & Carpenter, 1980; McConkie & Zola 1981).

Interactive theories

The interactive theories emerging in recent years are replacing the one-directional (bottom-up and top-down) theories of the reading process. According to Anderson (1981), interactive models emphasize the reader as an *active* information processor whose goal it is to *construct* a model of what the text means. Two aspects of the models are of primary importance: (1) the central role of background knowledge in constructing meaning from text; and (2) a number of dynamic processing strategies ranging from the specific aspects of decoding print to the metacognitive strategies of consciously monitoring one's processing of information. Comprehension proceeds from the top-down as well as from the bottom-up; that is, it is driven by preexisting concepts as well as by the data from the text. There are times when the information processor is largely data driven or text driven and is controlled by the visual data from the printed page. It seems then to be assuming a relatively passive role waiting for data from the text to activate and relate to preexisting concepts or schemata. At other times the processor seems to assume a more active role and seeks to predict the probable data ahead in the text. In contrast to this alternation of bottom-up and top-down roles, some models such as Rumelhart's (1977) interactive model suggest a constant and simultaneous generation of hypotheses about visual information and meaning both from data driven (bottom-up) and conceptually driven (top-down) sources.

The schema theory form of interaction theory uses a model similar to Rumelhart's with the added concept of schemata as organizing frameworks for preexisting knowledge. Anderson (1981) defines a schema as "a hypothetical knowledge structure, an abstract mental entity to which human information processors bind their experiences with the real world" (p. 606). He states that the abstract character of schemata is important because schemata are prototypic rather than specific, that is, one can have a schema for chair but probably not for every particular chair one experiences. When applied to objects and simple ideas, schemata are identical to what are called concepts or categories. But schemata can be constructed for all levels of knowledge from something as specific as a letter of the alphabet to something as abstract as a philosophy of life, and for such concepts as love, kindness, perseverance, and hope.

Thus, the schema concept provides a powerful tool for organizing knowledge into meaningful units which aids in acquisition, storage, and retrieval. The effect of meaning on memory functioning is well documented; words are easier to recall than unrelated letters, sentences easier than unrelated words, and so forth. In fact, any body of semantically related data is easier to retrieve from memory than any comparable body of semantically unrelated data. Schemata are the devices by which knowledge is organized into meaningful units and incoming data (such as from a text) are incorporated into the existing schemata, modify such schemata, or help form new schemata. And schemata, at various levels, are combined with related schemata into higher order, and usually more general, schemata.

TEXT VARIABLES

Vocabulary

The word is the basic semantic unit from which discourse is constructed. Anderson and Freebody (1979) have reported extensively on the primary role played by a large vocabulary in reading skill, readability measures, and intelligence testing. They concluded that people who do not know the meanings of very many words are most probably poor readers. Johnson, Toms-Bronowski, and Pittelman (1982) and Pearson and Johnson (1978) provide recently developed theories and models of how vocabulary is believed to develop in hearing individuals. Vellutino (1982) analyzed and synthesized a century of research data on word recognition and concluded that the unit of perception in word recognition is relative and depends on characteristics of the word stimulus, the context in which the word appears, and the skill of the reader. A substantial body of evidence (Anderson, 1981) seems to support the idea that letters are processed individually as units in word recognition rather than words being recognized by more global characteristics. A series of studies by McConkie (1982) and a group of colleagues, and many other studies, have shown that skilled readers process words down to their graphemic details. Finally, although there is clear evidence that lexical (word) access can take place visually (Kleiman, 1975), there is substantial evidence that speech recoding also commonly occurs in reading, although it might be of greater significance in syntactic processing than in word processing.

All of this evidence points to vocabulary development as being a major variable in language comprehension, including reading, and word processing as being a basic skill in reading development. Studies have shown repeatedly that problems in word processing are the best discriminators between good and poor readers (Biemiller, 1977), that beginning and poor readers tend to have poor word analysis skills (Graesser et al., 1980), and that beginning and poor readers tend to rely too heavily on context and higher mental processes becasue they lack efficient decoding skills (Anderson, 1981). Beginning and poor readers have to devote so much attention and working memory space to basic level processing of words, which is automatic in the skilled reader, that higher level processing (concentration on meaning, prediction, etc.) suffers. Evidence also indicates that, although skilled readers can rapidly access the meanings of words visually, they can routinely use orthographic and phonetic structure in word analysis when necessary (Just & Carpenter, 1980; McConkie & Zola, 1981). In other words, they seem to use elements of what are labeled in instruction as "look–say" and "phonics" approaches. This is not to say they were taught phonetic analysis directly. It is likely that many skilled readers acquire phonetic and graphemic analysis inductively. This is not likely for poor readers and the average beginning reader, however, who might have to be taught how to use such skills.

Syntax

The ability to *integrate* information across linguistic units seems to be the key factor in processing information at the sentence and intrasentence (phrases, clauses) level. Information from individual lexical items must be integrated with information from other lexical items according to syntactic rules to form semantic units corresponding to propositions, and propositions must be integrated with other propositions, both from within and across sentence boundaries, to form larger interrelated structures (Anderson, 1981). Many theorists have suggested that working memory capacity plays a critical role in reading comprehension (Just & Carpenter, 1980; Kintsch & van Dijk, 1978), and that its major influence might be on sentence and intrasentence processing. Both information storage and information processing take place in working memory and the more effort (and consequently space) that must be devoted to basic processing, the less is available for storage, and the smaller and less efficient will be the chunks of information that can be integrated in short-term memory.

The concept of limited capacity and time for processing information is particularly critical for deaf children. Whereas a hearing child from a typical middle-class home is likely to approach beginning reading with well-developed general language comprehension skills, the typical deaf child is likely to approach beginning reading with poorly developed general language comprehension skills resulting from experiential deficits, cognitive deficits, and linguistic deficits. These accumulated deficits are not due apparently to any lack of inherent ability in the deaf child (Quigley & Kretschmer, 1982), but simply to an impoverished early background due to lack of appropriate experiential and linguistic input.

Daneman and Carpenter (1980) showed that there are trade-offs between the storage and processing functions of working memory and that these affect the ways information is chunked by poor and by skilled readers. The recoding of many concepts and relations into a single chunk has the economizing effect of reducing the load on working memory and increasing the functional working capacity for subsequent processing. Mason and Kendall (1979) showed that these research findings have possible instructional applications. They found that separating the pausal units of complex sentences, or dividing complex sentences into several shorter sentences, resulted in better reading comprehension for less skilled readers. This chunking into smaller units seemed to allow the less skilled readers to spend more time and working memory capacity on higher level integrative processing at text intervals by reducing the amount needed for storage of information.

Jarvella (1971, 1979) and others have shown that clause and sentence boundaries seem to influence the chunking of information in working memory. Kleiman (1975), Levy (1977), and Baddeley (1979) have produced evidence that speech recoding plays a role in the storage of sequential information necessary for the comprehension of connected discourse. This type of processing might be important in comprehending particular syntactic constructions, such as embedded or interrupted constituents which require integration of information from the beginning and the end of a sentence, for example, medial relative clauses. Thus, working memory with its limited capacity for storing and processing linguistic information, and speech recoding as the form in which sequential linguistic information is temporarily stored seem to be critical in integrating information in sentences and connected prose.

Discourse

During the past decade, there has been a sharp increase in research on the pragmatic aspects of utterances, on their *use* in communication. This emphasis on pragmatics has focused research attention on larger units of discourse than words and sentences. One aspect of this research on discourse analysis, which is important in the reading process, has been the analysis of the underlying structure of whole texts, such as the analysis of the structure of stories through story grammars (Mandler & Johnson, 1977). Leaving aside differences in detail, all theories of text structure of various genres (stories, informative material, poems, etc.) attempt to provide an account of the underlying representation of events in the genre and a set of rules or transformations linking the underlying representation to the sequence of events in the surface structure of the text. Accumulated knowledge of the structure of various genres is then another form of prior knowledge that readers, particularly skilled ones, bring to the reading process and which aids their comprehension of a text. It is also knowledge which writers can use to make their writing more easily understood. Outlines, summaries, abstracts, and series of headings and subheadings can help guide a reader more easily through a text. So can the practice of conforming the surface structure to what the reader expects for a particular genre structure, except, of course, when the surface order is deliberately changed from the expected structure for a particular purpose or to achieve a particular effect.

Figurative language

For the student of English as a second language and for hearing impaired (deaf) English language learners, the difficulty of the language learning task is greatly increased by the profusion of figurative expressions in standard English. The language abounds with metaphors, similes, and idioms as well as less common forms such as irony, proverbs, allegories, neologisms, and so forth. And the beginning reader will encounter many figurative uses of language even in the very first books of commonly used basal reading series (Dixon et al., 1980). Research has revealed that even very young children have some control of figurative language, so the beginning reader often brings some knowledge of this important aspect of language to the reading process (Reynolds & Ortony, 1980; Winner et al., 1980). Research has also revealed that comprehension and explication of figurative language develop in an incremental manner. Ability to comprehend and to use the various forms of figurative language is essential to communication in English and presents considerable difficulty for deaf learners of English (Giorcelli, 1982).

READER VARIABLES

Three reader variables are of importance here: development of schemata, inferencing, and metacognitive strategies.

Schemata

Schemata are the building blocks of cognition, and adequate early cognitive development provides the base for all language development, including reading. A schema theory is a theory about knowledge and schemata are the units in which knowledge, and information about how to use the knowledge, is packaged. In interactive theories of reading, a central role is played by the preexisting knowledge of a topic that a reader brings to reading a text on that topic or related topics. And preexisting knowledge is assumed to be stored in the human information system in meaningful units. In schema theory, these meaningful units are schemata structures for representing in memory the generic concepts of knowledge and knowledge use. The reading of a text (even the reading of the title) will activate schemata in the reader's repertoire that are related to the text. All of the interrelated knowledge in those schemata will become available and permit the reader to relate text information to it by means of inferencing and to predict what lies ahead in the text, which will aid in fast interpretation of textual input. Thus, schemata are organizing frameworks for cognition which also serves a critical role in reading through influencing important top-down processes.

Inferencing

Inferencing is ubiquitous in reading. It is vital to text comprehension beyond the level of very literal texts, which means just about all material beyond a third-grade level and probably much that is below that level. The meanings of words, sentences, paragraphs are affected by the contexts in which they occur and by the prior knowledge of the reader about the material being read. Inferencing is the process of relating what is in the text to what is in the reader's knowledge store, or supplying from preexisting knowledge information that is only implied in the text. The importance of this process to reading serves to highlight again the critical role played by prior knowledge in the reading process. The more prior knowledge about more topics that a reader has stored in memory, the easier the reading of any text is likely to be.

Research studies have defined and traced the development of inferencing (Brewer, 1975; Omanson, Warren, & Trabasso, 1978; Spiro, 1977). Guszak (1967) has demonstrated that, in spite of the importance of inferencing to reading, teachers do not use inferential questioning very often in their classrooms. Several studies by Hansen and Pearson (1980), Hayes and Tierney (1980), and others showed mixed results of direct instruction on inferencing. There was a tendency toward positive results, however, indicating that inferential processes are susceptible to training. Inferencing, of course, is limited by an individual's prior knowledge of any topic being read and, unfortunately, improvements in prior knowledge seem attainable only by gradual assimilation of knowledge over a considerable period of time. This has important implications for reading instruction with deaf children. Because of lack of early childhood experiences and the cognitive and linguistic skills that arise from those experiences and from fluent interactive communication with parents, many deaf children reach beginning reading with very limited background knowledge in a variety of common topics.

Metacognition

Metacognitive skills are particularly important to advanced reading and to studying, although they have significance for all levels of reading. These skills are consciously applied techniques of planning, monitoring, self-questioning, and summarizing. Brown (1980) regards them as providing conscious control of knowledge which itself is largely unconsciously acquired. Brown and Day (1980) have shown that these skills have a developmental order in learning from text from simple deletion of unimportant details to summarizing and synthesizing information. They also showed that even students in graduate courses often have not acquired mastery of the advanced metacognitive skills of summarizing and synthesizing. Again, as with inferencing and other higher order reading skills, the development of metacognitive skills seems to be influenced by direct instruction (Brown, Campione, & Day, 1980; Day, 1980).

SOCIOECONOMIC AND CULTURAL VARIABLES

Socioeconomic and cultural influences have been shown repeatedly to be significant in learning to read (Labov, 1970; Troike, 1978) and the influence of various factors has been studied in detail. Various studies have reported a variety of mismatches between the backgrounds of children from homes of low socioeconomic level and the requirements of middle class oriented schools: mismatches between the language and dialect of teacher and student;

between the child's background and curricula, tests, and textbooks; and mismatches in background and schema knowledge.

A study by Durkin (1966) is of particular interest. She studied children who could read prior to attending school. One of her findings was that, while low socioeconomic level is usually associated with low reading achievement scores, the relationship is neither causal nor inevitable. Some children from homes of low socioeconomic levels learn to read very well and the significant factors seem to be lots of reading material in the homes, assignment of high value by the parents to learning to read, and encouragement and tutelage in reading by the parents. These findings emphasize again the importance of various experiences in infancy and early childhood for development of the cognitive and linguistic base which makes skilled reading possible.

AN INTERACTIVE SCHEMA THEORY OF READING

This quote from Brown (1980) illustrates the condition of skilled reading.

> Consider skilled readers, who can be characterized as operating with lazy processors. All their top-down and bottom-up skills are so fluent that they can proceed merrily on automatic pilot, until a *triggering event* alerts them to a comprehension failure. While the process is flowing smoothly, their construction of meaning is very rapid, but when a comprehension failure is detected, they must slow down and allot extra processing time to the problem area. They must employ debugging devices and strategies, that take time and effort. The difference in time and effort between the normal *automatic pilot* state and the laborious activity in the *debugging state* is the difference between the subconscious and conscious levels. (p. 455)

The differences between highly skilled readers of this type and less skilled and problem readers are perhaps that top-down and bottom-up processes are not always as fluent and automatic for the latter groups. Such readers encounter more comprehension failures and consequently spend more time in the debugging state than in the automatic pilot state.

Comprehension failures, for any type of reader, can occur at any level of the reading process: word recognition and processing, syntactic processing, figurative language processing, inferencing, incorrect schema activation, no schema activation, and so forth. Highly skilled readers will only rarely encounter comprehension failures. Perhaps they will encounter an unknown word which cannot be interpreted from context and will need to resort to a dictionary. Perhaps they will encounter unfamiliar subject matter and highly complex syntax, such as in legal documents, and must read very slowly with frequent recourse to dictionaries, other reference works, or experts on the subject matter (Anderson, 1981). But all of these are relatively minor failures of the knowledge base and are relatively easily remedied.

For less skilled and for problem readers, more serious deficiencies may be present in the knowledge base. This can create problems in schema activation, with either no cognitive schema or an inappropriate schema being activated, and in inferencing. Supplying material from prior knowledge through inferencing to make explicit material that is implicit in the text requires that the needed information be available in the knowledge base. The smaller the base, the less likely this will be, and reading comprehension will suffer. Problems can arise in the other processes also. As stated, problems at the word processing level have been found repeatedly to be the best single class of discriminators between good and poor readers. It has also been demonstrated that poorer and beginning readers rely too heavily on context and do not have the fluent bottom-up skills that skilled readers have. Finally, on this topic, skilled readers have been shown to fixate almost every content word when they read and to be capable of detailed phonic and graphemic analysis when required.

It is apparent here that all of the levels of information processing presented are important to reading and that problems with any of them will lead to reading difficulties. As described in the quote from Brown (1980), most of the processes become automatic and fluent in the skilled reader. LaBerge and Samuels (1974) and Stanovich and West (1979) have described how automaticity for these processes can occur. With most of the processes proceeding automatically, conscious attention can be devoted to comprehension of the text.

With all of these processes (bottom-up and top-down) having been demonstrated as important to reading, bottom-up and top-down theories separately can account for only part of the empirical data. This has led to the development of interactive theories which will allow both types of processes to occur and to interact. And the concept of schema has been added to develop a particular form of interactive theory with activated schemata as central elements. In this theory, the cognitive or knowledge base for reading assumes critical importance. Units of related knowledge or action items, packaged as schemata, are activated by the text being read. These schemata then guide inferencing from the text and prediction to the text ahead. As more information is acquired from the text, a schema can be modified or replaced to fit the incoming information. All of this, of course, requires that the bottom-up, text-based skills of lexical and syntactic processing are proceeding automatically and unconsciously. If so, fluent and skilled reading should result.

DEAF CHILDREN AND READING

The problem facing the teacher of reading to deaf children is that all or most of the multiple processes involved in reading, as described in the preceding section, are likely not to be developed to the same level by deaf as by hearing children by the beginning reading stage. Much of this may be a result of lack of appropriate environment and developmental procedures with deaf children in infancy and early childhood. Whatever the cause, however, deaf children are likely to arrive at beginning reading with a very limited knowledge base, inadequately developed cognitive and linguistic skills, and little or no comprehension of English figurative language. Any language they have internalized is likely to be a form other than English and in a mode other than aural. These differences will result in problems of decoding, inferencing, and predicting in the reading process. In short, deaf children are likely to have problems with every aspect of the reading process described in the previous section. There might be significant exceptions to this, such as highly intelligent deaf children of well-educated deaf parents, but the situation described is accurate for most deaf children.

Reading achievement levels

Although educators of deaf children have probably always been perfectly aware that the achievement levels of deaf students in reading English text are far below the levels of hearing students of comparable chronological and mental ages, it was only during the first and second decades of the present century that systematically collected quantitative data first documented the extent and nature of the deficits. Pintner and Patterson (1916) reported that deaf children of 14 to 16 years of age had median reading scores on the Woodworth and Wells Test for following directions that were usually attained by 7-year-old hearing children. Studies over the next 60 or more years have consistently confirmed these findings (Fusfeld, 1955; Goetzinger & Rousey, 1959; Myklebust, 1960; Pugh, 1946). National norms for reading levels of deaf children were supplied by Wrightstone, Aronow, & Moskowitz (1963) who administered the elementary level battery of the Metropolitan Achievement Test to 5,307 hearing-impaired students between the ages of 10½ and 16½ years. In a detailed analysis of the data from that study, Furth, (1966a) showed that only 8% of the national sampling of hearing-impaired students read above the fourth-grade level. Furthermore, reading grade levels for the sample increased from a mean of only 2.7 between the ages of 10 and 11 years, to only 3.5 between 15 and 16 years of age. This represented an increase of less than 1 grade level in 5 years.

The most comprehensive information on the reading achievement levels of deaf students has been supplied in a series of studies by the Office of Demographic Studies (ODS) at Gallaudet College. The ODS regularly collects and reports a wide range of educational and other data on most deaf students in schools in the United States. These national studies have confirmed and expanded the findings of the earlier studies cited. In one such study, DiFrancesca (1972) reported that, for approximately 17,000 students between the ages of 6 and 21 years, the average growth on the Paragraph Meaning subtest of the Stanford Achievement Test was only 0.2 grade levels per year of schooling. This is almost identical to the figure reported earlier by Furth (1966a) for the Wrightstone et al. (1963) data on the Metropolitan Achievement Test. In a more recent ODS study, Trybus and Karchmer (1977) reported reading scores for a stratified, random sample of 6,871 deaf students. They found that the median reading level at age 20 years was a grade equivalent of only 4.5 and that only 10% of the very best reading group (the 18 year olds) could read at or above the eighth-grade level.

Other studies have documented that these low reading levels and the slow rate of progress in reading are not unique to students or to the United States population. Hammermeister (1971) reported a significant increase in scores on the Word Meaning subtest but not on the Paragraph Meaning subtest of the Stanford Achievement Test for 60 deaf adults 7–13 years after they had left school. She interpreted these findings as indicating that the subjects' vocabularies had increased since they left school but their ability to read connected language had not. A number of studies reported in Conrad (1979) attest to the universality of the reading problems of deaf persons. Using the Wide-Span Reading Test (Brimer, 1972) with 468 deaf students in England and Wales between 15 and 16 years of age, Conrad found they had a reading age equivalent to 9-year-old hearing children. He also cited a number of studies conducted in Sweden, Denmark, and New Zealand which reported performances of deaf students at about 16 years of age as being no higher than the level of typical 10-year-old hearing children.

Quigley and Kretschmer (1982) have pointed out that national norms obscure the achievements of individual schools and that some schools might greatly exceed those norms. For example, Lane and Baker (1974) compared reading levels of 132 former students of Central Institute for the Deaf (CID; a private oral school), aged 10 to 16 years, with the reading levels of students of similar ages reported by Furth (1966a). The rate of progress in reading level was much higher for the CID students than for the national sample reported by Furth and also by the DiFrancesca (1972) study cited previously. Both Furth and DiFrancesca reported progress of about 0.2 grade levels per year of schooling whereas Lane and Baker reported 0.6 grade levels for the CID students. Lane and Baker attributed the more rapid reading progress and higher reading achievement levels of the CID students to continuous education in the same school with the same educational philosophy at all levels, maximum use of residual hearing, and oral communication in the school and in the home. Ogden (1979), who conducted a large follow-up study of students from the same school, also reported that the student body and their families were a socioeconomically elite group.

Even though studies of reading achievement levels consistently show greatly depressed performance by deaf individuals, there is evidence that the performance might be even more depressed than those studies show. Moores (1967) compared the reading performance of 37 deaf students with the performance of 37 hearing students using the cloze procedure. The two groups were matched on reading scores on the Stanford Achievement Test. Subjects read passages of 250 words each, selected from fourth-, sixth-, and eighth-grade reading texts, and were requested to replace words that had been deleted from the passages. Using measures constructed to indicate the subjects' abilities to use their vocabularies and syntax in replacing the missing words, Moores found substantial and statistically significant deficiencies in vocabulary and syntax for the deaf subjects as compared to the hearing subjects. Since the two groups had been matched on reading levels, it was reasonable to expect that their vocabulary and syntax levels would have been comparable. O'Neill (1973) found deaf students performed significantly lower than hearing students on the ability to judge the grammaticality of pairs of grammatical and ungrammatical sentences. As in Moores' study, the deaf and hearing subjects of the O'Neill study had been matched on reading achievement levels. These two studies suggest that the reading levels of deaf students might be even lower than the low levels obtained on standard reading tests.

The studies cited are only part of a much larger literature which indicates that deaf individuals do not perform well at any age level on tests of *general* ability to read standard English text. Some of the *specific* difficulties that deaf persons have in reading English text have been explored and are discussed here under the categories used to present the literature on the reading of hearing children—text variables, reader variables, and socioeconomic and cultural variables.

Text variables

Vocabulary

As stated in the section on the reading of hearing children, many studies have indicated that vocabulary knowledge plays a primary role in reading skill. This would seem to be the situation with deaf children also. In studies of educational achievement using such tests as the Stanford Achievement Test, a typical profile of performance on the various subtests has been found consistently. Deaf students usually have their lowest performance on the vocabulary or Word Meaning subtest with a typical pattern of better performance on the other subtests. Performance tends to be lower on any subtest involving meaningful language such as Word Meaning, Paragraph Meaning, and Arithmetic Reasoning and higher on subtests with lesser language involvement such as Spelling, Arithmetic Computation, and Language. (The Language subtest is simply a test of language mechanics such as capitalization and punctuation and not a test of meaningful language). The consistently lowest score for Word Meaning indicates the difficulties that understanding of English vocabulary poses for deaf students. The somewhat higher scores for Paragraph Meaning (and for Arithmetic Reasoning) probably reflect the well-documented facilitating effect of context on language comprehension.

Extensive studies of vocabulary development have been reported by numerous authors (e.g., Fusaro & Slike, 1979; Griswold & Cummings, 1974; Hatcher & Robbins, 1978; Kyle, 1980; Myklebust, 1960; Schulze, 1965; and various ODS surveys). All of them confirm that deaf students at all age levels typically comprehend from print substantially fewer words than hearing children and that the distribution of types of words such as nouns or verbs is different for deaf than for hearing children. Some of these studies have attempted to isolate various factors that influence vocabulary development in deaf children. Hatcher and Robbins (1978), for example, found that deaf children they studied had developed vocabulary and reading skills beyond the level expected from their knowledge of primary word analysis skills.

Walter (1978) conducted a study of vocabulary in deaf children that has diagnostic value beyond simple reporting of deficits in vocabulary level. He selected lists of words sampled from the *American Heritage Dictionary* (Carroll, Davies, & Richman, 1971) distribution of words based on their frequency of occurrence in texts widely used in schools in the United States. These lists were administered to a national sample of deaf children and scores obtained. Theoretically, it should be possible to use a deaf child's score on one of these tests to estimate, from the *American Heritage Dictionary* word frequency distribution, the approximate size and composition of the child's vocabulary. This has considerable educational value beyond simply knowing of the existence and extent of a vocabulary deficit.

Syntax

Although the pattern of subtest performance on educational achievement tests, and surveys of teachers' recommendations for special reading materials (Hasenstab & McKenzie, 1981), indicate that vocabulary is perhaps the area of primary concern in the reading development of deaf children, syntax has also always been a major concern to teachers and researchers. This has been true for the more than 200-year history of educational work with deaf students in France, the United States and other countries (Moores, 1978). The reason for this interest is apparent from study of the variance from standard English syntax of the written samples as shown in Chapter 1. Also, as discussed in chapter 2 on Cognition and Language the relation of short-term (working) memory and speech recoding to syntax might mean that development of English syntax presents special problems for deaf persons.

The study of syntax in deaf children's use of English has usually been influenced by the prevailing linguistic theories. In recent times that has meant the transformational generative grammar of Chomsky (1957, 1965, 1968) and generative semantics (Chafe, 1970; Fillmore, 1968; McCawley, 1968). A substantial number of studies have detailed the syntactic variance of deaf individuals use of English with these theories as frameworks. A series of publications by Quigley and a group of associates (e.g., Quigley et al., 1977; Quigley, Smith, & Wilbur, 1974; Quigley, Wilbur, & Montanelli, 1974, 1976), detailed the performance of a national stratified, random sample of deaf students between the ages of 10 and 19 years on tests of comprehension of various syntactic structures presented singly in sentences. Table 2 presents a summary of the findings showing (1) the order of difficulty of various syntactic structures for deaf students between 10 and 19 years of age, (2) the order of difficulty for the same structures for hearing students between 8 and 10 years, and (3) the frequency of occurrence of each structure in a reading series from Houghton-Mifflin (McKee, Harrison, McCowen, Lehr, & Durr, 1966).

Table 2
Summary of performance on syntactic structures and their frequency of occurrence per 100 sentences in the _Reading for Meaning_ series.

Structure	Deaf Students				Hearing Students	Frequency of Occurrence	
	Average across ages	Age 10	Age 18	Increase	Average across ages	Level at which structure first appeared	Frequency in 6th grade text
Negation							
be	79%	60%	86%	26%	92%	1st Primer—13	9
do	71	53	82	28	92		
have	74	57	78	21	86		
Modals	78	58	87	29	90		
Means	76	57	83	26	90		
Conjunction							
Conjunction	72%	56%	86%	30%	92%	1st Primer—11	36
Deletion	74	59	86	27	94		
Means	73	57	86	29	92		
Question Formation							
WH-Questions:							
Comprehension	66%	44%	80%	36%	98%	2nd Primer—5	6
Yes/no questions:							
Comprehension	74	48	90	42	99	1st Primer—5	3
Tag questions	57	46	63	17	98		
Means	66	46	78	32	98		

(Cont. over)

Table 2
Summary of performance on syntactic structures and their frequency of occurrence per 100 sentences in the *Reading for Meaning* series. (Continued)

Structure	Deaf Students				Hearing Students	Frequency of Occurrence	
	Average across ages	Age 10	Age 18	Increase	Average across ages	Level at which structure first appeared	Frequency in 6th grade text
Pronominalization							
Personal Pronouns	67%	51%	88%	37%	78%		
Backward Pronominalization	70	49	85	36	94	4th grade—1	0 (4 per 1000)
Possessive Adjectives	65	42	82	40	98	1st grade—4	27
Possessive Pronouns	48	34	64	30	99	3rd Primer—1	0 (3 per 1000)
Reflexivization	50	21	73	52	80	2nd grade—1	2
Means	60	39	78	39	90		
Verbs							
Verb Auxiliaries	54%	52%	71%	19%	81%	1st grade—1	18
Tense Sequencing	63	54	72	18	78		
Means	58	53	71	18	79		
Complementation							
Infinitives and gerunds	55%	50%	63%	13%	88%	2nd Primer—4	32

Table 2. (Cont'd)

Structure	Deaf Students				Hearing Students	Frequency of Occurrence	
	Average across ages	Age 10	Age 18	Increase	Average across ages	Level at which structure first appeared	Frequency in 6th grade text
Relativization							
Processing	68%	59%	76%	17%	78%	3rd Primer—2	12
Embedding	53	51	59	8	84		
Relative Pronoun referents	42	27	56	29	82		
Means	54	46	63	18	82		
Disjunction & Alternation	36%	22%	59%	37%	84%	1st grade—1	7

Source: Adapted from Quigley, Wilbur, Power, Montanelli, and Steinkamp (1976).

It can be seen from Table 2 that the average 8-year-old hearing student scored higher on the various tasks than the average 18-year-old deaf student. It can also be seen that there is a large gap between the age when deaf students comprehend various syntactic structures in single sentences and the typical age level when the same structures appear in the reading series. This would indicate a serious reading problem based on syntax alone. And when the typical vocabulary, conceptual, and experiential problems of deaf students are added, it would seem that commonly used reading materials might present serious reading difficulties for many deaf students.

Table 3 presents a list of distinctive syntactic structures that appear consistently in the written productions of many deaf students and citations of studies that have found the same structures in speakers of a variety of native languages who were learning English as a second language. It will be noted that almost all of the distinctive structures found in the written productions of deaf students are found also in the productions of some other population learning English as a second language. Thus, these distinctive structures are not unique to deaf individuals. What might be unique to deaf persons is that they probably have a greater variety of them, have them in greater profusion, and have much greater difficulty changing them than any other population.

The studies by Quigley and associates revealed that the distinctive syntactic structures which appear consistently in the written productions of deaf individuals are also accepted by them as grammatical when used in written tests. The use of these structures in written productions and their acceptance in reading suggests that they are part of the internalized language structure of deaf people. Deaf persons, in addition to showing great delay in the development of English syntax, also appear to have some rules which are not part of standard English. Some of these are in the distinctive structures listed in Table 3. Others have been described by Taylor (1969).

Hatcher and Robbins (1978) concluded from an intensive study of the development of reading skills in six primary and six intermediate grade deaf children that the essential skills for learning to read seem to be those related to comprehension of standard English syntax. In another study of 36 deaf students, 9–12 years of age, Robbins and Hatcher (1981) reached the same conclusion. They found that controlling for word recognition and training in word meaning did not improve performance in reading single sentences containing various syntactic structures. Their analyses revealed that passive voice sentences were the most difficult to comprehend, followed by relative clauses, conjunctions, pronominalization, and indirect objects. Active sentences were the easiest to comprehend. This order of difficulty is similar to that shown in Table 2.

Some studies have shown that deaf students seem to comprehend syntactic structures more easily in connected discourse than in single sentences (Gormley & McGill-Franzen, 1978) and that in some instances comprehension of a particular structure is not necessary for comprehension of a larger unit of discourse (Ewoldt, 1981). These will be discussed in the section on Discourse.

Table 3
Distinctive structures in the language of deaf children and the occurrence of these structures in other populations.

DISTINCTIVE STRUCTURE[1]	ENVIRONMENT	EXAMPLE	OTHER POPULATIONS USING STRUCTURE*
Placement of negative outside sentence	Negation	No Daddy see baby.	First language learners (Bellugi, 1967); Spanish-speaking, Chinese speaking (Dulay & Burt, 1972, 1974); (Cancino, Rosansky & Schumann, 1975)
Placement of negative inside sentence but not correctly marked	Negation	Daddy no see baby.	Same as above.
Non-recognition of negative marker	Negation	Reads negative sentence as positive.	Not found in literature review.
Object-Object Deletion	Conjunction	John chased the girl and he scared. (her)	Learning English regardless of first language (All ESL) (Richards, 1974)
Object-Subject Deletion	Conjunction	The boy hit the girl and (the girl) ran home	Not found in literature review.
No inversion in Questions	Question Formation	What I did this morning? The kitten is black?	First language learners (Klima & Bellugi, 1966); Norwegian-speaking (Ravem, 1974); Spanish-speaking (Hernandez, 1972); All ESL (Richards, 1974); hearing children of deaf parents (Jones & Quigley, 1979)
Inversion of Object and Verb	Question Formation	Who TV watched?	Not found in literature review.
Overgeneralization of contraction rule	Ques. Form. Negation	Amn't I tired? Bill willn't go.	First language learners (Bellugi, 1967); Spanish-speaking (Politzer & Ramirez, 1973)
Noun Copying	Ques. Form. Relativization	Who the boy saw the girl? The boy saw the girl who the girl ran home.	Not found in literature review.

(Cont. over)

Table 3
Distinctive structures in the language of deaf children and the occurrence of these structures in other populations. (Continued)

DISTINCTIVE STRUCTURE[1]	ENVIRONMENT	EXAMPLE	OTHER POPULATIONS USING STRUCTURE*
Pronoun Copying	Ques. Form. Relativization	Who he saw the girl? The boy saw the girl who she ran home.	Spanish-speaking (Politzer & Ramirez, 1973); Arabic-speaking, Persian-speaking, Japanese-speaking, Chinese-speaking (Schacter, 1978); Language-delayed (Haber, 1977)
by Deletion	Verb Processes	The boy was kissed the girl.	All ESL[2] (Richards, 1973); Arabic-speaking (Scott & Tucker, 1974)
Unmarked verb in sequence	Verb Processes	The boy saw the girl and the girl kiss the boy.	All ESL (Richards, 1974); Arabic-speaking (Scott & Tucker, 1974); Spanish-speaking (Cohen, 1975)
Be + unmarked verb (ing missing; ed missing)	Verb Processes	The boy is kiss the girl. The sky is cover with clouds.	All ESL (Richards, 1974); Spanish-speaking (Cohen, 1975); (Politzer & Ramirez, 1973)
Incorrect pairing of auxiliary with verb markers (Confusion of tense markers)	Verb Processes	Tom has pushing the wagon.	All ESL (Richards, 1974)
Omission of Verb	Verb Processes	The cat under the table.	Spanish-speaking (Cohen, 1975); (Politzer & Ramirez, 1973); Arabic-speaking (Scott & Tucker, 1974)
Be-Have Confusion	Verb Processes	The boy have sick. The boy is a sweater.	All ESL (Richards, 1974); Spanish-speaking (Politzer & Ramirez, 1973); (Cohen, 1975); Arabic-speaking (Scott & Tucker, 1974)
Omission of Be or Have	Verb Processes	John sick. The girl a ball.	Same as above.
Subject-Verb Agreement (Third person marker missing)	Verb Processes	The boy say "hi".	First language learners (Brown, 1973); All ESL (Richards, 1974); Spanish-speaking (Cohen, 1975); Lance (1970)

Table 3. (Cont'd)

DISTINCTIVE STRUCTURE[1]	ENVIRONMENT	EXAMPLE	OTHER POPULATIONS USING STRUCTURE*
Omission of conjunction	Conjunction	Bob saw liked the bike	Spanish-speaking (Cohen, 1975); First language learners (pause instead of conjunction—Cohen, 1975)
Omission of determiners	Determiners	Boy is sick.	First language learners (de Villiers & de Villiers, 1978); All ESL (Richards, 1974); Spanish-speaking (Politzer & Ramirez, 1973); (Cohen, 1975); Arabic-speaking (Scott & Tucker, 1974)
Confusion of determiners (Non-recognition of definite-indefinite distinctions)	Determiners	The some apples. . . A test friend. . . He was the bad boy.	Same as above.
Confusion of Case pronouns	Pronominalization	Her is going home. This he friend.	First language learners (Menyuk, (1963); (Hatch, 1969); Spanish-speaking (Cohen, 1975); (Politzer & Ramirez, 1973)
Wrong Gender	Pronominalization	They packed our lunch. (their) Sue is wearing his new dress today.	Spanish-speaking (Cohen, 1975); First language learners (Cohen, 1975); (Wilbur, Montanelli & Quigley, 1976)
Relative Pronoun Deletion (Object-Subject Deletion)	Relativization	The dog chased the girl had on a red dress.	Arabic-speaking (Scott & Tucker, 1974); Persian, Japanese and Chinese-speaking (Schacter, 1978); Spanish-speaking (Cohen, 1975)
Relative Pronoun + Possessive Pronoun	Relativization	The boy helped the girl who her mother was sick.	Same as above.
NP's	Relativization	The boy helped the girl's mother was sick.	Not found in literature review.
Extra *for*	Complementation	For to play baseball is fun.	Not found in literature review.
Extra *to* in POSS-ing Complement	Complementation	Joe went to fishing.	
Infinitive in place of gerund	Complementation	Joe goes to fish.	Spanish-speaking (Politzer & Ramirez, 1973); Arabic (Scott & Tucker, 1974)

Table 3
Distinctive structures in the language of deaf children and the occurrence of these structures in other populations. (Continued)

DISTINCTIVE STRUCTURE[1]	ENVIRONMENT	EXAMPLE	OTHER POPULATIONS USING STRUCTURE*
Omission of *to* before second verb	Complementation	Chad wanted go.	Spanish-speaking (Politzer & Ramirez, 1973)
Incorrectly inflected Infinitive	Complementation	Bill like to played baseball.	Spanish-speaking (Politzer & Ramirez, 1973); First language learners (Black English) (Bartley & Politzer, 1972)
Adjective following Noun	Relativization	The barn red burned.	Spanish-speaking (Cohen, 1975); (Politzer & Ramirez, 1973).
For + Ving or For + V for Infinitive	Complementation	The boy likes for fishing.	Arabic-speaking (Scott & Tucker, 1974)
Surface Reading Order Strategy	Verb Processes	The boy *was* kissed *by* the girl.	First language learners (Bever, 1970); (Bell, Bird & Burroughs-Keith, 1977); French-speaking (Ervin-Tripp, 1972)
	Relativization	*The boy who hit the* girl ran home.	
	Complementation	*That the boy hit* the girl surprised me.	
	Nominalization	*The discussion of* the party bored Bob.	

Source: King, (1981).

*All learners learning English either concurrently with another language or as a second language. Learners include both children and adults.

[1] Adapted from Quigley, Steinkamp, Power and Jones (1978). Each distinctive structure has been found in the language of deaf children and youth.

[2] Richards collected these errors from studies of English errors produced by speakers of Japanese, Chinese, Burmese, French, Czech, Polish, Tagalog, Maori, Maltese and the major Indian and West African languages (Richards, 1974, p. 173, 182–188).

It seems reasonable to conclude at this time, however, that English syntax presents problems for deaf persons both in reading and in writing.

Figurative language

As stated previously the difficulties for deaf children in learning English are compounded by the profusion of figurative expressions in the language. This applies to the written as well as to the spoken form of English. As Dixon et al. (1980) have shown, the beginning reader will encounter many figurative uses of language even in the very first books of commonly used reading series. In recent years, a number of studies have investigated some of the problems that figurative language presents for deaf children in reading English.

Conley (1976) compared comprehension of idiomatic expressions by 643 hearing and 137 deaf students. No significant differences were found in the performance of deaf and hearing students matched on reading levels from grade 2.0 to 2.9; however, significant differences in favor of the hearing students were found for reading levels above 3.0. Scores on the test of idiomatic expressions were significantly and positively related to reading for both groups of subjects. The results of the study may be confounded with variables other than idiomatic expressions. Some of the idioms, for example, were phrased in complex syntactic structures such as relative clauses, complements, and passive voice which have been demonstrated to present comprehension difficulties for deaf readers.

Iran-Nejad, Ortony, and Rittenhouse (1981) constructed metaphorical expressions which were controlled for vocabulary and syntax in accordance with reported comprehension levels for deaf students at various ages (Quigley, Wilbur, Power, Montanelli, & Steinkamp, 1976). In general, the deaf subjects at all age levels (9 to 17 years) scored high on literal comprehension and also at unexpectedly high levels on the metaphorical tasks. A related training study showed improvement in comprehension of metaphors with practice. The authors concluded that deaf children do not have any cognitive deficiency which prevents their comprehension of metaphorical English and that their subjects were able to interpret metaphorical language if their tendency to interpret literally was counteracted in practice sessions.

This study is important for two reasons. First, it attempted to control textual factors other than metaphorical expression (e.g., vocabulary and syntax) so that figurative language was the independent variable of study. Second, it is one of a very few studies to show relatively good comprehension of figurative language by deaf subjects. Problems are present in the design, particularly in how figurative language can really be expressed when vocabulary and syntax are controlled at very low levels, but it is important to note the conclusion that difficulties deaf children might have with figurative language are not due to cognitive deficits. This is in agreement with much of the presentation in chapter 2 on Cognition and Language.

A study by Wilbur, Fraser, and Fruchter (1981) also showed unexpectedly high levels of comprehension for figurative language by deaf subjects. In this case, the aspect of figurative language studied was idiomatic expressions. The authors speculated that at least some idioms might be memorized or learned as a whole so that vocabulary and syntax might not present confounding problems. Studies by Page (1981) and Houck (1982) concluded that deaf children are not impaired in their comprehension of idioms when there is sufficient contextual information in the written material and when "extraneous factors" are controlled.

It probably would be very difficult to convince experienced teachers of deaf children on the basis of any research study or group of studies that figurative language does not present major comprehension difficulties for deaf children in reading. Teachers seem to regard this as one of their major problems in language development, including reading. Some possible explanations for the contrary findings for some research studies are offered in the section on Discourse.

Two recent studies of figurative language produced findings which, along with those of Conley (1976) already cited, are probably close to teachers' perceptions of the matter. Giorcelli (1982) constructed a Test of Figurative Language consisting of 100 multiple-choice items. The test assesses 10 specific aspects of figurative language: analogical and syllogistical reasoning, associative fluency, linguistic problem solving, interpretation of anomaly, and discrimination between paraphrases of novel and idiomatic metaphors. Choices of idiomatic phrases, syntax, and vocabulary were carefully controlled. Isolated and short and long contextual conditions were used. High measures of reliability, validity, and usability were obtained for the test battery.

Three groups of 25 deaf subjects, each group ranging in age from 9 years, 9 months to 19 years, 11 months, and one group of 25 hearing subjects aged from 8 years to 9 years, 4 months were tested. Results were that the hearing subjects scored significantly higher than the deaf subjects on total test performance and on 7 of the 10 subtests. Performance for the deaf subjects improved with the addition of context but still remained well below the performance of the hearing subjects. The 18-year-old deaf subjects did not perform as well as the 9-year-old hearing subjects, which is similar to the findings for syntax by Quigley, Wilbur, Power, Montanelli, and Steinkamp (1976). There also was very little improvement in performance of deaf subjects beyond 13–14 years of age, which is similar to the plateaus in reading reported by DiFrancesca (1972) and others.

Payne (1982) studied the extent to which deaf and hearing subjects could understand verb–particle combinations of English. This structure is one of the most common means by which English is expanded. Verb–particle combinations can be literal, for example, "run up a hill" or idiomatic, for example, "run up a bill." Payne assessed his subjects performance on verb–particle combinations at three levels of semantic difficulty (literal, semi-idiomatic, and idiomatic) and in five syntactic surface structures with a written test of 64 items with vocabulary controlled to first- and second-grade level. He found that the hearing subjects scored significantly higher than the deaf subjects on all levels of semantic difficulty and for all syntactic structures.

Although there are contrary findings, extensive studies of figurative language lend support to the contentions of teachers that figurative expressions present a major problem in reading for deaf students. When added to the problems presented by vocabulary and syntax, and the obvious interactions among all of these, it is apparent that many textual variables contribute to the low performance of deaf students on standard reading tests. Some of the contrary research findings on figurative language raise the question of whether the problem is with the deaf person's lack of the form in which the figurative concepts are expressed, that is, the English language, or lack of the underlying concepts themselves. Some studies in discourse shed some light on this.

Discourse

Most of the research discussed in this category of textual variables has focused on single, controlled aspects of text—vocabulary, syntax, figurative language. The purpose has been to try to determine to what extent these various aspects of text contribute to the general low performance of deaf students on standard reading tests. Reading tests provide only a general measure of reading comprehension. Knowledge of the contributions of specific aspects of text, such as vocabulary and syntax, to the general measure and the general problem should provide more detailed understanding of the matter. It can be argued, however, that such an approach distorts the typical reading process. Studies by McGill-Franzen and Gormley (1980) and Ewoldt (1981) have taken this position and have attempted to investigate larger units of discourse than words and sentences.

McGill-Franzen and Gormley (1980) studied deaf children's comprehension of truncated passive sentences (e.g., The wolf was killed) presented in context and in isolation. Their results indicated that deaf children who could not comprehend a passive sentence presented in isolation could comprehend the same sentence when it was embedded in the context of a *familiar* fairy tale. The results were interpreted as demonstrating that deaf children could understand passives in context. The results of the study have been criticized by Robbins and Hatcher (1981) on the ground that the use of highly familiar material (known fairy tales) meant that probably very little knowledge about the stories was text dependent. In other words, given the topic of a passage, subjects probably could have responded appropriately to questions without even reading the passage. Furthermore, a study by Israelite (1981) found that the use of context did not aid in correct interpretation of passive sentences.

Ewoldt (1981) also stresses the contextual analysis skills of deaf children and claims that deaf children can bypass English syntax and move directly to meaning. Ewoldt conducted an intensive analysis of the reading of four prelingually deaf children aged 6 years 11 months to 16 years 11 months. The children read and interpreted 25 stories in sign language which were videotaped. Comprehension was assessed by Goodman's miscue analysis, cloze procedures, and retellings of the stories by the children. Ewoldt concluded that the subjects were users of language and were able to read and retell stories written in English by interpreting them into their own sign language. She reported that the subjects made extensive use of the syntactic and semantic cuing systems but did not "over-rely" on graphic information. This was interpreted as support for the top-down theory of reading and its use by deaf children. It will be recalled from the discussion of reading theories, however, that a top-down approach to reading is typical of beginning readers and poor readers who have not acquired automatic and unconscious control of bottom-up processing of text. This approach can enable the beginning reader and the poor reader to acquire a "general idea" of the meaning of a text without fully understanding it. It is difficult from Ewoldt's report to determine the extent to which context did allow her subjects to bypass the syntax of the stories. Only two examples are given and interpretations of those could be made other than that syntax was being bypassed.

A final study is of interest in the analysis of discourse. It will be recalled that Mandler and Johnson (1977) and others demonstrated that there is underlying intersentential structure to text which aids (and perhaps directs) reading comprehension. Gaines, Mandler, and Bryant (1981) have extended this type of discourse analysis to the reading of deaf children. They compared immediate and delayed recall of stories by hearing and deaf children. Three stories from Mandler (1978) were used: (1) The first story consisted of standard prose; (2) the second contained nonphonetic misspellings (e.g., "throgh: for "through"); and (3) the third contained confused anaphoric references. Six deaf and six hearing subjects were matched for reading age (Gates Vocabulary Test). Deaf subjects ranged from 14 years 3 months to 15 years 1 month (mean = 14 years 5 months); reading ages ranged from 11 years 6 months to 13 years 9 months (mean = 12 years 6 months). The deaf subjects were from an oral school. The very high reading ages and the high quality of the written English used by the deaf subjects on the recall tasks indicate that they were highly select individuals.

Results of the study revealed no significant differences between the deaf and hearing subjects in the amount of recall of story propositions on the normal prose story, but the deaf subjects had significantly higher amounts of recall for both of the confused stories. However, in accuracy of recall of story content deaf subjects made significantly more distortions than did the hearing subjects. Most of the deaf subjects' distortions were semantic confusions and there was no significant difference in the mean number of written syntactic errors between the deaf subjects (5.2) and the hearing subjects (3.5).

The investigators speculated that the deaf subjects used a "broad reconstructive 'top-down' schematic approach" to reading (p. 467). Thus, they were able to comprehend the overall meaning of the stories and recall an *amount* of story propositions similar to the hearing subjects; however, they did have significantly more semantic distortions than the hearing subjects.

This is typically what would be expected from hearing students who were beginning or poor readers. As stated, such readers can often get the "general idea" of a passage by the use of "top-down" strategies but will have a lack of understanding or misinterpret important details.

Reader variables

A number of researchers have attempted to define the personal variables which account at least partially for the performance of deaf readers. Jensema (1975) found (as have many investigators) that vocabulary and comprehension performance are inversely related to degree of hearing impairment; the greater the impairment, the lower the performance. Similarly, and also well known, age at onset of hearing impairment was related to reading performance— prelinguistically impaired students read less well than those impaired at later ages. Rogers, Leslie, Clarke, Booth, and Horvath (1978) conducted an extensive study of the factors influencing vocabulary and comprehension scores for a large part of the hearing-impaired student population in British Columbia. In addition to the factors reported by Jensema (1975), these investigators found that students who used oral communication performed better on both vocabulary and reading comprehension than students who used simultaneous (total) manual and oral communication, and students who wore hearing aids scored higher in comprehension than those who did not.

The three reader variables discussed in the section on the reading of hearing persons were development of schemata, inferencing, and metacognitive strategies. Research on schemata development with deaf children is almost nonexistent, although the study by Gaines et al., 1981 reported that highly literate oral deaf readers were using "a broad reconstructive 'top-down' schematic approach" (p. 467) to the reading process. As Kretschmer (1982) has pointed out, research into metacognitive processes with deaf readers has been limited to studies of judgments of grammaticality (Quigley, Wilbur, Power, Montanelli, & Steinkamp, 1976; Kretschmer, 1976). Kretschmer (1982) reports that research with deaf readers in metacognitive processes—ranging from what hearing-impaired children think reading is, to study skills approaches—might result in better ways to teach productive study skills to deaf students.

In the area of inferencing, there has been at least one extensive study conducted with deaf students. Wilson (1979) pointed out that many studies of reading achievement levels have shown that deaf students tend to plateau at about the third- or fourth-grade level, at 13–14 years of age, and their scores change very little from then through at least age 19. He speculated that this might be due to changes in the format and content of reading materials and tests at the fourth-grade level. Up to the third grade, most reading materials emphasize word analysis skills and vocabulary and reading tests assess those factors. Beyond the third grade, materials increasingly require the utilization of prior knowledge to infer meanings that are not explicitly stated in the text. As stated in the section on hearing children, inferencing becomes ubiquitous in the reading process. And its assessment becomes ubiquitous in reading tests. Wilson (1979) reasoned that if deaf children had problems with inferencing, this might account at least partially for their plateauing in reading at the third- or fourth-grade level.

Wilson (1979) constructed a series of short passages in which inferencing was studied in various syntactic environments and with vocabulary controlled. The purpose was to determine how well deaf students could understand material that required inferencing as compared to material that could be understood literally. For example, given the sentences (Wilson, 1979):

> The shirt is dirty.
> The shirt is under the bed.
> The cat is on the shirt.
> The cat is white.

it can readily be understood by most people that *The cat is under the bed* even though this is not stated explicitly in the text. Using these techniques, Wilson found that inferencing presented much greater difficulty for his deaf subjects than for his hearing subjects, and that inferencing was independent of type of syntactic structure. So here is another ability important to reading on which deaf students evidence lowered performance.

Another of Wilson's findings is important to note. His stories were administered in speech, signs, and writing and it was found that the hearing subjects scored highest with the spoken presentations, whereas the deaf subjects scored highest with the written presentations. This supports findings of other studies of efficiency and effectiveness of communication. Quigley and Frisina (1961) reported that reading appeared to provide a more stable means of communication for deaf students than the reception of speech or finger spelling. White and Stevenson (1975) similarly found reading print to be superior for receptive communication to reading speech or signs, and Stuckless and Pollard (1977) showed that children raised using finger spelling could process the written form more readily than finger spelling. A little reflection will reveal the unexpectedness and significance of these findings.

Socioeconomic and cultural variables

Just as socioeconomic and cultural influences have been shown repeatedly to influence the reading development of hearing children, so have they been shown to influence the reading development of deaf children. Brasel and Quigley (1977), Ogden (1979), and many others have shown that the standard measures of socioeconomic status, family income, occupations, and educational levels are related to language and reading development for deaf children just as they are for hearing children. The unique factor in this area for deaf children is whether they are actually members (or destined to be members) of a separate culture of deaf people rather than members of the general culture. If it is accepted that at least some significant portion of deaf children are members of a separate culture, and that American Sign Language is the language of the culture, then the approach to the development of reading could be significantly affected.

For hearing people, reading can be regarded as a parasitic function which is founded on the primary auditory based language developed during the first few years of life. In spite of the current emphasis on top-down processes, reading in the narrow sense can be regarded as the decoding of print. This is all that is unique to reading. All of the other factors of prior knowledge and inferencing are the result of experience and of linguistic development which occur as natural processes when an intact human organism raised in a reasonably responsive family interacts with its environment for the satisfaction of its needs and wants. Prior knowledge and inferencing develop as part of the total auditory based language process even if reading is never taught.

Most, probably all, methods of reading instruction with deaf as well as with hearing children assume the existence of an auditory based language in the prereading child. If such an auditory based language is not present, then how should reading be developed? And, more importantly, is it worth the effort to develop it at all given the meager results of 200 years of educational effort?

Educational variables

Instructional practices

As Clarke, Rogers, and Booth, (1982) have reported, there are very few texts on teaching reading to deaf children in contrast to the hundreds that exist for teaching hearing children. They list and describe some of the major existing works by Hart (1963), Streng (1965), the Clarke School for the Deaf *Curriculum Series on Reading* (1972), Truax (1978), and Blackwell et al. (1978). Examination of these approaches shows that they generally utilize adaptations of approaches used with hearing children, which are, of course, based on auditory language. Such approaches also usually assume that the prereading child brings much more experientially based internalized language to the beginning reading process than most deaf children do. Because of the prereading deaf child's great lack of a structured internalized language, the reading process also becomes a language learning process which must make an already difficult process even more difficult for many deaf children.

Given the importance of reading to the educational process and the difficulties of teaching reading to deaf children, it would be expected that reading instruction would be prominently featured in the preparation of teachers. This does not seem to be the case, however. Coley and Bockmiller (1980) conducted a survey of 122 residential schools to obtain information about (1) the extent of reading instruction in teacher preparation, (2) the current methods being used to teach reading to deaf children, and (3) the teachers' self-assessments of how well prepared they were to use a variety of methods to teach reading. About 72% of the questionnaires were returned in usable form. It was found that teachers had little formal training in teaching reading.

Approximately 20% of the teachers had no or only one college course in reading, and of those who had masters degrees (56.2%), almost 40% had no graduate course in reading. Regardless of their training, teachers overwhelmingly used basal readers for a large precentage of instructional time. More than 40% of the teachers reported spending more than 40% of their instructional time using basal readers. Given these figures, and recognizing the importance and difficulty of teaching reading to deaf students, it is obvious that much more research, development, and particularly training in reading and reading instruction are needed.

Special materials

King and Quigley (in press) devote a chapter to discussing the arguments for and against the development of special reading materials for deaf children and to describing some of the materials developed during the past 150 years. They state that materials constructed for problem readers, including deaf students, have typically taken one of three approaches: (1) rewriting of existing materials to an "easier" level; (2) modification of instructional techniques used with existing materials; and (3) writing of original materials to meet the needs of specific learners (Stowitschek, Gable, & Hendrickson, 1980). Regardless of the specific approach, however, the use of special materials and techniques has been controversial in many areas of special education, including the education of deaf children. King and Quigley (in press) offer the following quotations to illustrate the opposing points of view:

> No one questions the need for adapted materials for children with physical or sensory deficits. (Goodman, 1978, p. 93)
> [I]t is [not] advisable to simplify written materials. (Kachuk, 1981, p. 375)

Two basic positions have been taken in the use of special reading materials with deaf children: (1) those who support the use of special materials, at least for the beginning stages of reading instruction; and (2) those who see no value at all, and even harm, in the use of special materials. There does seem to be general agreement, however, that a major objective of any reading program for deaf children should be to enable them to read eventually the generally available literature (Clarke et al., 1982; Quigley, 1982). Also, the expressed or implicit goal of most special reading materials is "to develop reading skills to the extent that children can *successfully* use existing materials" (Quigley & King, 1981, p. 2, italics added).

King and Quigley (in press) draw three major conclusions from an extensive review of the research with various special populations on adaptations and special materials which are written to reduce language and reading demands. First, a number of variables have been identified which can contribute to text difficulty (e.g., vocabulary, syntax, inferencing), but the relative contributions of each of these variables and the interactions among them have not yet been determined. Further, while researchers have attempted to manipulate variables individually to determine their effects on reading comprehension, it has not been possible to uncover in what ways the individual variables actually increase difficulty or improve clarity in a text (Klare, 1976). Second, adaptations can actually be more difficult than the original, as well as uninteresting if the sole purpose of the adaptation is to attain some level of difficulty as measured by readability scores. The best adaptations are those which are guided by the desire to communicate meaningfully and by a thorough understanding of the properties and uses of language. Third, and most important, although reduction of the complexity of texts by rewriting apparently has little effect on the reading comprehension of older and more proficient readers (Charrow & Charrow, 1979; Johnson, 1981; Johnson & Otto, 1982), the effects of adaptations are generally positive for individuals with low reading and low language skills (e.g., Armbruster, Echols, & Brown, 1982; Beck, Omanson, & McKeown, 1982; Johnson, 1981). The research also indicates that the use of adapted or specially written materials is most beneficial at the instructional reading level (DiStefano & Valencia, 1980).

With reading levels typically no higher than fourth grade, most deaf children fit the category for whom specially written and rewritten materials are helpful, and studies with deaf children have shown positive effects from the use of such materials (Anken & Holmes, 1977; Heine, 1981). Heine (1981) used several stories from Level 5 of *Reading Milestones* (Quigley & King, Eds., 1981, 1982, 1983, 1984) to investigate the influence of higher order (more important) and lower order ideas on the comprehension of deaf children. *Reading Milestones* is a reading series prepared especially for deaf children and other types of problem readers. Heine did not find predicted differences between higher and lower order ideas, but he did find that deaf children comprehended literal information in the passages *as well as or better than* a comparison group of hearing children. Given that deaf children typically have much lower comprehension of regular materials than hearing children, this result provides support that the use of linguistically controlled reading materials can positively affect the comprehension of deaf children.

SUMMARY AND CONCLUSIONS

The hearing reader

Research to date with hearing children indicates that interactive theory which incorporates schema theory best explains at present the empirical data on the reading process and problem. Top-down and bottom-up theories provide only partial explanations of the existing data. Top-down notions are of major importance in reading. It is commonly accepted now that reading is part of a general language comprehension process and cannot be separated from it. Thus, infant and early childhood learning experiences, early schema development, cognitive and linguistic development, inferencing and figurative language abilities, and the knowledge base that will result from all of these provide the prereading child with all the major skills for reading except one—decoding of the printed word. They provide the child with the abilities to use context and prior knowledge for prediction in reading as part of the whole process of constructing meaning from text. But the bottom-up processes, the decoding or text-driven data, are also important. The studies of McConkie (1982), Rayner et al. (1980), and Zola (1981), among many, confirm that, contrary to claims of top-down theorists, skilled readers fixate almost every content word in a text and use individual letters and other graphemic (and phonic) knowledge and skills extensively in reading. In reading, letters and words are the basic data on which the human processor must work.

The issue of the place and form of decoding has been at the heart of a long-standing controversy in reading instruction (Chall, 1967; Flesch, 1955) as to whether emphasis should be placed on the whole word (look–say) approach or spelling–sound correspondences (phonics). Vellutino's (1982) exhaustive analysis of a century of research data on the unit of perception involved in word recognition concluded that both visual and phonic access to words are used by skilled readers and that persons who can use only one form of access often have reading problems. In support of Vellutino's conclusions, there is also the extensive body of data showing that differences in abilities at the level of letter and word processing are the single best class of discriminators between good and poor readers (Biemiller, 1977-1978; Graesser et al., 1980). Other investigators (Adams, 1980; Stanovich, 1980; Stanovich & West, 1979) have shown that reliance on top-down rather than bottom-up processing is characteristic of younger and less able readers. Such readers tend to apply their relevant prior knowledge, sight comprehension of some of the words in a text, some syntax from knowledge of word order, and slowly acquire a "general idea" of a text. This is probably similar to the process used by many deaf children in getting the gist or a "rough idea" of the meaning of a text. This is not skilled reading. It is not even adequate reading. Detailed testing or questioning will readily reveal the lack of detailed comprehension and the misunderstandings that result from this superficial form of reading, which is apparently due to lack of adequately developed word-processing skills.

Skilled readers have a thorough knowledge of orthographic redundancy and spelling-to-sound correspondences which they can use in reading when required. Such readers, however, usually utilize direct visual access to words. As Kleiman (1975) has demonstrated, speech recoding of printed words is not necessary for access to meaning, but speech recoding does occur after lexical access and facilitates the temporary storage of words for *sentence comprehension*. There is now considerable evidence for the point that speech recoding is *not necessary* for gaining access to *word meanings* (Baron, 1973; Kleiman, 1975), although it can be used for this purpose whenever required. There is also accumulating evidence that speech recoding *is* an important process in the *comprehension of sentences and intersentential text*. Speech recoding makes possible the temporary storage of words in working memory to comprehend complex syntactic structures and disambiguate sentences. This could be a critical factor in the reading problems of deaf children.

The picture of the skilled hearing reader, then, is one of automatic and unconscious use of word-processing (decoding) skills as demonstrated by LaBerge and Samuels (1974), which allows most of the reader's attention and working memory to be devoted to the higher order processes involved in text prediction and relation of text information to prior information (inferencing). Some of these higher order processes also become automatic (e.g., inferencing, prediction) and allow skilled readers to engage consciously in the metacognitive techniques of planning, monitoring, self-questioning, and summarizing.

The less skilled and problem readers present the opposite picture. Their bottom-up and top-down processes are not as fluent and automatic as for skilled readers. They also often have experiential and linguistic deficits from infancy and early childhood which impoverish the knowledge base and word-processing skills needed for fluent reading. On the basis of their performance on standard reading and other tests, most deaf children can be included in the category of less skilled or problem readers.

The deaf reader

National surveys, individual studies of reading achievement, and studies of specific aspects of the reading process all indicate that most deaf children have difficulty with reading the English language. Few of them become really skilled readers. This seems not to be due to any single factor (excepting, of course, deafness itself), but to problems with all of the factors involved in the reading process. Where the typical hearing child brings to the reading process a substantial knowledge base resulting from a wide variety of infant and early childhood experiences which have been internalized through the spoken language acquired by interaction with parents and significant others, the deaf child typically brings to the same process a very impoverished knowledge base. This is not always due to lack of exposure to early experiences, but often to the lack of a fluent language and communication system with which to signify and internalize those experiences in some manipulable code.

In addition to the lack of a substantial knowledge base, deaf children often are lacking in inferential skills and in figurative language and other linguistic skills which develop automatically in young hearing children. In short, they do not have the experiential, cognitive, and linguistic base needed to learn to read fluently. Because of this, learning to read becomes also a basic language learning process for deaf children.

In view of the many deficits the deaf child brings to the learning-to-read process, the wonder is that the child ever learns to read at all. Yet, some deaf children learn to read very well. There is a need to determine from studies of successful deaf readers just what factors account for their success. Studies by Conrad (1979), Lichtenstein (1983), and others have indicated that the ability to use speech coding and recoding is related to reading success. And Conrad (1979) has shown that even some deaf children who have unintelligible speech have acquired a speech code. This could be one factor accounting for success.

Speech recoding seems to be important for hearing readers not so much for access to word meaning as for temporary storage of words in working memory in order to comprehend clauses and sentences. This form of coding and storage involves temporal–sequential memory and, as discussed in chapter 2 on Cognition and Language, this is one aspect of memory where deaf persons have been found consistently to have shorter spans than hearing persons. These two facts, shorter temporal–sequential memory spans and lack of a speech code, could account for some of the language acquisition and reading problems of deaf children. They might also help explain why acquiring the syntax of English (and perhaps of any spoken language) seems to present extreme difficulty for many deaf persons.

Given the deficits deaf children bring to the learning-to-read process, it seems that the methods and the materials used with hearing children might not be appropriate for many of them. King and Quigley (in press) have provided an extensive analysis of the research on the construction and use of special materials with deaf children. Their conclusion was that special materials have value for less able and problem readers, including deaf children. There is a need with many deaf children to provide materials which will match their limited experience and limited knowledge of the vocabulary, syntax, figurative expressions, and other aspects of standard English and which will increase in difficulty at a limited pace. If language instruction is proceeding concurrently, such special materials could gradually be phased out until the deaf child eventually was using the regular reading materials of the general school system.

The methods of reading instruction used with deaf children generally are those used with hearing children with some concessions to the limited language base of deaf children (Clarke et al., 1982). These are methods based on spoken and auditory language which many deaf children do not have. Such methods might work for those deaf children who, by whatever means, have acquired a speech code (Conrad, 1979), but many deaf children do not acquire this code. It seems logical that teaching reading to those deaf children would require special methods based on visual language. The methods would have to take into account whatever form of visual language the child had internalized prior to the beginning reading process. This might be some form of manually coded English (MCE), some form of pidgin sign English (PSE), or a variety of American Sign Language (ASL). In order to teach reading to these children, the teacher needs to be able to determine which language or communication form the child typically used and use it as the base for teaching reading. This, in turn, requires that the reading teacher be fluent in ASL and other forms of visual language. The similarity of this process to the teaching of English as a second language is obvious and is discussed in chapter 6.

The need for special methods might be most pronounced for deaf children of well-educated deaf parents who have used ASL as the primary language with their children. These children bring to the beginning reading process all the experiential, cognitive, and linguistic skills that hearing children typically do, but in a language (ASL) different from English and in a communication mode (manual/visual) different from oral/aural. This might be considered a special case of the previously discussed group and declared a case of teaching English as a second language. But it also has been argued that for some of these children and for other deaf children also, the teaching of reading of print might simply deter their educational progress. Although reading has an almost revered status in the educational system, it basically is a means for transmitting and acquiring information. This can be accomplished by other means. For example, printed English material could be transformed to ASL on videotapes for use by deaf persons. This is analogous to "talking books" for blind people.

In spite of the problems deaf persons have with reading English, the studies by Quigley and Frisina (1961), White and Stevenson (1975), Stuckless and Pollard (1977), and Wilson (1979) cited earlier indicate that many deaf children find it a more effective means of receiving English than speech, signs, or finger spelling. In view of this, Stuckless and a number of associates at the National Technical Institute for the Deaf (e.g., Stuckless & Hurwitz, 1982; Stuckless & Matter, 1982) have used a computer and a stenotypist to produce on a screen and on paper printed versions of the spoken word while the word is being spoken. This is called real-time graphic display and has promise as an educational tool for deaf people. Although the equipment and the methods are not yet fully developed, they are far enough advanced to make feasibility virtually certain.

Even in the limited space of this single chapter, the rapidly developing research interest in reading for deaf people should be obvious. This research will increase and the next decade holds promise for greater understanding of the language and reading processes of deaf children and the application of research to the development of new teaching methods, new materials, and new devices. It could develop that different approaches, materials, and devices will have to be developed for different groups of deaf children. Some of those children, especially those who acquire speech coding, might simply need special uses of the materials and methods developed for hearing children. Others might need special materials and methods adapted to various forms of visual/manual English and perhaps the use of some of the techniques of teaching English as a second language. And still others might need to receive information in some visual form other than printed English (e.g., videotaped ASL). If this develops, a major research and educational program will be to determine which approach goes with which child, and since the determination needs to be made very early in life, it is a very knotty problem indeed. The alternative, though, is even worse. It is to swing from one basic language to another, oral English, manually coded English, or ASL, for *all* deaf children and base one set of reading approaches on the language of choice. The low reading performances of deaf children attest to the lack of validity of this approach and argue for more diversification of reading techniques based on the various language and communication approaches. And then there is the question of whether the teaching of the reading of print is feasible or a productive use of time at all for some, as yet undetermined, portion of the population of deaf children.

chapter 5

Written language

Until the recent great upsurge of interest in American Sign Language and manually coded English, much of the research on the language of deaf children was conducted on written language productions. This is in distinct contrast to hearing children where primary spoken language is usually the focus of interest. The reason was simply that the spoken language of many deaf children is extremely limited and often unintelligible and therefore not readily available for inspection and analysis. Reading and written language became the common denominators of educational programs for deaf children and the means whereby the progress of children and the status of programs are measured. There has been some shift in this now that ASL and MCE systems are being used with many young deaf children. Analysis of the language of children using these systems has begun and is reported in chapter 3. But it probably is still fair to say that educational programs use reading and written language, even though they are secondary language systems, as the major indicators of primary language development and progress in deaf children. Spontaneous written language productions are generally considered to be among the best indicators of a deaf child's level of mastery of English.

There are a number of problems associated with this use of written language productions, however.

1. Usually, some external stimulus is used to elicit a written sample—a picture, picture sequence, short film, request to write a story or letter, and so forth. The validity and reliability of these techniques often are unknown. If it is found that certain vocabulary items, morphological structures, syntactic structures, or other linguistic units of interest do not appear in the written samples elicited, there is no way of knowing whether this is due to the deaf child's inability to produce such structures, or whether it is merely that the stimulus used did not elicit them.

2. Some linguistic units (e.g., infinitival complements) might appear in the written productions, but in insufficient numbers or variety to allow for study and analysis.

3. Some constructions (e.g., some types of relative clauses) appear in linguistic environments such that it is difficult to understand them and their role in a sentence.

4. As probably every teacher of deaf children knows, the written language productions of many deaf children are often as unintelligible as their spoken language.

In spite of these problems of eliciting and analyzing written language productions, such productions are valuable indicators of a deaf child's grasp of English and of the internalized language structure with which the child is working. Bloom and Lahey (1978) have provided a systematic means of analysis of written samples and Kretschmer and Kretschmer (1978) have adapted it for use with deaf children. This form of language production is classified in this chapter as *free response*.

In addition to free response elicitation, written language can also be elicited by *controlled response* methods. According to Cooper and Rosenstein (1966), controlled response studies are those in which the investigator, in collecting data, attempts to control or manipulate the behavior of a subject or informant by holding certain linguistic variables constant. The linguistic method of presenting pairs of sentences which differ on only one structure and asking subjects for judgments of the sentences' grammaticality is one example. In free response language studies, in contrast, the data to be analyzed are obtained from freely produced samples of writing.

In addition to whether free or controlled methods are used to elicit language samples, studies also differ on the theoretical linguistic frameworks used to direct data analysis. The two major frameworks are labeled here as *traditional* and *generative*. Although dividing lines between free response and controlled response studies and traditional and generative frameworks are not always sharp, the categories serve adequately for grouping the data on the written language of deaf children. Thus, these data are presented here under two major headings: Free Response Studies; and Controlled Response Studies. Within each of these categories studies using traditional and generative analysis are discussed.

HEARING CHILDREN

In most of the chapters of this book, the practice has been to present quite extensive information on hearing children prior to the information on deaf children. That will not be done here for several reasons. First, the literature is too voluminous to present adequately even in very summary fashion. Second, the great gaps between the written language of deaf and hearing children are only too well known to teachers of deaf children and hardly need repeating. And third, it is more helpful to present information on hearing children's written language, where needed, along with specific studies of deaf children rather than generally. This is what is done here, except for the following few studies of hearing children.

It is worthy of note, that the study of written language with hearing individuals has progressed in directions not yet explored with deaf people. Past studies have tended (and many still do) to be concerned with the mechanics and problems of writing. For example, Harrell (1957), working within a traditional/structuralist linguistic framework, studied the oral and written language of hearing students 9–15 years of age. He reported extensively on the developmental pattern of sentence structure. Loban (1963), working within a structuralist linguistic framework, conducted a longitudinal study of language abilities, following the same students from kindergarten through high school. He, too, reported extensively on developmental patterns in sentence structure. Another group of investigators (Hunt, 1965; O'Donnell, Griffin, & Norris, 1967) used transformational generative grammar as a framework for analysis of the oral and written language of hearing students from kindergarten through 12th grade. They reported extensively on the development of specific syntactic structures and sentence-combining transformations.

Such studies provide helpful comparisons in studying the written language of deaf children and some similar studies with deaf students are discussed in this chapter. Recently, however, the interest of some investigators has shifted from studying the problems and linguistic structure of writing to studying the basic psychological processes involved in composing written discourse. A summary of the literature in this developing area has been provided by Black (1982). A study cited by Black (Cooper, Cherry, Gerber, Fleischer, Copley, & Sartisky, 1979) illustrates some of the variables in which this new area is interested. In this study of the entering class of 1979 at the State University of New York at Buffalo, it was found that major writing problems were present; however, they were not problems of written language mechanics. The conclusions cited by Black (1982) indicated that the students had nearly flawless control at the word and sentence level but that they had great difficulty creating written text that had adequate connections and relationships from sentence to sentence. They were unable to generate examples, anecdotes, and details to support generalizations. "In short the students are careful editors but poor composers" (p. 200). This area of research on written language has been largely unexplored with deaf students, and the study of intersentence aspects and creative aspects of discourse composition could be fertile areas for future research. Some preliminary studies at the intersentence level (discourse analysis) are presented later in the chapter.

DEAF CHILDREN

Free response studies

Typical free response studies consist of the analysis of written samples of language, usually within the framework of the prevailing grammar (linguistic) theory of the period. The language samples usually are obtained by asking the subjects to write in response to some stimulus such as a still picture, a sequence of pictures, or a motion picture. Many studies of this type have demonstrated deaf children's lower performance in written language in comparison to hearing children of even much younger ages, and the great extent to which deaf children's written language productions vary from stan-dard English (e.g., Heider & Heider, 1940; Ivimey & Lachterman, 1980; Powers & Wilgus, 1983; Stuckless & Marks, 1966). Following Cooper and Rosen-stein's (1966) lead, some of this work is summarized here under several headings: productivity, complexity, flexibilty, distribution of parts of speech, and types of errors. The presentations under these headings include extensive material from Quigley, Wilbur, Power, Montanelli, & Steinkamp (1976). In most of the sections one or two major studies are discussed in detail and smaller studies are cited as supporting resources.

Free traditional grammar studies

Productivity. The extensive analysis of Heider and Heider (1940) indicated that although their deaf subjects' compositions did not differ in total length in words from those of hearing children of the same age, the average length of single sentences was strikingly shorter than that of hearing children. Deaf children did not attain the average sentence length of 8-year-old hearing children until they were 17 years old. These results have been confirmed by Simmons (1962) and Myklebust (1964).

Complexity. Heider and Heider (1940) found that their deaf subjects were typically 17 years old before they used the same proportion of compound and complex sentences in their compositions as did 10-year-old hearing subjects. They were similarly developmentally delayed in their use of subordinate clauses of all types. In 1965 Hunt introduced a new "summary index" of language complexity in his *T-unit* ("one main clause plus all the subordinate clauses attached to or imbedded in it," p. 141). In a major study Taylor (1969) repeated Hunt's analysis on a corpus of writing of deaf children. She reported that several of Hunt's indices based on the T-unit (mean number of clauses per T-unit, mean T-unit length, and so forth), showed significant increases in the writing of deaf children from grade to grade, and confirmed several of the findings of previous "traditional index" studies. Part of Taylor's analysis was repeated by Marshall and Quigley (1970), who reanalyzed the corpus of writing collected by Stuckless and Marks (1966). They generally corroborated Taylor's findings about various T-unit indexes being sensitive indicators of maturity of language expression in deaf children to the extent that they showed signifi-cant increases over time. They also found the more traditional *subordination ratio* (number of subordinate clauses per main clause) to be just as good an indicator, but felt that T-unit analysis was more useful educationally, because the internal structure of the T-unit was more easily examined to determine the factors which contribute to its maturation.

The most extensive study designed to establish developmental indexes of language production phenomena in deaf children was that of Stuckless and

Marks (1966). They used mean teacher ratings of the "goodness" of compositions written by deaf children in response to a picture series as the criterion variable to establish a multiple regression equation. This equation used the objective predictor measures of *composition length, type–token ratio,* and a *grammatical correctness ratio* (based upon the number of correctly used words in the first 50 words produced by the child). Despite some reservations as to the objectivity of the *grammatical correctness ratio,* this would appear to be a useful "summary index" of deaf children's written language developmental level, although, as the authors pointed out, the large standard errors of estimate at various ages make it useful only for studying large groups of subjects. Norms of written language development were produced for children between the ages of 10 and 18 years.

Flexibility. It has been claimed that deaf individuals have a relatively rigid style and use many stereotyped repetitions in their written language. This claim was supported by Myklebust (1964), who found that deaf children use a much greater percentage of "Carrier Phrases" (*I see a* ___, *There is a* ___, etc.) than do hearing children of the same age, although this finding could be partially due to Myklebust's use of only one stimulus picture containing a number of different objects. This inflexibility of language was also reflected in Simmons' (1962) finding of much lower *type–token ratio* (TTR) in the written language of deaf than of hearing children. The TTR is the ratio of the number of different words to the total number of words in a language corpus, and is considered to be a measure of vocabulary diversity. In an extensive longitudinal study of deaf pupils in Benelux and United States schools, Tervoort (1967) found that the TTR increased with age, indicating increasingly flexible use of language. Categories which contributed most to this improvement were nouns and function words, with verbs, adverbs, and adjectives contributing less to his deaf subjects' increasing verbal sophistication. Simmons also found that deaf children in her sample all tended to use the same phrases. She cites the example of *They had an idea* used in 50 of 52 essays she examined. Her subjects also had a tendency to use adjectives only in predicate positions (*I see a car. The car is red*), whereas hearing children used them both as predicates and as modifiers (*I see a red car*). It has been argued (van Uden, 1977; Tervoort, 1967) that this stereotyped use of a limited number of phrases is due more to the effects of formal "constructivist" teaching methods than to any effect of deafness per se on language acquisition.

Distribution of parts of speech. Both traditional classifications of parts of speech (Myklebust, 1964) and Fries' (1952) structuralist based word classes (Simmons, 1962) have been used in this type of analysis. Both Simmons (Fries' classes) and Myklebust (traditional categories) found systematic differences in this area between deaf and hearing children. In general, (using traditional terminology) deaf children use more determiners, nouns, and verbs than hearing children and fewer adverbs, auxiliaries, and conjunctions.

Kinds of errors. Two studies representative of much work in this area are those of Perry (1968) and Myklebust (1964). Both authors presented pictures to samples of deaf children and asked them to write compositions about the pictures. Both analyzed the errors made in these compositions under roughly the same rubric. They reported that deaf children made errors of *addition* (of unnecessary words), *omission* (of words needed to make the sentence correct in standard English), *substitution* (of wrong words), and *order* (with word order of their sentences departing from that of standard English). The great impact of severe deafness on language development is demonstrated by the consistency of the findings between the two researchers. Myklebust in the United States and Perry in Australia each found that the most frequent errors made by deaf children were those of omission, followed by substitution, addition, and order errors. Neither author provided a detailed analysis of the kinds of errors in the various categories, or the implications of these errors for syntactic structure.

In summary, there is substantial support for Cooper and Rosenstein's (1966) conclusion that

> [D]eaf children have been found to be markedly retarded in their achievement test scores. Their written language, compared to that of hearing children, was found to contain shorter and simpler sentences, to display a somewhat different distribution of the parts of speech, to appear more rigid and more stereotyped and to exhibit numerous errors or departures from standard English use. (p. 66)

Free generative grammar studies

The 1960s saw the beginning of a new series of analyses that was more concerned with intrasentence and intraclause phenomena and with explicating the *rules* that children use to produce sentences at various developmental levels. The notion of the "generativity" of sentence processing is central to these new developments. The idea of language being "generative" refers to the fact that there is a limited number of highly abstract mechanisms used (at a subconscious level) for the processing (comprehension and production) of a theoretically infinite number of sentences. These abstract mechanisms are often described in terms of "rules" for sentence processing (production or interpretation).

Both the old and the new approaches are found in the transitional work of Hunt (1965), whose research has already been discussed in the preceding section. Hunt was concerned not only with providing a more valid "traditional" measure of language maturity (his T-unit), but was also concerned with describing intraclause phenomena such as complementation, nominalization, and so forth. He described systematic changes in these phenomena with increasing age and considered the major process at work to be one of *consolidation* of grammatical structures. Consolidation consists of the incorporation of a number of simple sentences into a complex sentence via conjunction and, more importantly, via processes such as complementation and relative clause formation, which embed one or more simple sentences within another to make a complex sentence, producing, for example, *I saw the boy who stole the car.* from *I saw the boy. The boy stole the car.*

It was noted earlier that both Taylor (1969) and Marshall and Quigley (1970) analyzed deaf children's language using the traditional aspects of Hunt's techniques. Both these studies also concerned themselves with intraclause and intra-T-unit development. They attempted to find phenomena internal to language structures that changed significantly over time in the written language of deaf children. Marshall and Quigley demonstrated that some intraclause phenomena increase in frequency of use most from 10 to 14 years of age (genitives, personal pronouns), others after 14 years (present participles, linking verbs, adjective clauses), while still others showed steady increase over the entire age range from 10 to 18 years of age (gerunds, past participles, infinitives), or fluctuated erratically (auxiliaries).

Along with the traditional quantitative analysis reported previously, Taylor (1969) pioneered a kind of analysis new for deaf children's written language, a transformational–generative analysis. One way of looking at the components of grammar for expository convenience is to divide them into four types (Russell, Quigley, & Power, 1976); phrase structure rules, the lexicon, morphological rules, and transformational rules.

Phrase structure rules operate to rewrite symbols to produce the deep structure of sentences; for most nontechnical purposes, the product of these rules can be seen as having the structure of one or other of the "simple" or "kernel" sentences of English. These rules are violated in such sentences as *Ran the girl home* (an *order* violation), *The boy to the park* (an *omission* violation), and *The boy ran to home* (a *redundancy* violation).

The lexicon is the speaker's subconscious listing of words and their characteristics—for practical purposes, roughly equivalent to a *dictionary.* The lexicon also includes components specifying *selectional restrictions,* that is, rules which specify which classes of words can co-occur with others and thus bar the creation of sentences like *The rock sang an aria;* and *categorical rules* which specify the functions of words in sentences and which categories of words may co-occur in certain sentence environments (rules violated, for instance, in such sentences as, *The boy said a sad,* where an adjective is used in noun phrase position) or which specify whether certain nouns must be preceded by a determiner (violated in *The man bought car*).

Morphological rules deal mainly with inflections and derivations of nouns, verbs, and adverbs. Inflectional rules (those which concern the addition of endings to words, especially verbs, to express grammatical relationships) are violated in a case like *The boy ranned home;* derivational rules (rules which typically change a word of one class to a word of another class, as adjectives to adverbs) are violated in, *John is a happily boy.*

Transformational rules manipulate (move, delete, or insert) the products of the phrase structure rules into surface structures which are the heard or seen expression of sentences. On the surface these may be either simple sentences or more complex ones constructed by conjoining two sentences or embedding one or more sentences inside another.

These four categories will be used in this review of previous research which has used transformational generative grammar theory as a model. Much of the research discussed in this section is from Taylor (1969). In this major study, Taylor had 35 deaf children at each of four grade levels write compositions in response to their viewing of an 8-minute movie on Aesop's fable of "The Ant and the Dove." Taylor presents an analysis of the errors her subjects produced, but there is a significant shift of emphasis in her work from previous work. She does not just catalog the frequency of occurrence of omissions and other errors; she uses such phenomena to describe the rules violated in the production of any variant or nongrammatical structures.

Phrase structure rules.

• 1. Omissions. Taylor found four major omissions in the writing of her sample of deaf children: those of prepositions (*The ant slept the bed*), determiners, (*The ant saw grasshopper*), direct objects (*A girl threw in the water*), and verbs (particularly copulas) (*The bird away*). Determiner omissions were the most frequent at all age levels, followed by prepositions, direct objects, and verbs, in that order. However, at age 10 verbs were the second most frequent omissions. These findings were apparently confirmed by Kates (1972) who did not, however, give a detailed analysis of the types of omissions made by his subjects. By age 12 verbs had become the least frequent omissions. This led Taylor to suggest that one of the earliest standard English rules mastered by young deaf children is that the predicate of a sentence must contain a verb; that is, $S \rightarrow NP + VP$: A sentence must contain a noun phrase and a verb phrase.

The frequency of occurrence of all omissions decreased with age, indicating that deaf students gain increasing mastery over this aspect of sentence production. One exception to this trend was omission of direct objects; the number of such omissions dropped between ages 10 and 14, but increased considerably again between ages 14 and 16. Taylor was able to provide an interesting analysis of these fluctuations in terms of the environments in which direct object omissions occurred.

• 2. Redundancy. Taylor found that the major type of redundancy in her data occurred with prepositions, in such forms as *The ant walked to home* and *He thanked to the dove.* The frequency of occurrence of such phenomena declined little over the age range she studied. In comparing the occurrence of omissions and redundant use of prepositions, Taylor was able to discern a pattern of development which has been held to be typical of language acquisition in younger hearing children (e.g., Cazden, 1968; Slobin, 1966): (a) the failure to apply a rule until it is learned, (b) the gradual acquisition of the rule and its increasingly correct use, (c) the subsequent "overgeneralization" of that rule to environments where it should not be applied, and (d) predominantly correct use. This finding was confirmed by Quigley, Wilbur, Power, Montanelli, and Steinkamp (1976) who showed also that it can be detected in other types of redundancies in more complex language structures of older children.

• 3. Order. Taylor found order problems to be relatively infrequent in her sample. Such as there were occurred mainly at about age 10. She felt that the order of English syntax might have been mastered by most deaf children before this, the earliest age represented in her sample. It seems more likely, however, that this conclusion is an artifact of collecting written samples in response to external stimuli. Results from other studies (e.g., Quigley, Wilbur, Power, Montanelli, & Steinkamp, 1976) indicate that order problems are quite frequent in deaf children's language competence, as exemplified in their performance with controlled testing on questions and passive sentences. Taylor's findings probably apply only to simple active declarative sentences.

The lexicon.

• 1. The dictionary. "Dictionary studies" of the language of deaf children have been largely confined to investigations of scores on vocabulary subtests of standardized achievement tests. Taylor made an interesting beginning to a somewhat different approach to deaf children's knowledge of vocabulary. Following her analysis of *selectional restriction* errors, she notes that her subjects made many other word choices that were impossible to classify.

> Some appeared to result from incompatible semantic features, some from incompatibility between the word chosen and the events that transpired in the stimulus film, and some from the students' unfamiliarity with English idioms. (p. 126)

• 2. Selectional restrictions. Very little information is available concerning deaf children's violations of selectional restrictions. Taylor found her data in this area very difficult to interpret. Errors that could confidently be attributed to violation of selectional restrictions were very infrequent. The only two categories that appeared to be clear were "combinations of determiners and nouns which were mutually incompatible with respect to the feature ($\pm$ count) e.g., *a water* and *the few grass,* or with respect to the feature ($\pm$ plural), e.g., *a scissors* and *a pliers*" (p. 124). (Notice that for some speakers of standard English the last two examples are grammatical because of reanalysis of the nouns as singular.) No discernible improvement in deaf children's performance in this area could be detected within the 10- to 16-year age range investigated by Taylor.

• 3. Categorial rules. Deaf children in Taylor's sample made few substitutions of one major category of English for another, but they did not noticeably improve their performance in this area across the age range she studied. Taylor felt that sentences containing such phenomena were not grossly variant, and could be readily interpreted by readers. She ventured the tentative hypothesis that variant structures such as *Mother table the food* are akin to such functional shift use of nouns as verbs in such expressions as *table the motion.*

Kates (1972) reported a study where deaf students were required to write a sentence in response to a stimulus word given to them (a total of 32 words was provided). He found the same as Taylor: "few subjects. . . made unaccep-table functional shifts, that used one part of a speech to perform the func-tion of another" (p. 45).

Morphological rules. Taylor found significant improvement with age in deaf children's ability to use correctly those kinds of morphological rules that she investigated. Most of the difficulties occurred in verb inflections, followed by singular–plural inflections and possessive inflections, in that order.

Verb inflection difficulties followed typical patterns found in much younger hearing children (Cazden, 1968). The most frequent were omission of inflec-tional endings, for example, *So she fly and get a leaf,* followed by overgeneraliza-tion of the correct form, as *The dove was scared and flied away,* or incorrect application of the correct rule as in *The circle broked.* The least frequent of verb morphological variances occurred as incorrect tense marking in sentences like *Dove saw ant can't swim* (where standard English would use *couldn't*).

Most singular–plural variances occurred in redundant use of the plural mor-pheme as in *The sheeps went to sleep,* followed by omission of the plural morpheme, *Six boy went to the party,* and use of such confused forms as *The leave was on the tree.* Taylor also found some confusion in her deaf subjects in the use of the possessive morpheme, that is, *'s* and *s'*.

Transformational rules. Taylor examined deaf children's use of three ma-jor types of transformational rules in her study. Compared with some other categories there were relatively few transformational variances; but Taylor con-sidered that this was not because deaf children performed well in this area, *but because they, in fact, rarely attempted to use complex transformations.* The students did not show a significant decline in the number of nonstan-dard transformational structures they produced with age, but Taylor felt that they showed some increased mastery of transformational rules, because while the number of variances did not decrease, the number of transformations at-tempted did increase significantly with age. Taylor examined three major transformational rules.

• 1. Conjunction. Attempts to join two or more sentences together using conjunctions (most commonly *and*) were the transformation most frequently found in Taylor's data. She found deaf children had two major problems in this area. The coordinating conjunction was often *omitted,* as in sentences like *A ant see a tree a bird and Ant walk found animals;* or *misplaced,* as in *The dove got out of the tree and took a leaf threw it down.* Many children placed a conjunction between every sentence conjunct, as in *The ant ran to its home and get the scissors and hit a man's leg.*

The other major problem deaf children had was in knowing what deletions were permissible in conjoined sentences. Taylor felt that many children operated thus: If the subject of a sentence is identical to any noun phrase in the preceding sentence, then that subject may be deleted and its predicate conjoined to the predicate of the preceding sentence (p. 104). This inferred rule was used to explain such sentences as, *The tool hurt the hunter and yelled* and *The hunter scared the dove and flew away.* This phenomenon was also extensively found by Quigley, Wilbur, Power, Montanelli, and Steinkamp (1976) and is reported as *object–subject deletion.* Quigley, Wilbur, Power, Montanelli, and Steinkamp also found evidence for what is called *object–object deletion,* where the object of the second conjunct of a conjoined sentence is deleted on identity with the object in the first sentence. Taylor also found this to be fairly common in her data, in such sentences as *The ant threw a ball on the ground and put in his room.* A further phenomenon reported by Quigley, Wilbur, Power, Montanelli, and Steinkamp as tense sequencing also occurred in Taylor's data. It was particularly common for deaf writers to mark tense only on the first verb of two conjoined sentences, thus producing things like *The ant went off and ride the dragonfly.*

• 2. Nominalization. Taylor found that her deaf subjects had great difficulty in this area—particularly in the correct use of nouns formed from verbs: gerunds (swimming) and infinitives (to swim). Confusion as to the correct use of these categories produced such errors as *The ant like to played with insects, The man began screamed,* and so forth. Other students seemed confused as to the correct environment for gerunds and infinitives, as in *He cannot know how to swimming* and *The hunter missed to shoot the dove.* The verb *see* also caused particular problems for deaf writers in such sentences as *The ant saw him what he was doing.*

Taylor summarized her findings on nominalization by saying that it would appear from her data that many deaf students never fully acquire the nominalization rules of English, that they have great difficulty in acquiring even some of them and that, if any are acquired, they are acquired quite late in the language development process. This was confirmed by the experience of Quigley, Wilbur, Power, Montanelli, and Steinkamp who found that it was not possible to include several tests of verb nominalizations in their final test battery, because pilot testing indicated that even most of the oldest pupils were completely unable to score on them.

• 3. Relative clauses. Few problems were observed in this area, *again largely because Taylor's deaf subjects rarely attempted the use of relative clause structures.* When they did, however, they almost invariably produced nonstandard English structures.

Three variant structure types were prevalent in relative clauses. One was the nonuse of the relative pronoun where it is obligatory in standard English, as in sentences like *The ant held the thing look like circle.* Other examples of errors given by Taylor appear to be instances of the *copying* phenomenon found by Quigley, Wilbur, Power, Montanelli, and Steinkamp. It occurs in such sentences as *There was a little hole underground which a smart ant lived in it.* The deep structure of this is: There was a little *hole* [$_S$ a smart ant lived in the hole $_S$] *underground,* where the bracketed sentence is embedded in the main sentence. In the standard English rule for forming relative clauses, *the hole* in the embedded sentence is replaced by *which,* which then moves to the front of the embedded sentence. In *copying,* however, *which* is simply inserted at the beginning of the embedded sentence and *the hole,* rather than being deleted, is pronominalized to *it.* Some deaf children also produced such structures as *the hunter man,* perhaps an analogy to *the old man.*

It can be seen from Taylor's research that deaf children's written productions, even at the age of 16 years, still vary considerably from standard English usage. In general, it can be said that at 16 they have achieved mastery over many aspects of the production of simple active declarative sentences. That is, they only infrequently make errors of substituting major categories incorrectly, as in *The boy played a happy;* rarely do they disturb the standard subject–verb–object order of the simple sentence; and very rarely do they violate selectional restrictions, as in *The rock sang a song.* However, even at this advanced age, they still have many problems with the morphology of English, particularly as regards verb and noun inflections. They still also have many problems in handling the determiner and auxiliary systems of English—indeed they have more problems in these areas than in any others. They make relatively few mistakes in producing complex transformations, but this is only because they rarely attempt such difficult productions. It would seem from Taylor's analysis that most 16-year-old deaf children know little about the relativization and nominalization rules of English, and that when they attempt usages of such structures, they produce many variant structures. They are, at this age, beginning to attain correct use of conjunction rules, but, even so, still produce many conjoined sentences that are not standard English. Although Taylor used the traditional terminology in speaking of examining the "errors" made by her subjects, it is clear from her analysis that these deaf children were not just making "errors" in producing English sentences, but were producing "correct" (for them) sentences from rules which, however, were not those of standard English.

The extensive studies of Quigley and a group of associates have been listed and discussed in chapter 4 on reading, and Table 2 and 3 provide concise summations of some of the major findings of those studies. Those and such studies as O'Neill (1973), Power and Quigley (1973), and Schmitt (1969) can be viewed as studies of comprehension (reading) of syntax as well as its production (writing). It was chosen to discuss the Quigley, Wilbur, Power, Montanelli, and Steinkamp (1976) studies in the reading chapter. Some aspects of those studies, however, are of interest also in the context of written language.

Besides examining the comprehension of specific syntactic structures by the use of specific tasks, Quigley, Wilbur, Power, Montanelli, and Steinkamp obtained written language samples from their stratified random national sample of more than 400 deaf students between the ages of 10 and 19 years. As reported in the various publications, only limited instances of the structures studied by the tests were found in the freely produced written samples. Brief summaries illustrate the findings.

The students' order of difficulty with respect to relative pronoun type and relative clause position as demonstrated by the Test of Syntactic Abilities (TSA) were confirmed by the analysis of the written language samples. Subject relative clauses outnumbered object relatives 5 to 1, with subject relatives comprising 84% of the total and object relatives only 16%. Nine percent of the deaf students produced one or more subject relatives, while those in object position were used by only 2% of the students. Similarly, approximately twice as many final relatives (68% of the total) were produced as were medial relatives (32%); 11% of the deaf sample used at least one final relative, while medial relatives were used by only 6%.

In the written language sample, conjoined sentences were the most frequent form of conjoined structure produced by deaf students: Thirty-one percent of all conjunctions were conjoined sentences; at age 10 they were produced by only 10% of the students, while at 18 they were produced by 84% of the students. Conjoined verb phrases accounted for 25% of the occurrences of conjoined structures, and were produced by 17% of the 10-year-old deaf students and 68% of the 18-year-old deaf students, generally at least two per student. Conjoined structures with *but* occurred only 119 times in the 472 writing samples, compared to 2,431 uses of *and*. At age 10, only 4% of the students used *but* in a conjoined structure at least once; the percentage increased gradually to 31% at age 17 and at 18 the figure was 22%. Conjunctions with *or* (i.e., alternation) occurred even less frequently, with just 36 uses. Two percent of the deaf students at age 10 (1 student) used such a structure and 10% (5 students) at age 18.

Analysis of the deaf students' written language samples revealed a general increase of complement usage over age. No subject complements were produced by any of the deaf students, although at least one object complement was used by 22% of the deaf students at age 10, increasing to 92% of the deaf students at age 18. *For–to* complements were used most frequently, followed by *that* complements, with only a few POSS–*ing* complements. Nearly all of the complements occurred with active verbs, fewer than 1% occurred with perception verbs, and none occurred with stative verbs. Fewer than 10% of the infinitive complements were incorrectly inflected.

Analysis of errors in the written compositions provided supplementary data on the students' actual use of the proper pronoun forms in their own writing. There were almost no instances of inappropriate case usage in the written samples. The absence of large numbers of such mistakes adds support to the finding of comparatively good performance of the deaf students on the pronominalization tests of the TSA. Number mistakes were even less frequent, with no mistakes at all at ages 10, 11, or 12, and a high of only .2% at age 14. In comparison, person mistakes (The family went on a picnic. They packed *our* lunch, rather than they packed *their* lunch) were more frequent, occurring approximately 5% of the time. This percentage of errors indicates uncertainty on the part of the deaf students as to the appropriate reference of the different person pronouns.

Both Wh-questions and yes/no questions were produced in the writing of only about 3% of the deaf students. This might have been partially a result of the task type: that of writing a *description* of a picture. For Wh-questions,

14 students produced just 20 uses; at least one Wh-question was used at each age except 17, while only the 18-year-olds produced more than this—6 uses by 4 students out of 50. Only one tag question occurred in the entire writing sample, produced by a deaf 16-year-old. Wh-questions, subject Wh-words, and object Wh-words were used equally frequently by the deaf students. *Subject–auxiliary inversion* was applied 47 times by just 14 students (3%); one 12-year-old applied it 20 times and one 18-year-old 10 times.

On the whole, the students appeared to have negative placement fairly well mastered in their productions, with correctly formed negatives accounting for 93% of the total; 101 students produced 182 correctly positioned negatives at all ages from 10 to 18, with only 3% of the students (13) producing just 14 sentences with the negative incorrectly placed. Ten percent of the deaf students (48 students) correctly contracted *not* to *n't,* with many of them doing so more than once. All instances of incorrect negative placement involved negatives placed within the sentence; no deaf students produced *Neg-S* or *S-Neg* structures. Also, there were no occurrences of *amn't* or *willn't,* despite the use of such forms as found in earlier studies.

The relative order of difficulty for the verb structures was seen to be the same in the production data of the written language sample as for the grammaticality judgments of the TSA. That is, present progressives were easiest followed by perfectives and then passives, the least used of the three. Progressive tense was very common in the writing of the deaf students, with 407 instances produced by 148 of the 469 students (32%). Usage increased with age, with 4 deaf students producing progressives at age 10, and 22 (out of 50) using them at age 18. Perfectives were seldom used, with only 25 occurrences; they were produced by only 22 deaf students, 5% of the total. One student at age 10, six at 17, and three at 18 each produced one perfective. Passive sentences were even less common, with only 11 uses of *be* passives by 10 deaf students (2% of the total). Five deaf students (8%) each used one *got* passive. Neither type of passive appeared at all before age 14. Auxiliaries were incorrectly deleted just 43 times by 30 deaf students (6%).

Controlled response studies

Controlled generative grammar studies

Despite the valuable insights that free generative grammar studies of corpuses have provided, there are major problems with this approach. The basic problem is that neither *natural* (informally recorded) corpuses nor ones elicited by pictures or other stimuli may call forth all that a child knows and can use of language. Several examples of this problem are available from the corpus of written productions of deaf children studied by Quigley, Wilbur, Power, Montanelli, and Steinkamp which have just been discussed. These writings were elicited in response to a series of picture sequences and not one example of a reflexive pronoun was found in a corpus of several hundred samples. It is thus not clear whether deaf children really cannot use reflexive pronouns or whether they simply were not elicited by this particular stimulus. Similarly, personal pronouns, although they occurred in those corpuses, appeared in insufficient numbers to allow adequate interpretation of their pattern of development. It has also been noted that Taylor found very few sentence *order* problems in her corpus, perhaps mainly because her stimulus was such that it called forth virtually no questions from her subjects—questions being an environment in which Quigley, Wilbur, Power, Montanelli, and Steinkamp found many instances of *order* problems. Further, some constructions in the language of deaf children are so variant that it is very difficult to disambiguate what the child "really meant" with the result that any analysis is necessarily subjective. Taylor found this to be the case in trying to decide upon the type of variance found in many of her categories.

For these reasons, and because careful manipulation of stimulus and response requirements can give clearer insight into the dynamics of language acquisition, production, and comprehension, many investigators have used controlled manipulation of linguistic variables. There is now a substantial body of research with deaf persons which is based on transformational generative grammar theory and which used controlled presentation of stimuli. For convenience, these studies are surveyed using the same framework as that adopted for the free generative grammar inspired research.

Phrase structure rules.

• 1. Omission. In her study of deaf children's understanding of the correct use of *phrase structure rules,* O'Neill (1973) developed a Test of Receptive Language Competence in which subjects were required to judge whether simple sentences generated by correct and incorrect rules were "right" or "wrong." In the *omission* section, her subjects (aged 9 to 17 years) made correct judgments on 75% (versus 84% for the hearing children) of the items and showed significant improvement with age. As in all her categories (the others were *order, redundancy*, and *selectional restrictions*), her deaf subjects did about as well as the hearing on correctly selecting "right" sentences as "right," but they had a tendency to call "wrong" sentences "right" much more often than did the hearing children. O'Neill found that her deaf subjects were much more likely to accept incorrect sentences where function words such as determiners, prepositions, and verb particles had been omitted than sentences where nouns, verbs, and adjectives (content words) had been incorrectly omitted. This finding is in close agreement with that of Taylor (1969) for free written production.

• 2. Redundancy. This category proved to be slightly more difficult than *omission* for O'Neill's deaf subjects (73% correct overall, versus 85% for the hearing subjects). A similar pattern of results to that for omissions was found, with sentences containing redundant determiners, prepositions, and verb particles being more difficult to judge than those containing redundant content words. It was also noted that her deaf subjects tended to accept sentences which contained a redundant verb (i.e., sentences like, *The children went walked to the park*).

• 3. Order. This category proved to be the easiest for O'Neill's subjects (90% correct, versus 86% correct for the hearing subjects). O'Neill comments "Only two grammatically incorrect sentences in the Order category were judged 'right' by these deaf subjects, which indicates that syntactic order, at least in these sentences, was not a great problem for the deaf subjects" (p. 92).

O'Neill's youngest subjects were 9 years of age with a reading age of at least the second grade. Using a test in which deaf children were required to move toys to indicate the meaning of simple sentences, Power and Quigley (1973) found that many deaf children did not have a good grasp of the implications of word order for the meaning of English simple sentences. Many of the deaf subjects appeared to idiosyncratically allocate subject or object positions to toys. For example, when given a sentence and asked to act out the sentence with toys a sentence like *The car pushed the tractor*, the same child sometimes had the car push the tractor, and at other times had the tractor push the car. Power and Quigley also reported that nonreversibility in such sentences as *The horse kicked the box*, helped the deaf subjects to correctly interpret sentences from the earliest ages on. The indication was that deaf children pass through a *semantic* or *presyntactic* stage where interpretation of sentences is based upon momentary (and perhaps idiosyncratic) relationships between content words, with no appreciation of the role of function words or word order for sentence interpretation. This is in striking confirmation of the findings of Schmitt (1969) whose study will be discussed in more detail later.

The lexicon.

• 1. Selectional restrictions. O'Neill (1973) had a subtest dealing with this area which proved to be the most difficult subtest for both deaf and hearing subjects (82% correct for the hearing, 69% correct for the deaf). She found that her subjects accepted as correct a wide range of sentences violating selectional restrictions on nouns and pronouns including the features ± animate, ± count, ± masculine, ± human, ± common, and ± concrete. For example, *The desk serenaded Matilda* is a violation of the restriction on animateness; *Milk are good for you* is a violation of the *count* restriction. Violations of preposition–noun and verb–preposition relations also occurred. There was little improvement in her deaf subjects' performance in this area with age.

• 2. Morphological rules. A major study of deaf children's morphological rules has been reported by Cooper (1967). As he noted, generalizability of his results could be in doubt, as his subjects were drawn from only one school, but Cooper's results can perhaps be taken as an approximate indicator of deaf children's performance in this area. Cooper used Berko's (1958) technique of nonsense pictures ("This is a wug. Here is another wug. Now there are two _____") and nonsense words in sentences ("Mary knows how to zugg. She zuggs every day. She knows a lot about _____ . Choose one of zuggy, zugged, zuggness, zugging"). Both receptive and productive knowledge of the forms were tested.

In general, Cooper's deaf subjects performed poorly on the test. They averaged overall only 25.3 points out of a possible 48, and even the oldest children (19 years of age) averaged only 29.2 points. Some improvement in scores with age was noted. Receptive knowledge of the forms was superior to productive in all cases.

Cooper found deaf children's knowledge of inflectional morphemes (endings which when added to a base morpheme express certain grammatical relationships; e.g., verb and noun singular/plural markings; the progressive aspect marker; the superlative marker for adjectives; the possessive marker) to be superior to their knowledge of derivational markers (endings which form a new word, usually of a different grammatical class, from an existing one—the *-ly* adverb ending; *-able* adjective ending; *-ness* and *-ing* noun endings). This is consistent with the difficulty deaf children have with derived nominals of various types. Cooper's data generally confirm and extend those found by Taylor (1969) in her free data-gathering situation.

Transformational rules. Taylor (1969) noted deaf children's problems with three major syntactic structures—conjunction, nominalization, and relativization. The extensive controlled studies by Quigley, Wilbur, Power, Montanelli, and Steinkamp (1976) of these and other structures will be reported later. A few other studies of specific structures are available.

- 1. Negation. As part of a broader study, Schmitt (1969) administered comprehension and production tasks involving the selection of one of four pictures to correctly match a given sentence. He found that his 8-, 11-, 14-, and 17-year-old deaf subjects performed quite well on this task, the pattern of results indicating that most of these deaf children understood the meaning implications of the negative marker *not* in English sentences. The one exception to this was a number of his youngest (8-year-old) subjects who failed consistently enough on this task for Schmitt to hypothesize that they were operating with what he called the *no negative rule*, "which specifies the ignoring of the marker 'not' and the treatment of negative sentences as equivalent to affirmative sentences" (p. 124). It might be that such a response is even more typical of the performance of deaf children younger than those Schmitt tested.

- 2. Passive voice. In English the meaning of a simple active sentence is provided by the subject–verb–object word order. However, the set of morphemes identifying the passive voice, the auxiliary *was*, the past participle of the verb (usually marked by the *-ed* ending—*pushed*), and the agent phrase introduced by the preposition *by*, indicate that the order of action is reversed to object–verb–subject. That is, a sentence like *The boy was pushed by the girl* means that the girl pushed the boy. Passive sentences are said to be *reversible* (If interchanging the subject and object results in a grammatical, meaningful sentence, for example, *The boy was pushed by the girl*), or *nonreversible* (*The car was washed by the boy*—compare *The boy was washed by the car*). Frequently, the agent *by*-phrase is deleted because the agent of the action is unknown or obvious (*The man was killed*).

It has been demonstrated that understanding of reversed word order occurs relatively late in hearing children, and might not be fully mastered until 8 or 9 years of age. Until this time some hearing children interpret passive sentences as if they were active. That is, for them *The boy was pushed by the girl* means that it is the boy who did the pushing.

It would seem that many deaf children persist in this incorrect interpretation of passive sentences until an advanced age. In the study noted previously, Schmitt (1969) had deaf children aged from 8 to 17 years old select the one of four pictures which correctly illustrated the action of reversible passive sentences. He also had his subjects "fill-the-gap" in sentences to produce passive sentences to correctly describe pictures. He found that few of the deaf children below age 14 could pass his tests, and that even at 17 years of age, many children still could not comprehend the meaning of passive sentences or produce them correctly.

Schmitt's work was extended by Power and Quigley (1973) who used three tasks to investigate the acquisition of the passive voice by a sample of prelingually deaf children. In their *comprehension* task children were required to move toys to show the action of the passive sentence. Three types of passive sentences were used—full reversible, full nonreversible, and agent deleted (which can be reversible or nonreversible). With the agent-deleted sentences a forced choice of one of two pictures which represented the action of the sentence was used instead of the toy movement task. The *production* task was the same as Schmitt's.

Power and Quigley concluded that even at age 17–18 years a majority of deaf children have a defective rule for the processing of passive sentences, namely "passive reversal of subject–object order to process meaning of such sentences is signaled only by *by*; tense markers are free to vary" (p. 76). It would seem that many deaf children are very strongly constrained to interpret all sentences in terms of the standard subject–verb–object order of the English simple sentence, even at an advanced age.

Some studies (Ewoldt, 1981; McGill-Franzen & Gormley, 1980) have disputed the findings of these controlled response investigations of deaf students' comprehension of specific syntactic structures. Those studies, in turn, have been challenged by other investigations (Israelite, 1981; Robbins & Hatcher, 1981). The arguments and counterarguments have been presented in chapter 4 on reading.

Generative grammar studies have shown that deaf students make little progress in school in acquiring control of even the "simplest" aspects of standard English rules of grammar. They do achieve some success in mastering the structure of simple sentences, as reflected in the use of *phrase structure rules* and the proper placement of certain constituents in the sentence, but they still tend to overuse certain categories of sentence constituents, even at an advanced age. Even at the age for leaving school, many deaf students have problems with correctly using English selectional restrictions. Correct use of morphological rules also prove difficult, even for many older deaf children.

It seems that many deaf students acquire good control of only the simplest English transformations (negation; conjunction using *and*). Complex embedding and sentence-reducing transformations of English do not often appear in their written productions, and when they do appear, deaf students make many errors in their use.

Quigley et al. (1978) provided data on the universality of syntax problems with deaf individuals and the similarities of those problems in other populations. Figure 2 shows data for deaf students from the United States, Canada, and Australia; normally hearing students from the United States; and hearing college students from various countries who were learning English as a second language. The similarities in the profiles of all of the groups are striking, indicating that the order of difficulty for the syntactic structures studied were almost identical for all of the samples. Nor was the degree of difficulty greatest for the deaf students. It can be seen in Figure 2 that the ESL students had greater difficulty with all of the structures than did most of the deaf students. It would appear from this that the syntactic problems of deaf individuals are not unique; they are shared by many other populations.

King (1981), as cited in Quigley and King (1982), has also shown that the distinctive structures found in the comprehension and production of language by deaf students are not unique to deaf individuals. Table 3 shows distinctive structures for deaf students as reported by Quigley, Wilbur, Power, Montanelli, and Steinkamp (1976). Also shown are studies which reported the same distinctive structures for other populations. Almost every distinctive structure found in the language comprehension and productions of the deaf individuals was found in other populations. The data in Figure 2 and Table 3 indicate that the syntactic problems of deaf individuals are not unique. It can be speculated from this that the research and practice in ESL and other populations can perhaps be utilized in the teaching of deaf children as discussed in chapter 6.

Discourse analysis

As stated earlier, language research with hearing individuals has moved from sentence and intrasentence (word, phrase, clause) analysis to intersentence analysis, and from interest in language mechanics to language composition. Black (1982) and Freedle and Fine (1982) provide good summaries of the work in this area with hearing populations. As Freedle and Fine point out, discourse theory is in its infancy and many of the problems being studied (such as structures at different levels of a text) are at the very first stage of a science—the categorization phase. Work in this area has been heavily influenced by schema theory as discussed in chapter 4 on reading.

The published work in discourse analysis with deaf individuals is as yet very limited, but it will undoubtedly grow rapidly during the next decade and provide additional information on, and insights into, the language processes and problems of deaf persons. Wilbur (1977) reported on data from the Quigley,

Figure 2. Comparison of Mean Scores on the *TSA DIAGNOSTIC BATTERY* for Five Groups of Students

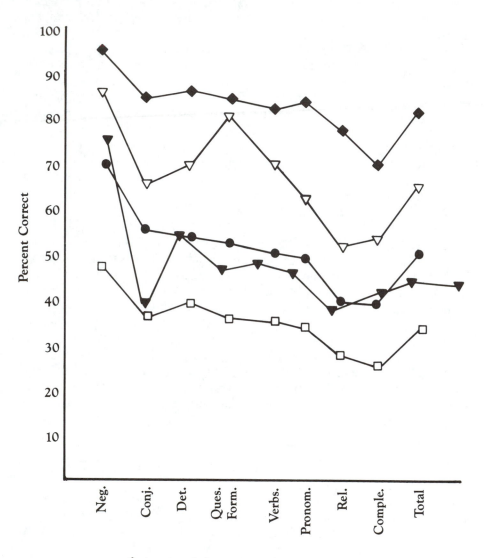

◆ American College Level Deaf Students

▽ American Normal Hearing Students (C.A. 8 - 13 Years)

● American Deaf Students (C.A. 10 - 18 Years)

□ Australian Deaf Students (C.A. 10 - 15 Years)

▼ College Level Hearing ESL Students

Wilbur, Montanelli, and Steinkamp (1976) studies to show how the appropriate use of articles, pronouns, and verb tense is related to understanding how sentences are related in a text. Wilbur argued from her data that deaf students' comprehension and usage of various structures could only be understood by analysis beyond the sentence level. McGill-Franzen and Gormley (1980) and Ewoldt (1981) have presented additional evidence of the importance of inter-sentence considerations and analysis. Most of this type of analysis to date with deaf children has been concerned with reading rather than written language and is discussed in chapter 4. Also, discourse analysis of written samples as proposed by Kretschmer and Kretschmer (1978) is discussed in chapter 7 on assessment and instruction.

SUMMARY AND CONCLUSIONS

Each time there is a shift in the understanding or perception of language which results in some new theoretical linguistic formulation, reexamination and reanalysis of the language, particularly the written language, of deaf children usually occurs. This is not, as it might seem, continual reinvention of the wheel. The changing theories (traditional grammar, structuralist grammar, transformational generative grammar, generative semantics, case theory, discourse theory) provide new ways of examining and analyzing the language of deaf children which often increase knowledge and understanding and provide new insights into the language processes and problems of deaf children. It is reasonable to state that there is a considerably larger body of knowledge and better documented understanding of those processes and problems now than there was 50 years ago. It is not reasonable to state, though, that this has led to greater mastery of the English language by deaf students. The record does not support such a claim.

Thompson's (1936) extensive analysis of 16,000 language samples from 800 deaf children provided detailed information on the numbers and types of "errors" (variances) in the written language of deaf students that is still current. Thompson also indicated the controversy between natural and analytic methods in language development by stating that it appeared necessary for teachers to spend more time and effort on the right use of words rather than on the treatment of structural grammar, because the written expression of deaf children is more likely to be mechanically correct than it is to have the words correctly used. This concern of teachers with vocabulary usage was also documented for the present time by Hasenstab and McKenzie (1981). The unfortunate tendency to think in *either–or* terms in relation to language approaches (natural and analytic) and communication forms (OE, MCE, ASL) is reflected in Thompson's statement. As stated in the Preface and in the concluding chapter of this book, each language approach and each communication form probably has a place in the education of deaf children; and the eclecticism of teachers and clinicians usually embraces elements of various approaches. This was documented by the recent survey of King (1983).

Thompson's (1936) large study was reinforced by another large one by Heider and Heider (1940) of 1,118 compositions written by 817 hearing students and 301 deaf students. These two studies provide for students and practicing teachers and clinicians a wealth of information on the written language of deaf children analyzed within the framework of traditional grammar. These extensive early studies in the traditional mold are supported by the more recent traditional analyses of Myklebust (1964), Perry (1968), and Stuckless and Marks (1966). The Stuckless and Marks (1966) study goes beyond the reporting of types and numbers of variances and provides a useful summary index of the quality of written compositions in terms of an equation involving measures of composition length, type–token ratio, and a grammatical correctness ratio.

Marshall and Quigley (1970) and Simmons (1962) are examples of structuralist and structuralist/generative oriented studies which formed a transition between traditional and transformational generative analysis of language. They provide information on variances in the written language of deaf children in terms of form classes (Fries, 1952) and clause and sentence combining transformations (Hunt, 1965). These were followed by the extensive transformational analyses of Taylor (1969) in free response and Quigley, Wilbur, Power, Montanelli, and Steinkamp (1976) in controlled response studies. These studies provide extensive information on the problems of deaf students with the syntactic structure of English. Other studies have tended to support the findings of Taylor and of Quigley, Wilbur, Power, Montanelli, and Steinkamp (e.g., Ivimey & Lachterman, 1980; Powers & Wilgus, 1983).

Major studies have not yet been reported with deaf children within the framework of discourse theory, but they probably will be during the present decade. Specific studies by Ewoldt (1981), McGill-Franzen and Gormley (1980), and Wilbur (1977) are based more on data on reading than on written language but they indicate the form of things to come. These investigators have reported essentially that the whole is greater than the sum of its parts; that is, at least some of the problems that deaf children have with various parts of language do not hinder their understanding of the whole, such as a whole text in reading. That might be true, to an extent. But in any area of knowledge, complete understanding of the whole usually requires full understanding of its parts. And it is difficult to accept that the massive problems that deaf children have with the various aspects of standard English (vocabulary, syntax, figurative language, etc.) as documented throughout this book have little consequence for the deaf child and that detailed knowledge of them has little value for teacher and clinician.

It was possible in the chapter on reading to show that data collected over the past 60 years (from Pintner & Patterson, 1910, to Trybus & Karchmer, 1977), revealed no significant advances for deaf children in general on scores on reading tests. The lack of standard assessment techniques makes the same longitudinal comparisons more difficult for written language. But examination of language samples in studies from Thompson (1936) to Quigley, Wilbur, Power, Montanelli, and Steinkamp (1976) and examination of the quantitative data reported in those studies indicate that there has been no general improvement in written language either, in spite of the much greater knowledge and understanding now available on the matter. This is discouraging considering the great increase in resources that have been devoted to the education of deaf children in recent times. Some possible reasons for the lack of progress and some implications are presented in the concluding chapter.

The linguistic theories of the past 20 years, particularly of structuralist and transformational generative grammar, have led to applications in the teaching and development of language with deaf students. The *Apple Tree Program* (Anderson et al., 1980), based on structuralist grammar, enjoys widespread use in educational programs. *Sentences and other Systems* (Blackwell et al., 1978) is based on transformational generative grammar and is also used in a number of programs. The *TSA Syntax Program* (Quigley & Power, 1979) was constructed as a structured and remedial teaching companion to the TSA (Test of Syntactic Abilities) and based on the research of Quigley, Wilbur, Power, Montanelli, and Steinkamp (1976). It is too soon to tell if these various techniques and materials will significantly affect the reading and written language (both of which, of course, are reflections of the internalized language) of deaf students.

chapter 6

Bilingualism and English as a second language

In recent years, investigators have suggested that English be considered a second language for deaf children and that the techniques and research in bilingualism and second-language learning be explored for possible means of providing improved language and educational development for deaf children (Cicourel & Boese, 1972a, 1972b; Hatfield, Caccamise, & Siple, 1978; King, 1981; Luetke, 1976; Stokoe, 1972). It has been proposed that deaf children be exposed to ASL and English concurrently in infancy and early childhood (bilingualism) or that ASL be developed first in a normal interactive manner and English developed later (second-language learning). Even a brief survey of the literature on bilingualism and English as a second language (ESL) reveals, however, that the field has as many and as deep differences in theory and practice as does the education of deaf children. In order to discuss the bilingualism and ESL approaches to educating deaf children, it is necessary to examine some of the theory and practice of these approaches with minority-culture hearing children and to understand some of the problems in the field.

DEFINITIONS

The first issue that must be confronted is that there is disagreement about what constitutes bilingualism and second-language learning. Bilingualism implies the use of two languages; however, this seemingly simple notion has produced a great deal of confusion in the theoretical and research literature. McLaughlin (1978) argues that the presence of two languages before the age of 2 years leads to simultaneous acquisition (bilingualism), whereas acquisition is successive (second-language learning) if the presence of a second language is delayed until the age of 3 years or later. Another perspective on the distinction between bilingualism and second-language learning has been offered by Lamendella (1977) who argues for adoption of the following terminology: *primary language acquisition, secondary language acquisition,* and *foreign language learning.* Lamendella refers to primary language acquisition as the normal language learning process occurring up to the age of about 5 years regardless of the number of languages involved and the manner in which they are introduced to the child. Secondary language acquisition, which can also involve learning two or more languages simultaneously or successively, is considered to occur in a naturalistic setting and manner after the period of primary language acquisition (after about 5 years of age). Foreign language learning, according to Lamendella, occurs in the formal classroom setting and is cognitively different from secondary language acquisition. In considering Lamendella's definitions, it should be remembered that the time period of primary language acquisition (the first 5 years or so of life) is not universally accepted. This issue, known as the critical period hypothesis, is still being debated (Krashen, 1973; Selinger, 1978).

A question that needs to be considered in the problem of defining bilingualism is whether a particular code or symbol system is, in fact, a language. The defining criteria for identifying a distinct language are not unequivocal. Some German universities, for example, have separate departments for the English (British) and American languages (Ferguson, 1977). Norwegians do not agree whether they have two languages or one (Haugen, 1956). This is an issue in considering the language of deaf children. Some researchers (Crystal & Craig, 1978; Namir & Schlesinger, 1978) question whether ASL is a bona fide language or a secondary signal system like a Morse code. Others cite evidence that it is a rule governed language (Lane & Grosjean, 1980; Siple, 1978; Stokoe, 1960, 1972; Wilbur, 1979).

This issue of the status of ASL as a language is complicated by the existence of systems of manually coded English. These systems are the ones most commonly used at present in the education of deaf children. The situation is further complicated by the fact that, besides two languages, ASL and English, these are two modes of communication, oral and manual. English can be coded either orally or manually, so bilingualism for deaf children can consist of exposure to ASL and manually coded English, ASL and oral English, or ASL, manually coded English, and oral English. Exposure to oral English and manually coded English would not constitute bilingualism but simply two coding forms of a single language—English.

It is likely that most modern proponents of bilingualism for deaf children support the use of ASL exclusively during the first few years of life until it is firmly established as the primary language and that English then be taught as a second language. There is still the question of whether this will be manually coded or oral English or both. Given the considerable technical requirements of developing speech and speech reading in deaf children, this is a difficult question to resolve. Also, as Marmor and Pettito (1979) and Reich and Bick (1977) have shown, oral and manually coded English might be incompatible to at least some extent.

Another issue related to the problem of defining bilingualism and to determining how to approach bilingual and secondary language teaching is the relation between bilingualism and biculturalism. The possession of two stylistic or dialectical variations of English (or sign language, see Tervoort, 1978) is not necessarily associated with cultural variation. In many cases, however, possession of two languages might reflect interaction and knowledge of distinct cultures, and thus many of the effects commonly associated with bilingualism might actually reflect concomitant biculturalism (Baker & Cokely, 1980; Lane & Grosjean, 1980; Wilbur, 1979). Many ESL programs for hearing students tend to ignore the cultural factor (biculturalism) and to concentrate on the language factor (bilingualism).

THEORETICAL MODELS

In addition to variation in definitions of bilingualism and second-language learning, there is a diversity of theoretical models in the literature: the balance theory, the interdependence theory, the additive/subtractive model, the societal factor model, the threshold model, the developmental interdependence model, and others. These models and theories reflect different interpretations of the data in the research literature, some of which are presented in a following section.

The balance theory (Macnamara, 1966), sometimes termed the genetic inferiority or verbal deprivation theory, suggests that a person has a fixed amount of language learning ability which must either be divided among two or more languages or devoted entirely to one. Balance theorists claim that most people are unable to learn two languages simultaneously as well as monoglots (monolinguals) learn one by itself. They point to a large body of data which demonstrates inferior performance of bilinguals in one language (usually, the majority or dominant language of society), suggesting that the other language interferes with the learning process. This deficiency in the majority language is claimed to be reflected in lowered performance in all academic areas.

An opposing model, the interdependence theory, is espoused by Lambert (1975) and Lambert and Tucker (1972). These theorists argue that, under certain learning conditions, access to two languages can positively influence the development of some cognitive processes which can consequently lead to higher IQ and academic achievement. These theorists also argue that in order for these positive effects to be detected by research studies, certain confounding factors must be controlled; for example, socioeconomic status, gender of subjects, and degree of bilinguality. Even when these factors are controlled, however, the evidence in the research literature is still contradictory. There is substantial support for the balance theory and for the interdependence model. Consequently, a number of recent theoretical models have been proposed to explain the contradictions.

The additive/subtractive theory has been proposed by Lambert (1975) as a corollary to his interdependence model. Lambert attributes the contradictory research findings in the literature to differences between bilinguals in an additive environment and those in a subtractive environment. According to this theorist, an additive educational or social environment is one which poses no threat of replacing the first (L_1) or home language of the speaker with a second (L_2) or majority language of the culture. Contrariwise, a subtractive environment aims to supplant the minority, home, or first (L_1) language with the majority one. Lambert further argues that bilinguals in an additive environment usually possess a first language which may be the dominant or majority language of the culture. These students (usually from middle or upper SES classes) become balanced bilinguals when they add another language (either a majority or minority one) and consequently perform at least as well as matched monolingual speakers of either of the two languages involved. On the contrary, the inferior skills of many of the bilingual subjects reported in other studies were probably due to the fact that these subjects were in a subtractive environment, which posed a threat to the first language. In addition, some of the contradictory research findings might be due to studies failing to (1) control for the bilingual subjects' level of competence in either L_1 or L_2, and (2) acknowledge that subjects might have had less than nativelike skill in both their languages (due to the fact that they came from low SES environmental background).

A somewhat similar model to the additive/subtractive one is the societal factor theory. Like the additive/subtractive theory, proponents of this model argue that a home–school language switch results in high levels of functional bilingualism and academic achievement in majority language children but leads to inadequate command of both languages and poor academic achievement in many minority language children. These theorists (e.g., Bowen, 1977; Cohen, 1976; Paulston, 1976; Tucker, 1977) have argued for an emphasis on the determining role of societal factors. Bowen (1977) remarks that the choice of medium of instruction should be determined by social conditions and not by a preconceived notion that the mother tongue (home language) should *per se* be used. Tucker (1977) similarly maintains that social rather than pedagogical factors will probably condition the optimal sequencing of language (i.e., which one should be used initially). Cohen (1976) has delineated a variety of social and attitudinal factors (e.g., community support for the school program, relative prestige of the languages involved, teacher expectations and attitudes) which provide explanations for the differential success of some programs (e.g., immersion programs) over others (e.g., submersion programs). In essence, the societal factor theory rejects axiomatic statements regarding the medium of instruction and assigns a fundamental causal role to societal or sociocultural factors.

Another theory presented as an explanation for the contradictory findings in the research literature is termed the threshold theory (Cummins, 1977, 1978). Cummins, the major proponent of this theory, argues that the cognitive and academic effects of bilingualism are mediated by the levels of competence attained in both languages regardless of whether the subjects possess a majority or minority language as a first language. This theorist further argues that there might be threshold levels of linguistic competence which a bilingual child must attain (i.e., in the two languages) both in order to avoid cognitive disadvantages and to allow the potentially beneficial aspects of bilingualism to influence cognitive functioning. The threshold model assumes that those aspects of bilingualism which might positively influence cognitive growth are unlikely to come into effect until the child has attained a certain minimum or threshold level of competence in the second language.

Another model, termed the developmental interdependence model, proposes that the development of skills in a second language is a function of skills already established in the first language (Skutnable-Kangas & Toukoman, cited in Cummins, 1978). In situations where the first language is inadequately developed, the introduction and promotion of a second language can impede the continued development of the first. This inadequate development of the first, consequently, will limit the development of competence in the second language. Contrariwise, a highly developed L_1 (prior to the introduction of L_2) will contribute to a high level of development in L_2 at no cost to L_1 competence. The developmental interdependence model emphasizes the importance of the continuing development of the first language.

The last theories to be discussed are those concerned specifically with the development of language and reading in the second-language learner. One of these, the vernacular advantage theory, asserts that the best medium for teaching a child in a bilingual situation is in the mother language or first language (Modiano, 1968; Rosier & Farella, 1976). In actuality, this theory is only intended for children whose first language is a minority language. Proponents of this theory argue that instruction through the medium of the first language or mother tongue for minority language children in the early grades is a prerequisite for equality of educational opportunity. Furthermore, when instruction is through the medium of a second or majority language and the school makes no concessions to either the language or the culture of the minority language child, the result is frequently low levels of competence in both languages and academic failure. In addition, it is argued that reading should be introduced in the learner's first language (the native language approach). In this approach, the sequential language skills of listening, speaking, reading, and writing are taught in the language (i.e., the mother language) for which the child has already acquired the sound system, structure, and vocabulary. Subsequently, when the student achieves an independent reading level in the first language, this student can then begin to read in the second language. It is further argued that the acquisition of reading skills in the first language leads to an efficient transfer of skills, and thus, faster acquisition of second-language reading (Gamez, 1979).

There are various studies, however, which seem to suggest that the direct approach to reading is the most efficient; that is, reading should be introduced initially in the second language. Most of this evidence seems to be from students whose first language or home language is the majority language or one that is as equally prestigious as the second language. This issue of the most efficient way to transfer skills from one language to another in reading is at present an area of intense research (Chun, 1980; Clarke, 1979). In addition, it has brought the debate on the theories of reading (i.e., top-down, bottom-up, and interactive) into the realm of research on reading in the second language. A question now is whether there are universal reading skills across all languages or whether readers must learn a new set of skills uniquely attributed to a specific language.

RESEARCH APPROACHES

The research on the various theories and programs of bilingualism and ESL is voluminous. Only two areas are discussed briefly here as bearing most directly on the ASL/ESL issue with deaf children: (1) research on cognitive and intellectual functioning, and (2) research on the effectiveness of various educational programs.

Cognitive and intellectual functioning

There are marked similarities between the research on the cognitive and intellectual development of minority culture hearing children involved in bilingualism and second-language learning and research conducted with deaf children as presented in chapter 2. In general, research perspectives in both areas usually have been influenced by the current thinking on the relationship between language and thought (cognition), and the subsequent thinking concerning the nature and appropriateness of tests of intelligence and cognitive abilities.

Studies prior to the 1960s inferred the nature of the cognitive abilities of hearing bilinguals from the findings of selected tests of intelligence. Saer (1923), for example, interpreted the inferior performances of bilinguals on a verbal intelligence test as indicative of the bilinguals' state of mental confusion resulting from the interference of one language with the other. In general, these early studies interpreted the inferior performance on selected tests of intelligence as a function of inferior cognitive processes. The nature of the intelligence tests and the conflicting findings in the literature have led to a reinterpretation of the earlier studies, however. It was noted, for example, that some of the studies reported equal or superior results for bilinguals when compared to matched monolinguals on the *nonverbal sections* of intelligence tests. As a consequence, debate ensued on the relationship between the two types of tests of intelligence; that is, verbal and nonverbal or performance. It has been argued that nonverbal or performance intelligence tests are more suitable instruments for assessing the basic intellectual ability of bilinguals (Cordasco, 1978). The reason for this is that it is assumed that nonverbal and performance tests of intelligence have little dependence on language. Such tests, therefore, offer bilinguals the opportunity to use one language or the other, or both, or no language at all. Similar arguments have been made in the literature on deaf children (Quigley & Kretschmer, 1982). Quigley and Kretschmer warn, however, that not all nonverbal tests are in fact nonverbal; some mediation in a linguistic system might be occurring.

Most of these earlier studies seemed to support the balance theory (Macnamara, 1966) which predicts inferior performance of bilinguals when compared to monolinguals in all academic areas; however, in addition to the verbal/nonverbal tests issue, certain flaws in the designs put the results in question. In Saer (1923) and Morgan (1957), for example, two distinct flaws existed: (1) lack of control for the SES factor, and (2) biased tests resulting from the lack of standardization on the minority groups tested. This lack of control for SES and test standardization exists in most of the studies which reported detrimental effects of bilingualism (Jones, 1960; Jones & Stewart, 1951; Lewis, 1959; Macnamara, 1966). More recent analysis of the early studies has suggested that the general trend warrants the conclusion that bilinguals are handicapped on verbal tests (i.e., linguistically) but not on performance tests. Results of recent studies seem to support this contention, (Bowd, 1974; Cummins, 1978) especially when such factors as SES, gender, level of competence, and standardization of the tests are either controlled or accounted for.

More recently, researchers have directed their attention to studying performance on specific cognitive abilities of bilinguals. Most of these studies have reported favorable effects of bilingualism on selected tasks of concept formation and analogical thinking. It has been inferred from the favorable results that bilingualism leads to greater awareness of the arbitrary nature of the word–referent relationship, greater cognitive flexibility, and precocious cognitive development (Ben-Zeev, 1977; Cummins, 1978; Feldman & Shen, 1971; Ianco-Worrall, 1972). These results, when coupled with those reported by Peal and Lambert (1962), seem to provide support for the interdependence theory.

Contradictory evidence has been presented which neither the balance nor the interdependence theories can adequately explain. A few of the more recent theories (e.g., additive/subtractive, societal factor, threshold, and the developmental interdependence) attempt to account for the contradictory evidence by placing more importance on sociocultural factors; namely, attitudes toward the languages involved, type of education program, SES, and quality of input from the environment. Two theories, in particular, deal with the interactions between linguistic factors (e.g., level of competence) and sociocultural factors (e.g., quality of input from the environment); the threshold and the developmental interdependence theories. The threshold theory (Cummins, 1977) suggests that adequate initial development of L_1 is indispensible to development of L_2; the developmental interdependence theory asserts that the continued development of L_1 is instrumental for the development of a high level of L_2 skills. Both of these theories also assert the importance of sociocultural factors in the development of either language.

Program models

In addition to having a variety of theoretical models, the fields of bilingualism and second-language learning have a number of program models. Bilingual education programs can be established for majority language students and for minority language students, and the goals of the two types of programs can be quite different (Cohen & Swain, 1976; Genesee, 1979; Swain, 1981). Bilingual programs for majority language students in the United States are a recent and limited occurrence (Hornby, 1980), whereas such programs are extensive and of long standing in other countries, notably Canada (Swain, 1981). Bilingual programs for majority language students could increase substantially in the United States in future years, but the programs of direct interest here, analogically, are the programs for minority language students.

In order to counter the high prevalence of academic failure among minority language students, educators in the United States and elsewhere have instituted various types of bilingual programs for these students. Controversies which have arisen about the appropriate goals and procedures for these programs are strikingly similar to some of the controversies in the education of deaf children. For example, there is disagreement as to whether the goal should be to make the minority language student a fully participating member of the majority culture even at the expense of the student's minority culture (assimilation) or to preserve and maintain the student's native culture even if this means lessened participation in the majority culture (language and cultural separatism). The various types of programs are related to the goals and vary from complete submersion in the general educational system with limited or no support in the student's native language and culture to separate education in the student's native language and culture and gradual submersion in the general educational system. These controversies over goals and procedures are similar to those surrounding whether deaf children should be educated to function largely in the general society and whether ASL or English should be the initial and primary language of instruction.

Bilingual education programs for minority language students can be divided into three general types: submersion, transitional, and maintenance models. The maintenance models can be further subdivided into static and developmental maintenance programs. In submersion programs the student is plunged into the regular education classes with no or limited special assistance (this is comparable to some mainstreaming programs for deaf children). In transitional programs (Cummins, 1977; Otheguy & Otto, 1980), the child's minority language (L_1) is typically employed in the initial stages only (first few elementary grades) to allow the efficient assimilation of curriculum content while the majority language (L_2) is being learned. The L_1 is not seen as functional in the child's academic or cognitive development and no attempt is made to promote or maintain competence in that language. The only major difference between transitional and submersion modes (termed the sink-or-swim model) is that in the transitional model temporary concessions are made to the child's home language and culture. In general, both models employ similar curricula, but ESL instruction is present in the transitional program whereas it might or might not be present in submersion type programs. Instruction in ESL typically includes about an hour daily of lessons in the grammar of English. In submersion or regular education programs, the minority language student might be exposed to similar English instruction as other students or might be placed in *special classes* (Title I, remedial English classes) or in ESL type classes (still considered remedial). The submersion and transitional models have also been termed the *assimilational models* (Hornby, 1980).

Similar to the transitional model is one type of maintenance model, termed static maintenance (Otheguy & Otto, 1980). Static maintenance refers to the process of preventing the loss of minority language students' L_1 skills while promoting proficiency and literacy in L_2. In both static maintenance and transition programs, reading is typically introduced in the L_2 mode. Proponents of these models typically endorse the balance theory of bilingualism. Four basic arguments are presented: (1) Instruction in or on L_1 subtracts from instruction for developing L_2 skills; (2) development of L_1 competes with L_2; (3) minority language students already possess competency in their L_1, thus, it is not necessary to teach L_1; and (4) reading skills are best developed in L_2 by employing the language of L_2 not L_1. In general, these proponents argue that the best way to teach English to limited English speakers is simply to teach them English (Troike, 1981).

Another model is the developmental maintenance program (Otheguy & Otto, 1980). The major aim of developmental maintenance programs is to develop a high level of competence in both languages. These have also been named the *integration models* (Hornby, 1980). They can refer to programs involving total or partial immersion in a second language or to programs in which the two languages are employed more or less equally (50/50) for instructional purposes (Cathcart, 1982). Total or partial immersion programs are typically established for either majority language students or students in a culture where two languages (or more) are equal in status; whereas programs in which two languages are employed in an equal or nearly equal pedagogical manner are typically established for minority language students. One of the languages in these programs is typically the dominant language of the general society. In general, proponents of the 50/50 programs endorse the vernacular advantage theory whereas total immersion programs endorse the direct approach; that is, teaching the content areas and reading initially in the second language. It has been suggested that positive effects of bilingualism for minority language students are more likely to appear in bilingual developmental maintenance models resulting from the formal instruction of both languages in these programs (Eddy, 1978).

Program effectiveness

A review of the literature suggests that positive effects of bilingualism for minority language students are most likely to appear in bilingual developmental maintenance models (Eddy, 1978). Success for majority language students can occur in either total or partial immersion programs with higher levels of fluency in the second language occurring only in total immersion programs (Edwards, Fu, McCarrey, & Doutriaux, 1981; Swain, 1981). In addition, it has been claimed that current ESL models are not producing favorable results for minority language students due to the employment of behaviorist theories of language acquisition (Legarreta, 1979).

One of the most comprehensive studies providing direct evidence of the effects of different program models on the language development of minority language students is that of Legarreta (1979). This study is discussed at length here to exemplify various program models and their educational effects. Legarreta examined the effects of five different programs on both acquisition and maintenance of English by monolingual, native Spanish-speaking kindergarten children.

Program 1:   The Traditional Method (submersion)—a regular curriculum was followed and only English was employed in the classroom.

Program 2:   The Traditional Method plus an ESL component—same as the first group with daily, sequenced lessons in English structure and use.

Program 3:   The Bilingual Method—each language (Spanish and English) was employed equally throughout the day. Staff was bilingual and the classroom environment was bicultural.

Program 4:   The Bilingual Method—the curriculum content and concepts were presented totally in Spanish for half a day and in English the other half. Staff was bilingual and the classroom environment was bicultural.

Program 5:   The Bilingual Method—same as group 3 plus an ESL component as in Group 2. Staff was bilingual and the classroom environment was bicultural.

Legarreta remarked that two programs (2 and 5) exemplified the behaviorist theory of language acquisition due to the use of formal audio lingual ESL training. The audio-lingual method is employed in the teaching of foreign language to adults and is the direct precursor of the ESL model currently in use (Hornby, 1980; McLaughlin, 1982). In this method, the students are trained to imitate language drills or dialogues exactly and to repeat them until memorized. In addition, they practice patterns in phonology and syntax based on a contrastive analysis of the target language and their home language (see the discussion in Hakuta & Cancino, 1977). Language acquisition in this pedagogical method is seen as simply a set of learned verbal habits in the conditioned response paradigm of behaviorist psychology.

Programs 3 and 4 exemplify a generative view of language acquisition. In these programs, the child is allowed to abstract rules concerning the structure of the language (either the first or second) based on a natural input in a variety of contexts. This generative approach, based on a transformational view of language structure, has as yet no clearly defined pedagogy or curriculum model (Hakuta & Cancino, 1977). Specifically, Legarreta attempted to isolate the effects of formal audio-lingual ESL training on Spanish-speaking children in traditional and bilingual classrooms. The identification of the optimal program model for facilitating English acquisition by Spanish-speaking children, while maintaining their home language, was also expected. It should be noted that analyses revealed that instructional time of each language was 50/50 in Program 4 and 28/72 in Program 3.

Subjects were 52 five-year-old kindergarten children identified as monolingual Spanish-speaking from 17 kindergarten classrooms. Subjects were equated on cognitive abilities and Spanish dominance. A battery of four measures was administered to each child in the pre- and posttesting sessions. Essentially, these were (1) measures of English and Spanish oral comprehension; (2) tests of vocabulary in Spanish and English in different settings (e.g., home or school); (3) a story-retelling task for oral production in Spanish and English; and (4) a communication competence task.

Data analyses consisted of comparing subjects' gain scores on each of the language measures in each of the five groups. Results indicated that the bilingual groups (3,4,5) produced significantly greater gains in English oral comprehension than the traditional groups (1,2). Group 3, however, produced the largest gain in English oral comprehension and communication competence in Spanish and English. In addition, those programs without the ESL component (1,3,4) produced significantly higher gains in Spanish vocabulary. The results appear to suggest that bilingual program models with a 50/50 utilization of each language produce the most benefits. Finally, Legaretta argued that the results demonstrate that the employment of formal audiolingual ESL training, exemplifying a behaviorist view of second-language acquisition, is useful only in enhancing basic English comprehension skills; whereas, communicative competence, which requires more complex skills, is best achieved in models without ESL instruction.

ASL and ESL FOR DEAF CHILDREN

Not all deaf children in the United States are exposed to English as a first language. Some are exposed to ASL, others to various forms of manually coded

English or pidgin sign English, and still others to various spoken languages which are the native languages of their hearing parents. Deaf children of deaf parents in many but not all, instances (see Brasel & Quigley, 1977; Corson, 1973) are probably exposed first to some form of ASL or pidgin sign English. It should be noted that these children are not necessarily exposed to a homogeneous language. Several investigators have discussed ASL as a diglossia (Stokoe, 1972) and as a continuum (Woodward, 1973; Baker & Cokley, 1980), both of which allow for a wide range of sophistication in ASL usage. Increased recognition of the critical importance of infancy and early childhood in language development, and the increasing popularity of manually coded English systems in the education of deaf children under the rubric of total communication, have led some hearing parents to learn and use those systems with their preschool deaf children. Just how many parents have done this and what systems they use are not known, but a number of investigations have reported on this situation (Babb, 1979). Given the intricacies of these systems, it is possible that in practice they become forms of pidgin sign English rather than strict manually coded English (Marmor & Pettito, 1979; Reich & Bick, 1977). Finally, some deaf children in the United States have hearing parents whose native spoken languages are not English. The largest group here is probably Hispanics. Luetke (1976) has estimated that there are between 3,000 and 5,000 deaf children with Spanish surnames. It has also been estimated that approximately 60% of these children come from homes in which Spanish is the only language used.

It is not possible in this chapter to discuss all of these potential bilingual or ESL situations and various combinations of them (e.g., English, Spanish, ASL). The main matter of interest is the increasing contention that ASL should be the first language developed with all deaf children and that English (or some other spoken language where appropriate) be developed later as a second language. This will be explored in some detail. However, a section is devoted to the situation of deaf children from Spanish-speaking homes because of the substantial and increasing number of these children and because a few studies have recently examined this population.

OE, MCE, and ASL as linguistic input

It seems reasonable to assume that the intelligibility, quality, and fluency of language input to a child, hearing or deaf, in infancy and early childhood are important factors in language acquisition. And the various language inputs used with young deaf children (oral English, manually coded English, and ASL) can be compared on these factors. It has been pointed out repeatedly that oral English presents the deaf child with only a partial representation of the language. Only about 50% of speech sounds are visible on the lips (Jeffers & Barley, 1971) and the children defined in chapter 1 of this book as deaf will receive only limited, and probably distorted, auditory input even with good amplification. The combination of visual and amplified auditory input has been shown repeatedly to provide greater information than either alone (Jeffers & Barley, 1971), but the result still falls far short of the intelligibility and fluency of auditory input to the hearing child. It would seem, therefore, that oral English for deaf children provides the least intelligible and least fluent of the three major systems. It should be born in mind, however, that this is "armchair theorizing." The study by Ogden (1979) has shown that, in spite of these "logical" deficiencies of the system, when practiced in its best form it can educate at least some deaf children to be socially and occupationally very successful in the general society. This affirms the need for greater educational experimentation to test the various "logically" supported communication and language systems proposed for use with deaf children.

A number of attempts have been made to supplement oral English input with manual cues to make the input more visually intelligible and fluent. The best known system in the United States and a number of other countries at present is cued speech (Cornett, 1967). This system was in widespread use in the United States during the 1960s, diminished in use during the 1970s, and is having a minor resurgence during the 1980s. As with other systems, the waxing and waning seems to be due to lack of a data base and experimental studies to support the "logical" arguments for the effectiveness of the system. Experimentation with the system is warranted to determine if the addition of manual cues can make oral English a visually intelligible, fluent, and easily learnable linguistic input for deaf children.

Manually coded English systems have been developed on the grounds that they provide deaf children with visually intelligible and fluent forms of linguistic input and that they conform to the syntactic (including morphologic) structure of English. The major systems in use are SEE I, SEE II, and pidgin sign English, although there are few data on the extent of use of each system and the faithfulness with which each is used. Some studies have indicated that SEE I and SEE II are cumbersome to use exactly and often evolve in (and on) the hands of practitioners into forms of pidgin sign English, although usually without the elements of ASL structure often found in true pidgin sign English (Marmor & Pettito, 1979; Reich & Bick, 1977). These various systems, though, do provide visually intelligible communication through signs which also are easily made manually in comparison to the fine and intricate motor movements required in speech. Thus, reception and expression seem "logically" to be easier, more intelligible, and more fluent for deaf children than oral English.

ASL can claim the same advantages as manually coded English systems on the factors of visual intelligibility, fluency, and ease of motor production. It differs significantly, however, in the claims that it is a language in its own right, separate and distinct in structure as well as form from English and all other spoken languages. It is probably fair to agree, at this stage of knowledge, that the claim has been reasonably substantiated by linguistic research as well as by ASL's persistence as the language of choice of many deaf adults (Moores, 1978; Quigley & Kretschmer, 1982). Only when ASL is involved concurrently with English, or is used to precede English, with deaf children can a true bilingual or ESL situation be claimed to exist. It is these situations that are the focus of attention here. Oral English and manually coded English systems are attempts to establish English in either oral/aural or manual forms as the *first* language of deaf children, although MCE can be used as an ESL system.

ASL as language

The pioneering work of Stokoe (1960, 1972) provided the modern basis for consideration of ASL as a genuine language with a systematic cherology of sign cheremes (analogous to the phonology and phonemes of spoken languages) and a syntactic structure different from the structures of spoken languages. His work has been expanded by other linguistic investigations. Cicourel and Boese (1972a, 1972b) state that native signers (usually deaf children of ASL-using deaf parents) are capable of doing with signs just what speaker–hearers are capable of doing with speech; namely, to develop signs related to objects and events in the environment; but in contrast to oral language, the signs begin as simulated iconic representations and then become more abstract with use. They also argue that deaf persons are able to monitor their own signs and the signs of others as well as facial expressions, body movements, and various subtleties of signs. These subtle sign movements and body and facial movements are analogous to the intonational and other suprasegmental aspects of speech. Extensive reviews of the linguistic and psycholinguistic studies of ASL are provided by Lane and Grosjean (1980) and Wilbur (1979).

Not only do many investigators argue for the use of ASL as the first language for deaf children, some also argue against the use of manually coded English systems (Baker & Cokely, 1980; Kluwin, 1981). They argue that the signed codes are visual–gestural in nature and English is aural/oral in nature and that signs cannot adequately represent an aural/oral language. There is some support for their contention in the research of Lichtenstein (1983) and others which indicates that the syntax of English is heavily dependent on possession of a speech code. As discussed in chapter 2, ASL syntax might have developed in conformity to the requirements of visual coding. In contrast, it can be pointed out that deaf people have evolved and used a manual English system of signs, a form of pidgin sign English, to communicate with people who have vocabularies of signs but do not know ASL syntax.

Earlier, it was pointed out that adequate acquisition of a second language by hearing children presupposes mastery, or at least reasonable control, of a first language. With deaf children acquiring English as a second language, a similar situation exists: ASL must have been acquired in early childhood by a natural interactive process. But this is true only for a small number of deaf children—usually, deaf children of deaf parents, and not even for all of them. Some deaf parents use only oral English with their deaf children (Corson, 1973), and some use a form of pidgin sign English, or manual English (Brasel & Quigley, 1977). It is likely, however, that most deaf children of deaf parents are exposed to some form of ASL as a first language in infancy and early childhood. A question of importance is, what form? Hearing children with English-speaking hearing parents are exposed to a wide range of English input, depending on socioeconomic and educational levels of families and other factors. The same factors apply to deaf children of deaf parents, but the almost universally depressed educational and language levels of deaf adults means their deaf children are probably exposed to a wider range of ASL input, with only a small percentage at the upper end of the range. This situation has led Stokoe (1972) to describe the situation as a diglossia.

The term diglossia was proposed by Ferguson (1959) for those situations in which two or more varieties of a language are used differentially within a single geographic region. Stokoe (1972) adopted the term to delineate two varieties of signing; a *high (H)* and a *low (L)* variety. According to Ferguson's usage (1959): (1) *H* contains grammatical categories not present in *L*; (2) *H* has an inflected system of nouns and verbs which is much reduced or totally absent in *L*; and (3) the bulk of the vocabulary of *H* and *L* is shared. In effect, the two forms differ much more in their grammar than in their vocabularies. Stokoe (1972) contended that this was similar to the situation for signing with high and low varieties existing in the deaf population.

Since the appearance of Stokoe's (1972) article, other investigators have attempted to create a concept of a sign language continuum linking the *H* and *L* varieties (Baker & Cokely, 1980; Woodward, 1973), rather than a diglossia. This continuum represents a scale of all the varieties of ASL and English produced by deaf and hearing signers. The continuum places ASL at one extreme and English at the other. The intermediate varieties (either signed and spoken simultaneously, or signed only) have been termed pidgin sign English (PSE). PSE is said to use varying degrees of the grammatical structures of both English and ASL and the position of any form of PSE on the continuum is determined by the relative proportion of grammatical structures from each language.

This continuum concept appears to offer an efficient means of categorizing the variety of communications used by signers. Lee (1982), however, argues that there should be two PSE continua: a PSE_d produced by deaf signers and a PSE_h produced by hearing signers. PSE_d is likely to have more ASL grammatical structures and to omit English inflections. PSE_h tends to have greater English influence and rarely approaches the ASL extreme of the continuum. It is argued further that these two continua do not intersect, but are distinct. For example, a PSE_h signer might decide to use the ASL sign (actually, the English gloss for the ASL concept) for FINISH in order to communicate the English sentence, *I want to finish my work*. The English phrase, *to finish my work,* means to continue until the work is finished. Two examples of PSE_h signing of this sentence are these:

1. I WANT FINISH MY WORK.
2. I WANT TO FINISH MY WORK.

In ASL, the sign/concept *finish* means any of the following: (1) a past tense marker, (2) a conjunction, or (3) a completed act (Baker & Cokely, 1980; Humphries, Padden, & O'Rourke, 1980). A PSE_d signer might interpret Statement 1 to mean, *I wanted my work*. Statement 2 is much more complex; however, given the meanings of the sign *finish* in ASL, this sentence too could be misinterpreted by a PSE_d signer.

Lee (1982) discusses several other points which seem to support the notion of a diglossic situation (two languages) with signers rather than diglossia (two varieties of the same language). First, L signing is invariably acquired by children in a natural interactive manner similar to the way hearing children acquire a spoken language, whereas H signing is usually learned in a formal educational setting. Most deaf signers, however, do not acquire L (or ASL) in infancy or early childhood (Woodward, 1978, 1980; Woodward & Markowicz, 1975). Some deaf children of deaf parents acquire it early in the same manner as hearing children acquiring a spoken language, but most deaf children acquire ASL (or L) from their peers at school and some acquire it only after entering special colleges for deaf students. These deaf signers often achieve near native competence in ASL, but they are not true native signers. Lee (1982) also argues that some deaf signers have competence in H (either spoken and/or signed) but no competence in L (strictly only signed), and some are competent in L but not H. He claims these deaf signers are really members of different linguistic communities. In sum, according to Lee, Stokoe (1972) and others could have been describing a bilingual community using ASL and some form of PSE in a diglossic situation.

It can be seen from this brief survey that there is considerable disagreement and some confusion about the exact form and status of ASL as a language. This is not surprising, however. Formal study of ASL is very recent in origin and limited in extent. Although a considerable number of books on ASL have been published during the past decade, they have drawn on a very small data base, usually studies of only a few language samples from only a few informants. This likely will be corrected in time as more and larger studies are conducted and the resulting data help to settle disagreements of interpretation and clarify confusions.

At present, investigations seem to support several conclusions pertinent to the purposes of this chapter. First, ASL has the characteristics of a genuine language; that is, it has its own cherology (phonology), syntax, and semantic network, all of which might be influenced by other languages but nonetheless are distinct from them. Second, there is either a continuum of signing from ASL to English with a variety of PSE forms in between or a dichotomy or diglossic situation of two languages, ASL and manually coded English. A corollary of this is that there might be two continua of PSE, one common to deaf signers PSE_d and one to hearing signers PSE_h. Third, there is a wide range of competence among deaf and among hearing signers in their use of ASL. All of these points are relevant to the issue of ASL/ESL with deaf students. Some relevant research also exists on the development of ASL in young deaf children and on the use of ASL as an educational tool.

Research studies of ASL/ESL

Retrospective Studies

There are very few studies dealing with the English linguistic abilities of deaf children who were supposedly exposed to ASL in infancy and early childhood. Most of these are studies of deaf children of deaf parents. Some of these studies were retrospective (e.g., Brasel & Quigley, 1977; Meadow, 1968) and used various means for determining the form of language used with the deaf subjects in infancy and early childhood. Even the best techniques, however, leave some doubt when respondents (deaf parents) are reporting on events that took place as much as 10–15 years previously. Some studies actually were conducted during the infancy and early childhood of the deaf subjects (Schlesinger & Meadow, 1972) and there is greater certainty of the language these parents were using with their children, but assurance is not complete. Interpretations of the findings of studies of deaf children of deaf parents have usually attributed the findings of superior academic performance (as compared to deaf children of hearing parents) to early use of ASL by the parents and children. It seems to be assumed that the language input was relatively homogeneous for these children. As the preceding section has shown, this is not necessarily the case. As these kinds of studies become more refined in their experimental techniques, there likely will be more detailed reporting of the child's early language environment. In the meantime, some caution must be exercised in interpreting them. In addition to the variation in signing documented previously, there is also the problem of bimodalism. Schlesinger and Meadow (1972) and Collins-Ahlgren (1974) have reported that some deaf parents simultaneously use speech and ASL signs with their deaf children. This not only involves bilingualism (ASL or PSE and spoken English) but also bimodalism (signing and speaking).

Most of the studies involving deaf children of deaf parents do not deal directly with the issues of bilingualism and ESL and have been reported elsewhere in this book. Only a few studies which seem to relate to the bilingualism/ESL issues are discussed here to illustrate the complexity of the issue.

Charrow and Fletcher (1974) investigated the possibility that deaf children learn English as a second language by comparing the performance on a test of English as a second language of two groups of deaf students (one group having deaf parents and the other having hearing parents) with each other and with a group of hearing students learning English as a second language. Three hypotheses were tested: (1) Deaf children of deaf parents should outperform deaf children of hearing parents; (2) the performance of the students learning English as a second language should resemble the performance of the DCDP group more than it resembled the performance of the DCHP group; and (3) the performance by the DCDP group on a test of English as a second language and on a standard test of English skills should resemble each other less than should performances by the DCHP group on the same tests. The two tests used were the Test of English as a Foreign Language (TOEFL) and the Stanford Achievement Test.

Results supported the first hypothesis: DCDP performed significantly better than DCHP on most of the subtests and on the total score on the TOEFL. In addition, DCDP performed significantly better than DCHP on the Paragraph Meaning and Language subtests of the SAT. Ambiguous results were reported, however, for the second and third hypotheses. With respect to the second hypothesis, it was found (as predicted) that the performances of the DCDP group resembled those of the foreign hearing students more than the DCHP group did on two of the TOEFL subtests (English Structure and Writing Ability) but on other subtests (Vocabulary and Reading Comprehension) it did not. Findings were similar for the third hypothesis. The hypothesis was supported by performances on some subtests of the SAT and not on others.

Charrow and Fletcher (1974) concluded that the issue of whether deaf children typically are learning English like a second language might be too broad to investigate. Based upon the mixed results for the second and third hypotheses, they argued that some aspects of English are learned by deaf students like a second language and some not. In the absence of logical or research support for such differences among various aspects of English, the interpretation should be treated with caution.

In another study, Charrow (1975) sought to identify, and provide normative data for, the nonstandard features of English language usage by deaf students which she labeled "Deaf English" (DE). This term implies that deaf persons might have a dialect of English which is different from standard English. Charrow argued that deaf individuals have typical patterns of variant structures in their use of English that are consistent. This was also reported in detail by Quigley, Wilbur, Power, Montanelli, and Steinkamp (1976) as discussed in chapters 4 and 5. These variances tend to become frozen or crystallized and to persist despite education and/or age. Charrow argued that these variances alternated with some standard English features to produce a simplification or pidginization of standard English. In essence, according to Charrow, the range of grammatical forms, standard English and nonstandard, appear to parallel the "pidgin continuum" found in the speech of pidgin English speakers.

Charrow (1975) studied this issue by comparing a DCDP group, a DCHP group, and a group of hearing subjects on their responses to 50 "Deaf English" (DE) sentences written by deaf teenagers and 50 standard English (SE) sentences that were judged equivalent in meaning to the DE sentences. Sentences were presented in random order to the subjects, individually, and they were required to write the sentences on an answer sheet from memory, one sentence at a time. Results were that the deaf subjects found the DE sentences easier to remember and recall than did the hearing subjects. It was also found that there was no significant difference in the deaf subjects recall of the DE and the SE sentences. Finally, there were no significant differences between the DCDP group and the DCHP group. On the basis of her findings, Charrow concluded that deaf students acquire most, if not all, the rules of standard English syntax but apply them in an inconsistent manner. She further concluded that many of the variances from standard English, such as omission of articles and past tense markers, that are found in the written language of deaf students are not results of interference from ASL but represent redundant, nonessential features of English that are difficult to learn and easy to overlook. In sum, this study and the study by Charrow and Fletcher (1974), found little evidence that deaf children are learning English as a second language. These are very indirect studies of the problem, however, and certainly do not settle the issue.

Table 3 from King (1981) as cited in Quigley and King (1982) lists a large number of consistent variant syntactic structures found in the written language of deaf students and which those students often accept as correct in testing situations. Also listed in the table are other populations in which the same structures have been found by other investigators. Most of these populations consisted of students from various first-language backgrounds who were learning English as a second language. It can be seen that almost all of the variant structures found in the written language of deaf students are found also in the English productions of populations learning English as a second language. This could be interpreted as support for the concept that English is functioning as a second language for many deaf persons; however, such interpretation should be made very cautiously. Given the rules of English, only a limited number of variations can take place, other than purely random variations, and so there are bound to be considerable overlaps in those variations among different populations.

Hatfield et al. (1978) investigated whether ASL interfered with MCE. The study had two purposes: (1) to determine if sociolinguistic data could be used to ascertain levels of ASL proficiency, and (2) to ascertain competency in ASL and MCE and examine some relations between ASL and MCE. Only the second purpose is relevant here. The subjects, 219 students at the National Technical Institute for the Deaf, were administered two videotaped stories. One story was presented in ASL and the other in MCE and subjects were tested on their understanding of the stories. It should be noted that the system of MCE used in this study was that typically used by deaf signers who have a good command of English, rather than one of the recently constructed systems such as SEE II. It involved primarily ASL signs used in English word order with certain function words (e.g., articles) and important affixes of English either signed or finger spelled. In addition, linguistic and paralinguistic features of ASL such as the use of space, directionality of sign movements, and questioning techniques were employed.

Results seemed to indicate that many of the deaf students were bilingual in that they were competent in both ASL and MCE. As a group, those subjects performing best on the ASL story also made the fewest errors on the MCE story. These findings were interpreted by the investigators as supporting the hypothesis that knowledge of ASL does not interfere with the development of English language skills. This in turn provides some indirect support for the bilingual development of ASL and MCE or the initial development of ASL and later development of ESL with deaf children. Hatfield et al. (1978) caution, however, that high performance on the MCE story by subjects skilled in ASL might be a result of the similarities between ASL and the type of MCE used in the study. It should also be noted that the students were probably a very select group intellectually and educationally and possibly were generously endowed with a general language ability which might have permitted them to acquire ASL, MCE, or standard English with equal ease in childhood. This might not hold true for most of the population of deaf people.

Primary bilingual development

Two studies have reported on deaf children reared in a bilingual home environment; that is, their parents used both ASL and spoken English (Collins-Ahlgren, 1974; Schlesinger & Meadow, 1972). It should be noted this situation is also bimodal and that these studies again demonstrate that not all deaf parents (who know ASL) use only ASL with their children. The deaf parents studied were themselves born of deaf parents. They use ASL signs and spoken English simultaneously. It could be argued that the simultaneous combination of "ASL-like" signs with spoken English produces a communication system that is different from ASL; that is, it might be a variety of manually coded English. Nonetheless, these two studies are steps in the right direction in obtaining data on the bilingualism and ESL issue with deaf children.

Schlesinger and Meadow (1972) described the primary linguistic development of four deaf children, each from a different family with either deaf or hearing parents. Only one child, who had deaf parents and two sets of deaf grandparents, is reported here. The subject, a girl, was diagnosed as deaf (due to heredity) at the age of 3. Her hearing threshold averaged 85 dB (ISO) across the speech frequencies in the better ear. Her parents used ASL and speech simultaneously with her from her birth, thus providing a bilingual home environment. It should be remembered that no formal assessment of the parents' competency, either in ASL or English, was conducted.

The researchers observed the child from age 8 months to 22 months. At 8 months, the child engaged in vocalization and gestures to convey emphasis and emotions. By the end of 12 months, she executed (approximately) the formal adult signs for pretty and wrong, and she understood the command "come here." By the 20th month, her sign vocabulary totaled 142, and she knew 14 letters of the finger spelled alphabet. The researchers concluded that the subject had a sign vocabulary that "compares very favorably with the spoken vocabulary of hearing children" (p. 60).

Schlesinger and Meadow also described the use and meaning of the subject's first individual signs/words which were similar to the one-word utterances of hearing children. A one-word/sign can have one of several functions: (1) It can express a feeling, (2) it can label or name an object, or (3) it can fuse the label with the feeling about the object. This one-word/sign can also be classified according to a single feature. For example, the sign *dog* was appropriately used by the deaf child for pictures of dogs, real dogs, and the *Doggie Diner Restaurant*; and it was inappropriately used to refer to all animals, or even to all animal objects not resembling the parents. It was found that the child acquiring sign language did not use all aspects of a sign (i.e., shape, movement, and placement) in the adult form, which was similar to hearing children who must mature in order to reproduce the sounds of language in their more adult forms. The most interesting finding reported was that the child's vocabulary of 117 signs at 19 months was greater than the typical range of normal hearing children's words which has been estimated to be more than 3 and fewer than 50 (Lenneberg, 1967).

Collins-Ahlgren (1974) analyzed recorded expressive language samples of a deaf girl from her 16th to her 44th month of age. The etiology of the subject's hearing impairment was heredity. She had been exposed to speech and signs simultaneously since her 8th month by her deaf parents, who were college graduates and were informally judged to be competent in English and ASL. It should be borne in mind that the subject might have been exposed to more ASL-like signing (with speech) in the earlier months with the emergence of English (a second language according to the researcher) occurring between the ages of 3 and 4 years. After various grammatical and semantic functions became productive through the sign forms, standard English forms (e.g., articles, auxiliaries, and inflections) were introduced through "signed" or "manual English" techniques.

This subject's expressive language revealed a diglossic continuum ranging from her own invented and imaginative signs through ASL, to signs used in English syntactical order without inflections, to signs with some English markings, and finally to signed standard English. An example is the manner in which the subject demonstrated awareness of the present progressive function. Initially, she utilized the ASL form *NOW*; for example, *I GO NOW* (these words are the English glosses for the ASL signs). Then, the auxiliaries and *-ing* forms were presented to her. Continuing with the example: *I AM GOING* (in this case, the sign, *NOW,* would be dropped unless the English sentence is: *I am going now*). A transitional stage with partial omission occurred prior to the time the full form became productive. In sum, Collins-Ahlgren concluded that this subject was developing a language equivalent to that of her hearing peers. The investigator also argued that if the educational signed or manually coded English systems *are taught as a second language* to children of both deaf and hearing parents, these systems can "build on a native language foundation, and it should prove helpful for English reading and for communication with the hearing world" (p. 493).

Teaching English as a second language

Very little research exists in the area of teaching English as a second language. Only two methods have been delineated: the use of ASL and the use of the written mode of English. Both of these methods assume that English is not the first language. The ASL method assumes that ASL is the first (or functionally dominant) language of most deaf children, and proponents of teaching English as a second language through writing are not concerned with the nature of the first language.

Stokoe (1975) argued that there is a difference between the use of signs and the use of a sign language (e.g., ASL) in teaching English as a second language. A sign language is a linguistic system similar to other languages in that it contains its own grammatical rules. If the signs of this language (e.g., ASL) are taken out of the language context and used in manually coded English systems, then they operate in a different manner. In fact, the signs employed in some MCE systems violate the phonologic (cherological) and semantic aspects of the signs as they are employed in ASL (Wilbur, 1979). In essence, Stokoe argues that signs used in MCE systems are part of a code which is employed to teach English structure, not to teach English as a second language. In addition, Stokoe argues that the prolific use of these MCE systems might cause the deaf child to become incompetent in either language, English or ASL. It should be born in mind that the rationale behind these codes is to teach English as a *first* language (Moores, 1978; Quigley & Kretschmer, 1982).

Crutchfield (1972) offered some insights on teaching English as a second language through the use of ASL. One example provided was that of utilizing the count features of English and ASL. The count features refer to words similar to *much, many, few,* and so on. If the count features in ASL are different from those in English, the first step is to bring the ASL-like features to the student's attention. One example is: *much boy left school.* Even with ASL-like signing, this sentence should be rejected by the students (those familiar with ASL signing). The student should be required to correct these unacceptable utterances utilizing ASL-like signing. Thus, the student would sign: *MANY BOY LEAVE FINISH SCHOOL;* the English glosses for this would be: *Many boy left school.* Next, the teacher would write this sentence on the board and explain that some utterances unacceptable in ASL may also be unacceptable in English, and that some acceptable utterances in ASL may also be acceptable in English—providing *boy* is given a plural inflection (which is another lesson). This writer states that the main purpose in this lesson (and all initial lessons) is to show similarities of acceptability and unacceptability in ASL and English. Subsequently, the instructor can proceed to those structures in English which are different from those in ASL and those in ASL which are different from English.

Jones (1979) provides another perspective on an issue previously discussed: the interference of a signed language in the written English of deaf students. This investigator attempted to delineate the interference aspects of a signed language for the purpose of incorporating them in the teaching of written

English. Jones argued that research on ASL has delineated nonmanual as well as manual aspects (Baker & Padden, 1978). The following illustrates some functions of nonmanual aspects.

Syntactic—yes/no question

A. brow raise

B. head and body forward

Syntactic— a relative clause

A. brow raise

B. backward head tilt

Jones adjudged the signing competence of deaf students at California State University to be that of PSE_d (see the earlier discussion of this term). This researcher argued that deaf students, in writing nontechnical prose, tend to translate into English only the manual signs of ASL that they would use if rendering the same passage in PSE_d. In essence, the nonmanual aspects, which supply very important information, are not signed and thus are omitted in the writing of English. Consequently, the writings of the students do not express enough of the intended message to be comprehensible to a fluent native speaker of English.

Jones further argued that if the writing included information from both manual and nonmanual aspects, it would become more comprehensible. In order to ameliorate this problem, the students must become aware that some signed information is absent in their writing. Informal interviews with native and nonnative users of ASL by the investigator indicated that both manual and nonmanual "signs" are important; neither is of primary importance (ASL, however can be executed without the nonmanual aspects). This is unlike spoken communication (e.g., English) in which non-oral activity is secondary to oral activity. Jones argued that the influence of English has caused deaf students to feel that their native language must have only a primary channel and their writing of English must reflect the fact that English has a primary channel. The result is that these students write only English glosses of the manual signs. (It is assumed, of course, that the students are proficient in English). Jones described the writing style as one very similar to the attempts of a hearing foreigner writing English imperfectly learned. He proposed two methods for ameliorating this condition: (1) Inform the students that they are translating manual signals only and are ignoring the other, nonmanual components of sign communication which contain information (semantic), and (2) demonstrate to the students that a "signed" version of what they have written contains much more information. Jones suggested that the second approach might be more beneficial in getting the students to include the nonmanual information "without making them overly self-conscious about either language" (p. 278).

Goldberg and Bordman (1974, 1975) described an ESL program offered for deaf students at the Tutorial Center of Gallaudet College. These writers argued that samples of writing by their deaf students indicated that most had reached adulthood without a command of English, and had difficulties in expressing themselves which were similar to those of speakers of other languages in ESL classes. Due to the inability of the students to hear, and their concomitant problems with English structure as well as with the concepts expressed, two major modifications were made in ESL procedures: (1) All language practices were conducted in writing (i.e., on the board, overhead projector, paper); and (2) steps were invented to compel students to express the concept involved. Due to the inconclusive evidence regarding the educational effectiveness of the various sign systems and/or communication modes, these writers argued that English must be presented exclusively in the written form to ensure that these students know, with certainty, the *words* that are being addressed. The "sign system" or communication mode prefered by the students is employed by the instructors *to communicate with the student, not to teach the students written English.* In addition, it was suggested that the serious English structure problems of these students are interwoven with the deeper problem of not knowing the concepts which these structures expressed, and not knowing when to use them. Thus, in their attempts to learn English, these students are in a situation similar to that of hearing speakers of ESL who do not make certain concept distinctions fundamental to English. For example, these hearing speakers may feel no need to distinguish between: *They eat sandwiches* and *They are eating sandwiches.* In sum, these writers state that there is a need to design materials which consider the above issues.

Deaf children of Spanish heritage

Very little research exists on deaf children of Spanish descent (King, 1981). It has been reported that from 1972 to 1977, enrollment increased 25.4% for Spanish deaf students in residential schools, and this group of children now accounts for approximately 9.4% of the total hearing-impaired population (Luetke-Stahlman & Weiner, 1982). The few special programs that exist for these students are based on models of education taken from the field of bilingual education.

In general, the proponents of bilingual education for Spanish-speaking deaf students advocate that these children, like hearing Spanish-speaking children, should be educated in their native language initially and then gradually transitioned into English. The major problem becomes the determination of a first language on which to develop English literacy skills. Whether or not Spanish functions as the first language for deaf children of normally hearing Hispanic parents may be dependent upon (1) the usefulness of the residual hearing, (2) the nature of the use of oral Spanish, oral English, and/or the nature of the signs, and (3) the assimilation of the family into the English-speaking society. Consequently, the language employed as a first language in the bilingual education model could be a combination of Spanish, English, and/or any of the number of sign languages and/or systems.

Luetke (1976) argued that to provide this group with a bilingual, bicultural education requires research investigating the culture, attitudes, expectations, and perceptions of the parents. This investigator designed a questionnaire, containing both English and Spanish versions, to gather information from parents regarding (1) family relationships, (2) involvement with the children, and (3) their knowledge and acceptance of their deaf child's education and educators. Only 27% of the 96 questionnaires sent out were returned. There were 28 children and 22 families represented in this study. The overall result indicated that the parents acquiescently accepted the education and educators of their children. Their reluctance to be actively involved seemed to be based on their perceptions that the monolingual teacher tended to disregard parental goals of bilingual–bicultural education. The results also indicated that these parents were of low socioeconomic status and were predominantly Spanish speaking and that the mother was the primary person for language education in the home environment. It was also reported that these families (1) had little or no opportunity to learn sign language, (2) had little or no functional use of English, and (3) depended on their child's lip reading ability to communicate. Only about 6% of the studied children were instructed in Spanish at school even though 27% of the studied parents desired this type of instruction and 20% of the other parents would prefer bilingual instruction. In sum, it is apparent that there was a discrepancy between the goals of the Spanish-speaking parents in this study and the goals of the schools in which their children were enrolled.

Luetke-Stahlman and Weiner (1982) conducted a study employing Spanish deaf children to determine whether or not there is a "first language" that should be selected in teaching language concepts to Hispanic hearing-impaired children whose parents were Spanish speaking and/or members of the Spanish community in the United States. In addition, these investigators were interested in determining if the children were homogeneous with respect to their first language (Spanish) and thus could be grouped together in the same classroom utilizing similar teaching methods. Five language/systems (L/S) were delineated: (1) oral English; (2) English and signs; (3) oral Spanish; (4) Spanish and English signs; and (5) signs only. Three Spanish deaf females were used as subjects. Subject 1 was 4 years 4 months of age with a bilateral, profound, sensorineural hearing impairment. Subject 2 was 3 years 5 months old and possessed a bilateral moderate-to-severe sensorineural hearing impairment. Subject 3 was 4 years 11 months old and had a moderate-to-severe sensorineural impairment. These subjects were taught a receptive vocabulary of nouns, verbs, and adjectives in each of the five L/S. Acquisition curves were constructed for each subject's performance on each of the form class of vocabulary words.

Results indicated that Subject 1 performed best in the English and signs, Spanish and English signs, and signs only. The greatest improvement in this subject's scores was determined to be due to the use of signs. Subject 2 performed best in oral English and signs only. Subject 3's results were mixed. For the noun category, the greatest improvement occurred in Spanish and

English signs and signs only; for the verb category, the greatest improvement occurred in English and signs, Spanish and English signs, and signs only; for the adjective category, the greatest gain was observed using the signs only L/S. Similar to the others, these gains were determined (by results on a pre- and posttest measure) to be due to the effects of training. From the results of this study, these researchers concluded that the choice of a language in educating Spanish deaf children should not be based solely on either heritage or etiological classification. It should be born in mind that only subject 1 would be considered *deaf*; from the description of her hearing impairment, it could have been 90 dB or greater in the better ear (the words *profound, prelingually* were used).

In essence, these investigators proposed that the choice of language is dependent on a combination of factors: (1) The language and/or communication system of the principal caretaker; (2) the amount of exposure to sign language and/or systems; (3) the degree of usable aided hearing ability; and (4) the language and/or system demonstrated to be most effective for learning. One possible inference that can be drawn from the results is that heritage might not dictate that a specific language be used by *deaf* Spanish students of hearing Spanish-speaking parents/caretakers. Consequently, the variable of cultural identity might not be significant in educating this group of students. Finally, it is interesting to note that the results demonstrated that *signs alone* might be the most beneficial instructional input mode for the instruction of prelingually, Spanish deaf students.

These results should be interpreted with caution. First, the sample size was small and employed females only. Second, each subject probably represented a different classification of hearing threshold level; thus, the results were probably based on a *n* of one. Finally, these investigators neglected to report hearing threshold levels in dBs and the age at onset. The employment of such terms as *profound* and *prelingual* have been shown to be ambiguous in the research literature; these terms should not be used in lieu of numerical data for hearing threshold levels and age at onset of the hearing loss.

Research by King (1981) also employed Spanish deaf students. This researcher utilized qualitative and quantitative measures; however, the focus was on qualitative measures since she was interested in shedding some light on the issue of whether the process by which deaf children acquire language is *different from* or *similar to* that of hearing children. This study also provided some insights for bilingual education since it employed deaf students exposed to Spanish as a first language. One component of language (syntax) and one mode of language (reading) were considered. The instruments utilized in the study were the Screening test and four individual diagnostic tests of the Test of Syntactic Abilities (TSA). Forty deaf subjects between the ages of 8 and 13, and 40 hearing subjects between the ages of 8 and 11 participated in the study. Twenty hearing and 20 deaf subjects were classified as L_1 learners (i.e., learned English as a first language); 20 hearing and 20 deaf subjects were classified as L_2 learners (i.e., learning English as a second language). The L_1

subjects were exposed to English in the home and had no formal foreign or second-language instruction. The L_2 subjects were Puerto Rican Americans of Spanish descent. The subjects were matched on language, type of school attended, amount of exposure to English, and type of instruction received; that is, all subjects attended schools in which English was the primary language and had received English instruction in content areas.

Results indicated that the order of difficulty on syntactic tasks were similar for both groups of hearing and deaf subjects. This led the investigator to conclude that deaf children acquire syntactic structures in the same order as hearing children. Results of the error types, which should be viewed as tentative according to the researcher, seemed to indicate that the types of errors were similar for both groups. The most interesting finding, for present purposes, was that on the effects of possessing another language. This factor appeared to have no effect upon the English language abilities of hearing children on a quantitative level. Implications of similar findings were presented in the section on hearing children and this seems to suggest no positive advantages for bilinguals, at least linguistically in the area of syntax. Contrariwise, the effects of another language on the abilities of deaf children were reported to be equivocal. The researcher proposed two explanations: (1) one of the two deaf L_2 groups might have been atypical; (2) deafness overrides any effect (positive or negative) of being exposed to two languages. Some support can be found for the second argument in the study by Luetke-Stahlman and Weiner (1982) in the case of the one subject who was classified as *"profoundly, prelingually deaf."* It is interesting to note that King (1981) reported that all deaf subjects used little or no English upon entering school.

A case for bilingualism and ASL/ESL

The rise in interest in bilingualism and ASL/ESL for deaf children has followed and paralleled a similar movement for hearing children whose native spoken language is not English. These have been chiefly Hispanics of various national origins (Mexican, Puerto Rican, Cuban, etc.), although other nationalities and linguistic communities have been involved. The early part of this chapter dealt with some of the philosophical, theoretical, program, and research issues involved in this movement. It was pointed out that there is great similarity between those issues and the bilingual and ASL/ESL situation with deaf children. There are, however, some important differences that should also be pointed out.

Hispanic children and those of other national and linguistic origins who come from homes where English is not the commonly used language, come also from established cultures different from the Anglo cultures of the United States. Those cultures have their own traditions, customs, literature, art, music, and so on, as well as their own language. This has resulted in the movement toward bilingual/bicultural programs for Hispanic and other non-English-speaking children rather than just bilingual programs. An argument has been made for a similar approach with deaf children (Hatfield et al., 1978; Luetke, 1976) but it seems strained, at best. There are no established bodies of traditions, customs, literature, art, that are unique to deafness and deaf people. The great common factor that binds most deaf people together as a distinct group is sign language. The arguments made on behalf of biculturalism for deaf people seem to be arguments for the creation of a culture rather than the protection of an existing one.

As Quigley and Kretschmer (1982, p. 108) have pointed out, most deaf children are assimilated into deaf communities rather than being born into them. This is another major difference between deaf children and hearing children from non-English speaking families. The latter are born to languages and cultures distinct from English. Only deaf children of deaf parents, and not even all of those (Brasel & Quigley, 1977; Corson, 1973), are born into homes where some form of ASL might be the native language. More than 90% of deaf children have two hearing parents and the first language to which they will be exposed is the spoken language of their parents.

When hearing children of non-English speaking parents are taught English as a second language, they are exposed to a bilingual but unimodal situation. Both their native languages and English are receptively and expressively aural/oral. But the deaf child exposed to ASL and English might be in a bimodal (aural/oral and visual/manual) as well as a bilingual situation (Schlesinger & Meadow, 1972). This has important implications for primary language development, but also for the secondary forms of reading and writing which are based on aural/oral primary language.

These differences are enough to demonstrate that the analogy between the bilingual/bicultural situation of non-English speaking hearing children in the United States and ASL/PSE using deaf children is imperfect. It is a useful analogy but the cautions made concerning it should be borne in mind. The case presented here eliminates the bicultural part of the analogy. It is this part which is generating the most controversy presently in the situation of non-English speaking hearing children, focusing on whether the basic objective should be assimilation of the minority culture member into the majority culture, linguistic and cultural separatism, or some degree of assimilation between these extremes. The presentation here is concerned only with the bilingual aspect, with whether ASL should be (or is) the native language of deaf children with English to be regarded as a second language.

A number of authors (e.g., Lane & Grosjean, 1980; Stokoe, 1972; Wilbur, 1979) have made extensive arguments for exposing deaf children to ASL in a natural manner and developing English later as a second language (ASL/ESL). A more limited presentation by Quigley and Paul is followed here. Quigley and Paul emphasize three points in favor of the ASL/ESL approach (1984).

First, it has been argued that the other approaches do not permit communication to take place in the easy and fluent manner which will permit visual language to be unconsciously absorbed by deaf children in infancy and early childhood as auditory language is by hearing children. Second, it has been argued that manually coded English systems and oral English are incompatible, especially since many practitioners do not adhere strictly to English structure in the manual component of the systems (Marmor & Pettito, 1979; Reich & Bick, 1977). Third, it is claimed that long use of the other systems has produced only limited results.

As has been pointed out previously, fewer than 50% of speech sounds are visible for speech reading. Even with the amplified use of residual hearing, the aural/oral input presents an imperfect signal for the deaf child. The use of cued speech might improve on this, but evidence for that is lacking as yet. In addition to providing an imperfect input signal, speech as an expressive act requires fine motor movements and coordination which are not under automatic auditory control by the CNS as they are for hearing children, but require conscious effort and control by the deaf child which results in a laborious and distorted output. Observation in almost any purely oral program will attest to the difficulties and limitations for this communication form. It should be remembered, however, that it has been used very effectively with students in some schools (Ogden, 1979).

The charge of incompatibility between oral English and manually coded English has some empirical support. Studies by Marmor and Pettito (1979) and Reich and Bick (1977) were cited earlier as showing that many users of MCE do not adhere strictly to English structure so that the MCE systems tend to become pidgin sign English. In order to achieve fluency with MCE systems many users seem to have to abandon parts of the systems. There is also the unanswered question of how well a child can attend to an English system on the lips and another on the hands of a communicator.

Perhaps the most telling criticism is that OE and MCE approaches have achieved only very limited educational results. The studies discussed in chapter 3 showed that OE seems to require special conditions of program and student for success and that those conditions are difficult to match in many programs and many students. Quigley and Kretschmer (1982) have summarized many of the studies of MCE and PSE that have been conducted during the past 20 years or so and have concluded that the results have been disappointing. Concern is with the educational results of those approaches and not with the contention that deaf children should be permitted to use any communication form that is natural and comfortable for them. That is a separate issue. But it was stated in the Preface that this book accepts that the main function of schools is to educate—to impart to children sets of skills and bodies of knowledge that will enable them to participate successfully in the general society. It is on these skills, such as reading and writing, and bodies of knowledge, educational achievement, that the effects of various communication methods must be judged. And it is in these areas that MCE systems have produced much more limited results than was probably expected by their originators. Quigley and Paul (1984) have stated that results of most of the studies are about on the order of what is often produced by the Hawthorne effect in educational studies.

One extensive study of a MCE system (SEE II) did show very substantial gains when the system was used in the home as well as in the school, but little progress was made by a group that used it only in school for 10 years, and so the source of the progress is in doubt (Babb, 1979). A study by Meadow (1968) also showed very substantial superiority for a group of deaf children of deaf parents as compared to a matched group of deaf children of hearing parents. The superiority was ascribed to use of manual communication in the homes by deaf parents, probably in some form of ASL. Brasel and Quigley (1977) reported equally impressive results for a select group of deaf children of deaf parents who were exposed to early communication in what the authors termed "Manual English." This was probably a sophisticated form of PSE or *H* in Stokoe's terminology. Corson (1973) also obtained impressive results for a group of oral deaf students who were communicated to by their oral deaf parents only in oral English. So the studies with impressive educational results (differences or gains of two or three grades in educational achievement) do not seem to support any single communication approach. Their commonalities seem to lie in (1) the groups of students studied were select in IQ, SES, and similar important factors, and (2) the groups had parents who, although using widely varying communication approaches, were literate, loving, and deeply involved in the linguistic development of their children. Most other studies of MCE and PSE approaches, as Quigley and Kretschmer (1982) have summarized, have produced only very modest results.

The case being made for ASL/ESL so far is based largely on negatives of other approaches. More positive arguments are presented by Lane and Grosjean (1980), Stokoe (1972), and Wilbur (1979). Some obvious positive points can be made. First, granting that ASL can be or is a sophisticated language, it can provide the intelligibility and quality that are needed for fluent communicative interaction among child, parent, teacher, and significant others. Signs are large and easily visible as input and ASL seems to have all the characteristics of a genuine language. Second, the signs of ASL are gross motor movements that can be made by deaf children much more easily than the fine motor movements of speech. Third, ASL might have a syntactic structure better adapted to visual coding than the structure of oral English. The research by Lichtenstein (1983) and others discussed in chapter 2 raises this as a potentially important issue. Fourth, the initial use of ASL followed by ESL (at least in manually coded English form), is a close analogy to bilingualism and ESL with hearing children from non-English-speaking homes. Thus, it could benefit from the large amount of research and practice accumulated with the hearing children situation.

There are at least a couple of obstacles to wide-scale use of an ASL/ESL approach with deaf children. First, ASL is not the native language of the parents of most deaf children. These are hearing people whose native language is usually English, or in a minority of cases, some other spoken language. There is an immediate problem as to how these people are to become proficient enough in ASL quickly enough to use it fluently with their deaf children in very early childhood. The only alternative seems to be to turn the development of their children over to others in infancy, something many parents might be understandably reluctant to do. Second, if English is to be introduced to deaf children, just how will this be done: with MCE, OE, or both in succession? If OE is used, the situation becomes bimodal as well as bilingual. If MCE is used, when, if ever, will the child acquire speech? Given the great effort and skill needed to develop oral communication (see Ling, 1976; Ling & Ling, 1978), this is a major matter. Third, how will reading be developed? Present methods seem to be based to some extent on internalized auditory language and the research of Lichtenstein (1983) again and that of Conrad (1979) indicate possession of a speech code might be required for fluent reading by deaf children also.

None of these obstacles is insurmountable, but they require consideration in the initiation of ASL/ESL programs. They also argue for a careful research approach to the issue rather than another unsupported change in linguistic forms with deaf children. It so happens that conditions exist that provide the opportunity for such a research approach. About 3% of deaf children have two deaf parents and another 5 or 6% have one (Rawlings & Jensema, 1977). The parents of many of these children might welcome the establishment of experimental ASL/ESL programs. It should be possible to identify enough infants and very young children to select groups with deaf parents at various educational and SES levels to evaluate longitudinally the use of ASL/ESL from infancy into the school years. The cooperation of willing, ASL-using deaf parents could provide the most favorable conditions for a trial of this approach. The programs might also fill a present gap in educational programs for deaf children. Hearing parents who provide an intensive early oral environment for their children can find school programs, public and private, that will continue this approach. Parents who use some form of early MCE input can also find school programs that use this approach. But parents who use ASL with their deaf children, usually deaf parents, can rarely if ever find similar programs in the schools. The option should be available. And if longitudinal research studies of the ASL/ESL approach were conducted with these deaf children of deaf parents, data on the effectiveness of the approach could be provided. It is possible, as seems to be true with the other approaches, that ASL/ESL programs will be found to work for some deaf children and not for others. If so, the important research and practical questions would then become concerned with which children go best with which approach and how can the determination be made in infancy and early childhood when language is most readily developed.

SUMMARY AND CONCLUSIONS

Bilingualism and ASL/ESL have received increasing attention in the literature during the past decade (Luetke, 1976; Stokoe, 1972; Wilbur, 1979) and it is likely that interest will continue during the next decade. It is also likely that attempts will be made to put bilingual and ASL/ESL concepts into practice and it is argued here that this can and should be done in a controlled experimental manner rather than wholesale with little or no empirical research justification. The history of language approaches to the education of deaf children is one of great enthusiasm for a particular approach at a particular time followed eventually by almost as great disillusionment— an almost constant waxing and waning. This may be the result of lack of reasoned initiation of an approach, careful evaluation of it, and establishment of a data base on it from which judgments can be made.

The ASL and PSE approaches reigned supreme in the United States educational system for deaf children during most of the 19th century. Some inroads were made by purely oral approaches when the Clarke School for the Deaf was established in 1869 and what is now the Lexington School for the Deaf shortly thereafter, but little real change took place until after the International Congress at Milan in 1880. The greatest impact of the change was in the day schools and day classes for deaf children which increased greatly in enrollment from the turn of the century until the present. Oral programs became established in residential schools also, but primarily for the young age groups. Older children often still had instruction through PSE or ASL and these were the common language forms for most of the children and their caretakers outside of the classroom. The important point is that this vast change took place in the late 19th century with no reasoned initiation, no careful evaluation, and no data base. It ensued from the repeatedly articulated arguments and beliefs that deaf children had to acquire both the communication mode (oral) and linguistic form (the spoken language of the general society) in order to attain adequate academic achievement and to participate at least adequately in the general society.

Another large swing took place in the 1960s and 1970s in the United States when disillusionment with the results obtained by purely oral methods led to a swing toward manually coded English, first in the form of "Neo-oralism" from the Soviet Union (Morkovin, 1960; Quigley, 1969) which was similar to the Rochester method (finger spelling and speech) established at the Rochester School for the Deaf by Zenos Westervelt in 1878; then in the newly constructed MCE systems such as SEE I and SEE II (Gustason, Pfetzing, & Zawolkow, 1975). Other innovations during this period were cued speech (Cornett, 1967) and "Verbotonal Audiometry" (Guberina, 1964). Of these approaches, SEE II seems to have become the most commonly used (Jordan, Gustason, & Rosen, 1976). Again, this swing took place with no reasoned initiation, no careful evaluation, and no data base.

It seems at least possible that another swing is about to take place—a swing to ASL as the initial or native language for deaf children with English to be established bilingually or as a second language, *if at all*. What is presented in this chapter is a case for bilingual and ASL/ESL (and primarily the latter) approaches to educating deaf children. It is proposed that this involve reasoned initiation, careful evaluation, and establishment of a data base rather than another sharp swing in linguistic and communication forms.

If ASL/ESL approaches are tried systematically with deaf children, they can draw on the large body of research and practices in bilingualism and ESL that exist for minority culture hearing children. The brief survey early in this chapter indicated that there are great similarities in issues, research, and practice between the educational situations of deaf children and minority culture hearing children. Research and theory with minority culture hearing children indicate that the interdependence theory espoused by Lambert (1975) and Lambert and Tucker (1972) might be the most applicable to the situation of deaf children. This theory holds that, under certain learning conditions, access to two languages (e.g., ASL and English) can positively influence the development of cognitive processes which in turn can lead to higher IQ and academic achievement. The certain learning conditions mentioned seem to include a positive (or additive) environment which involves good community support for the program, equal prestige for the two languages involved, and positive teacher expectations and attitudes.

Legarreta's (1979) research on five types of bilingual/ESL programs indicated that the most successful models were the developmental maintenance models that used a generative approach to language development and a bilingual program with a 50/50 utilization of each language. Such programs require, of course, that instructors be fluent in both languages. In the case of deaf children it could reasonably be argued that the instructors should be bimodal as well as bilingual, that is, that they should be proficient in oral English as well as manually coded English and ASL. Given the large body of research and practice with minority hearing children to draw from in establishing ASL/ESL programs and the probable willingness of deaf parents to have their deaf children involved in such programs, it should be possible to initiate the programs carefully, evaluate them experimentally, and establish a data base on their effectiveness. This would represent significant progress from the unsupported swings that have occurred from one approach to another during the past 200 years.

chapter 7

Assessment and language instruction

Barry W. Jones

As Quigley and Kretschmer (1982) have indicated, the primary goal of education, generally, is "to develop the ability to read and write the common language of the general society" (p. 65). This is also the goal of most programs educating deaf individuals. Quigley and Kretschmer (1982) also stated "that most deaf students...do not attain even adequate ability to read and write English" (p. 66). Even though the abilities to read and write are considered to be secondary receptive and expressive skills, developed upon the bases of the primary skills of listening and speaking (including the expressive abilities of the various forms of manual communication), one can state that the primary language skills of most deaf students do not enable them to use efficiently the common language of U.S. society, English. It should also be stated that the extent to which deaf individuals cannot use the common language of society is the extent to which they will be limited in their vocational, economic, and social opportunities. With these concerns in mind, therefore, it is incumbent upon educators to provide deaf individuals with the language skills to enable them to participate in the activities of life with as few limitations as possible.

There are two essential elements in any language instructional program— assessment and instruction. Obviously, the information gained from one's assessment procedures should suggest the instructional procedures to be utilized. In this chapter these elements individually and materials and techniques associated with each element are discussed.

ASSESSMENT

Assessment can be likened to the cornerstone of a building. The cornerstone, in terms of the total structure, occupies a very small space; yet, in terms of its function, it is indispensible. The same is true for assessment. A carefully planned assessment program should occupy only a small portion of the allotted instructional or therapy time, and also should provide teachers or clinicians with valuable information on students' entry level skills and their progress toward achieving instructional goals and objectives. Indeed, without assessment, one would have an instructional program based on factors other than students' needs and no way of ascertaining the efficiency of instruction. Returning to the analogy, without cornerstones, structures are weakened and apt to collapse.

Some important factors in assessment are (1) reliability considerations, (2) validity considerations, and (3) methods of language assessment and current practices in language assessment with deaf individuals.

Reliability

The concept of reliability is related to the consistency with which a test instrument or technique assesses individuals and groups. The concept has usually been associated with standardized (norm-referenced) tests. In terms of language assessment the concern of reliability with norm-referenced tests has been addressed by Bloom and Lahey (1978) and Kretschmer and Kretschmer (1978). The philosophical rationale for considerations of reliability is, however, essential for all assessment techniques and should not, therefore, be limited to standardized tests. If, indeed, one cannot depend on the consistency of either a test or a technique, one cannot assume that the obtained results will approximate the student's true performance on the trait being assessed. In a classic work on reliability, Thorndike (1951) wrote "that as the reliability of a score decreases, the low reliability makes tentative any judgment which is based on that score, and that as the reliability approaches zero, basing any judgment on it becomes impossible" (p. 219).

The most frequently used methods for determining the reliability of assessment tools and techniques are considered in this section. These include, for norm-referenced tests, (1) alternate form procedures, (2) test–retest procedures, (3) internal consistency measures. Additional procedures (inter- and intra-examiner reliability coefficients) address the issues of more informal assessment techniques. Each of these procedures involves the calculation of correlations between equivalent sets of measurements.

Reliability procedures for formal tests

Alternate form procedures. In those situations where test developers have made more than one form of the test available, the calculations of a correlation coefficient between the two forms of the test should serve as a reliability coefficient. The test user or developer should, however, ascertain that any correlational figures are, in fact, based upon the concepts of equivalence between test forms (Thorndike & Hagen, 1961). There are two primary problems related to test development that could lead one to challenge the equivalency of parallel forms. The two tests could differ in content and form to such an extent that the concept of equivalence would not be valid and the reliability coefficient could be underestimated. Conversely, the two forms could be so closely matched in content and form that the correlation coefficient would overestimate the reliability. When, therefore, test developers provide equivalent forms the test users should, whenever possible, investigate the logic and the subsequent procedures behind the test author's development of the instrument. The test user should also verify that a sufficient amount of time (a few weeks) has elapsed between the administration of the two test forms.

Test–retest procedures. Although test–retest is a less desirable method of determining the reliability of an instrument since the universe of items is more restrictive than when alternate forms of a test are available, the correlation coefficients may be higher than those for alternate form procedures. The test user or developer should also, however, be aware that the students' recall of responses (and, hence, repetition of responses) may contribute to the higher correlation. An additional factor which could lower the correlation is the attitude of the individuals being tested. If the examinees should become annoyed with the repetition of identical tests, they could provide haphazard responses resulting in correlations between sets of valid and invalid data (Thorndike & Hagen, 1961).

Internal consistency measures. In order to save time and to eliminate the problems associated with repeated measurements, test users and developers often utilize methods to determine the reliability of an instrument from a single administration of a test. The procedures utilized usually involve dividing the test into two equal parts and correlating the students' scores on the respective parts. The manner in which the test has been divided will, however, have an impact on the reliability coefficient. If, for example, the first half of the test is correlated with the last half, the factor of time (if the test is timed) may significantly decrease the reliability. Additionally, if the items have been arranged in a sequence of increasing difficulty, the second half of the test would not be equivalent to the first and hence, the correlation would be lowered. In contrast, if the test is divided on an odd–even numbered item basis, the difficulty and timing questions should be virtually eliminated. There is, however, the issue of similarity of content between items which could provide spuriously high correlations.

An additional measure of internal consistency for untimed tests utilizes analysis of variance techniques among items (Thorndike, 1951). One formula for calculating this correlation coefficient (Kuder–Richardson 20) estimates the "reliability from the relationship of total test variance to item variance" (Thorndike, p. 236), and takes factors that contribute to the variance such as difficulty levels of items, item variances, and intercorrelations into account. The Kuder–Richardson 20 (KR–20) formula will, however, provide a higher estimate of reliability than reliability measures obtained from the multiple testing procedures previously described.

Reliability procedures for informal techniques

Whereas the aforementioned reliability coefficients depend on correlations between examinees' responses on normed tests, the procedures to be discussed in this section depend on correlations between and within examiners. These procedures are appropriate for use with more informal assessment techniques such as the collection of spontaneous language samples. The data (the language sample) remains the same; the criterion of interest, therefore, becomes the extent to which independent analyses of the data will agree on the students' level of performance.

Interexaminer procedures. This type of reliability coefficient is based on the degree of agreement between independent evaluators looking at identical data. Generally, the evaluators are trained to use the evaluation techniques associated with the tests; this helps to reduce the variance and, hence, raises the correlation coefficients between examiners. This procedure is, for informal assessment techniques, analogous to internal consistency measures for standardized tests. If a number of evaluators can, after training, consistently arrive at closely similar conclusions regarding an individual's language sample, one could assume that the scoring procedures and instructions were sufficiently consistent to provide one with dependable interpretations. If, on the other hand, there is not a consistent sense of agreement between independent evaluators, the interpretations are, at best, suspect.

Intraexaminer procedures. These procedures are analogous to the test–retest techniques associated with standardized tests. Although these methods are not widely used, they can be utilized to determine the consistency of a single evaluator. The evaluator is presented either identical or highly similar data after a period of time has elapsed to ascertain the extent of agreement between the two interpretations. If there is substantial agreement, one could assume that the evaluator consistently applies the same criteria for interpretations. If the interpretations are not consistent, one could assume that the evaluator has analyzed the data in an arbitrary fashion.

Validity

The concept of validity addresses the issue of whether tests or techniques measure the variables they were intended to measure. If, for example, a test purporting to measure the variable of English syntax contained a large number of items requiring the students to select the appropriate definitions of words, one should question whether the test was measuring what it was intended to measure. There are three basic types of validity that are addressed in this section: (1) statistical validity, (2) content validity, and (3) construct validity.

Statistical validity

This type of validity involves ascertaining that the test under consideration measures similar variables as other tests. Thus, if a test was designed to measure vocabulary, it could be compared to another vocabulary test for the purpose of establishing statistical validity. Although this type of validity is important, one could argue that the rationale for content validity is more appropriate.

Content validity

This type of validity, more so than statistical validity, requires the establishment of a philosophical model within which one can place the variables of interest. The process is one of rational thought in which the test users must be aware of the assumptions of the test developers and the literature relating to the variables of interest. To establish the content validity of a comprehensive test for English morphology, for example, one would need to ascertain that the test included items assessing free morphemes, inflectional and derivational morphemes, and representative samples of items containing prefixes, suffixes, and infixes (Russell, Quigley, & Power, 1976).

Construct validity

Whereas statistical and content validity address different aspects of the same problem—the extent to which a measure assesses what it was intended to measure—construct validity procedures combine the two for the purpose of examining the degree to which the instrument reflects some theoretical construct (Ventry & Schiavetti, 1980). Thus, if a theory predicted differences in language behaviors between deaf and hearing individuals and the measurement did, indeed, verify those differences, then construct validity would have been established for the variable of hearing status.

ASSESSMENT METHODS

The types of information one can obtain from language assessments of individuals depend, to a large extent, on the methods utilized to acquire the data. In this section are discussed the strengths and limitations of controlled and free methods and the instruments or procedures associated with each format. Test instruments are discussed in relationship with controlled methods, and test and analysis procedures are considered with free methods.

Controlled methods

Controlled methods are usually associated with normative tests. In a practical sense this usually means that the test stimuli and the range of alternative responses are controlled in terms of content, presentation procedures, and subject selection (Wardrop, 1976).

Strengths and limitations

There are several general advantages to utilizing controlled methods. First, controlled methods permit examiners to investigate language phenomena that might infrequently or never appear in spontaneous language samples. The work of Taylor (1969) and particularly that of Quigley, Wilbur, Power, Montanelli, and Steinkamp (1976), indicate that language samples may not always contain sufficient evidence for one to conclude that an individual either had or had not acquired a particular linguistic principle. If, for example, an individual's language sample did not contain any conjoined sentences could one conclude that the individual had no knowledge of the structure? The answer is obviously no. Controlled methods, however, permit one to structure test stimuli in such a way as to elicit responses that provide examiners with opportunities to look at specific linguistic units.

Second, controlled procedures provide investigators with the flexibility to design tests that address specific issues of interest. There is no question that a teacher of deaf students or a language clinician would desire a measurement instrument that would provide information on a student's or client's phonologic, morphological, syntactic, semantic, and pragmatic skills. If one considers the nature of the task, however, it becomes apparent that test developers must concentrate on single-factor tests and that test users must utilize a variety of test instruments. In other words, it would be unreasonable to expect that a single test would evaluate two or more of the linguistic components listed above. Alternatively, one can receive detailed information on a student's or client's specific disorders only to the extent that the specific disorders have been assessed. One should, therefore, have instruments available to assess each language component.

Third, there is usually more objectivity in the analyses of test results from controlled methods than is present in analyses of data collected by free methods. The developers of controlled test procedures directly specify the methods by which their instruments should be interpreted. If, therefore, the content of the test measured the language variable of interest and the subjects who participated in the normative sample were representative of the students or clients being assessed, the test user should be able to depend on the interpretation procedures outlined by the test developers.

Fourth, the obtained results from controlled methods can be more easily compared with those of other students or clients who have similar characteristics. It is incumbent upon test developers to specify the characteristics of the population upon whom their tests were normed. If, therefore, one assessed a profoundly deaf client with a test instrument normed on other profoundly deaf clients possessing similar characteristics, one could assume that the results obtained from the assessment could be compared with those of the normative sample.

Fifth, the factors contributing to reliability and validity can be more easily managed. By controlling the test stimuli, the available responses, and the characteristics of the normative sample the amount of variance related to external factors can be reduced, and as a result, the validity and particularly the reliability coefficients can be enhanced. If, therefore, the reliability is high for a particular measurement instrument, the test authors have exercised care in planning the content of the test, and the subjects being assessed possess similar characteristics to those who made up the normative sample, one could be reasonably assured that the test was measuring what it was intended to measure in a precise manner for the subjects under investigation.

There are also limitations to the use of controlled methods. Perhaps the primary limitation is associated with the second advantage; even though examiners can obtain detailed information on a specific aspect of language, they cannot make judgments on an individual's overall language ability. An examiner should not, therefore, administer a test designed to measure syntax and expect it to provide information on morphology, semantics, and pragmatics. In order to gain these broader perspectives one must use a combination of other instruments designed to measure these other aspects of language and/or analysis procedures designed for interpreting spontaneous language samples.

A second limitation involves the nature of the tests; when investigators control the test stimuli, the testing environment, and/or the responses they cannot assume that the results are indicative of an individual's language behaviors in more naturalistic settings. It is, therefore, best for one to compare the results obtained from the controlled measure with those obtained in a more naturalistic manner.

Test instruments

The order of presentation for the tests described in this section is such that the tests developed for hearing-impaired students are presented initially. The other tests discussed in this section were developed for use with hearing individuals and have been used for describing some aspect of language for hearing-impaired students. Prior to any discussion of particular tests, however, the positive and negative aspects of comparing a normative sample of hearing-impaired individuals with other hearing-impaired individuals and comparing samples of hearing-impaired individuals with normally hearing individuals should be addressed. When one derives a percentile, age equivalent, or grade equivalent score from a student's test performance one is comparing that individual's score with those on whom the test has been normed. If, therefore, the test was normed on deaf individuals and another deaf individual scored in the 99th percentile one could assume that the examinee possessed superior abilities on the variable being measured among deaf individuals. One could not, however, assume that the individual's high percentile ranking would generalize to the performances of individuals with normal hearing. When, therefore, tests are used which were normed on hearing-impaired individuals the examiner must be aware of the limitations one must place on the interpretations.

On the other hand, if a deaf individual achieved a high percentile score on a test normed on individuals with normal hearing one could assume that the person had skills that were higher than those of individuals with normal hearing. It is incumbent upon the examiner, therefore, to assure that correct test interpretations have been made in relationship to the sample on which the tests have been normed.

Test of syntactic abilities. The Test of Syntactic Abilities (Quigley et al., 1978) is a comprehensive battery of 20 diagnostic tests and two forms of a screening test assessing profoundly deaf students' abilities to either select grammatically correct sentences in English or to comprehend them. The 20 diagnostic tests of the Test of Syntactic Abilities (TSA) were normed on a sample of 411 students who met five characteristics:

1. All subjects were between the ages of 10 years and 18 years 11 months.
2. All subjects had an IQ of 80 or higher on the performance scale on a recognized IQ test.
3. All subjects possessed a hearing loss of at least 90 dB (ISO) within the speech range (500, 1,000, and 2,000 Hz).
4. All subjects acquired the hearing loss prior to the age of 24 months.
5. No subject displayed evidence of multiple disabilities.

Although data have been collected and reported (Quigley et al., 1978) on students with normal hearing, Australian deaf children, college level deaf students, and hearing-impaired students from Canada, the data were normed on students who met the five criteria described above.

Table 4 depicts the nine structures assessed by the TSA, the type of task associated with each of the 20 diagnostic tests, and the internal consistency reliability coefficients for 19 of the 20 tests. From the table it can be seen that only two of the nine structures (Determiners and Pronominalization) do not have comprehension items and that the internal consistency reliabilities range from .94 to .98. Wardrop (1976) has stated that reliability coefficients of .80 or above are sufficient for making decisions about specific individual's performances; the individual tests of the TSA were developed, therefore, with sufficient precision to make decisions on individual students. The developers of these tests (Quigley et al., 1978) have also demonstrated content validity for the battery. The content validity has been further documented by Owens, Haney, Giesow, Dooley, and Kelley (1983).

Each of the 20 diagnostic tests of the TSA contains 70 multiple-choice items written, in terms of vocabulary, at approximately the first-grade level. The time required for administration of a single test ranges from approximately 35 to 60 minutes. Since the administration time for the entire battery requires 10 to 20 hours it is obviously impractical to administer all of the tests on a regular basis. For this reason the authors of the TSA developed two forms of a screening test which can be administered in approximately 1 hour.

Each of the screening tests of the TSA contains 120 items assessing, generally, the nine syntactic structures which constitute the domain of structures for the total test battery. The internal consistency reliability coefficients (KR–20) for the two tests are .98 and the coefficients for each of the nine structures range from .80 to .87. The reliability indices for each of the nine structures on the screening tests are sufficient for that purpose only—screening. It is suggested, therefore, that examiners administer the screening test initially and

TABLE 4. STRUCTURES, TYPES OF TASKS, AND INTERNAL RELIABILITIES FOR THE TSA

Structure	Type of Task	KR-20 Reliability
Negation	Recognition & Comprehension	.98
Conjunction		
Conjunction	Recognition & Comprehension	.97
Disjunction &		
Alternation	Recognition & Comprehension	.96
Determiners	Recognition	.96
Question Formation		
Wh-words	Recognition	.96
Answer Environments	Comprehension	.96
Yes/No Questions	Recognition	.97
Verb Processes		
Verb Sequence in		
Conjoined Structures	Recognition	.97
Main verbs, Linking		
verbs, & Auxiliaries	Recognition	.95
Passive Voice	Recognition & Comprehension	.97
Pronominalization		
Possessive Adjectives	Recognition	.96
Reflexives	Recognition	.96
Possessive Pronouns	Recognition	.96
Forward & Backward		
Pronominalization	Recognition	.97
Relativization		
Comprehension	Comprehension	.94
Relative Pronouns		
and Adverbs	Recognition	.93
Embedding	Recognition	.96
Complementation		
That-Complements	Recognition & Comprehension	.94
Infinitives &		
Gerunds	Recognition	.94
Nominalization	Recognition & Comprehension	Not available

determine those structures, following the procedures specified in the test manual (Quigley et al., 1978), on which the examinee has exhibited some difficulty. On the basis of this interpretation, examiners can then select the appropriate tests of the diagnostic battery to administer to the examinee.

Once the appropriate tests of the diagnostic battery have been administered the examiners have access to both formal and informal interpretation procedures. On a formal basis one can determine the student's percentile rank, percentile range, and age equivalent score. On a more informal basis one can calculate the percentage of correct responses for the types of tasks associated with each structure (recognition or comprehension) and the types of substructures associated with each of the nine structures assessed by the TSA. As an example, examiners can determine the percentage of correct responses on the Conjunction test for unreduced conjoined sentences (John went to the store and Mary went to the movies) as well as for reduced conjoined sentences such as conjoined subjects (John and Mary went to the movies), conjoined objects (I painted the house and the barn), conjoined verb phrases (Bill paints houses and washes cars), and conjoined verbs (I painted and cleaned the house).

There is an additional interpretation feature of the TSA which deserves special attention. The distractors (incorrect responses in terms of standard English usage) are representative of structures found to appear consistently in the language productions of deaf individuals. When, therefore, a student selects incorrect responses the examiner can, with information provided in the test manual, determine if the student consistently selects a deviation from standard English usage commonly found among deaf students. This information can be valuable for remediation purposes.

Grammatical Analysis of Elicited Language. The Grammatical Analysis of Elicited Language (GAEL) was developed at the Central Institute for the Deaf. The GAEL is currently available for three levels of analysis: the GAEL-P (Moog, Kozak, & Geers, 1983) for the presentence level, the GAEL-S (Moog & Geers, 1979) for the simple sentence level, and the GAEL-C (Moog & Geers, 1980) for the complex sentence level. The GAEL-P assesses readiness for language and one, two, and three-word combinations in comprehension, production, and imitation tasks given adequate prompts. The test was administered to 75 subjects with normal hearing between the ages of 2 years 6 months and 3 years 11 months; it was normed, however, on 150 hearing impaired children between the ages of 3 years and 5 years 11 months. Test–retest reliability procedures, based on 20 hearing–impaired students tested after an interval of 1 month, resulted in coefficients of .97 for the comprehension task, .95 for the prompted production task, and .93 for the imitation task. It should be noted that the authors of the test defined their hearing–impaired sample as "educationally hearing impaired" since their subjects were too young to provide consistent audiological data for analysis.

The GAELS consists of 94 pairs of identical sentences to assess the students' abilities to produce and, subsequently, imitate specific syntactic structures given adequate prompts. The structures assessed by the GAELS were selected from the Lee Developmental Sentence Scoring (Lee, 1974) and Language Sampling and Analysis (Tyack & Gottesleben, 1974) and include articles, adjectives, quantifiers, possessives, demonstratives, conjunctions, pronouns, nouns in subject and object positions, Wh-questions, verbs and verb inflections, copulas and their inflections, prepositions, and negatives.

The test was normed on 200 hearing children between the ages of 2 years 6 months and 5 years in the St. Louis, Missouri area and 200 deaf children between the ages of 5 and 9 years from 13 oral programs for hearing–impaired children across the United States. Additional criteria for the sample of hearing–impaired subjects include:

1. Hearing loss greater than 70 dB in the better ear in the speech range (500, 1,000, 2,000 Hz);
2. Hearing loss acquired prior to the age of 24 months;
3. No additional handicapping conditions of educational significance.

The authors of the test reported a test–retest reliability coefficient of .96 for both the prompted and imitated tasks for 20 hearing–impaired subjects retested after a 30-month interval. The validity of the instrument was demonstrated, primarily, through analysis of variance and trend analysis procedures to substantiate the effects of age on the linguistic variables assessed.

The GAELC consists of 88 pairs of identical sentences assessing the production and imitation of complex sentences given adequate prompts. The syntactic variables included in the analysis include articles, noun modifiers, nouns in subject and object position, noun plurals, personal pronouns, indefinite and reflexive pronouns, conjunctions, auxiliary verbs, first-clause verbs, other verbs and verb inflections, infinitives and participles, prepositions, negatives, and Wh-questions. The test was normed on 120 severely hearing–impaired students (hearing losses between 70 and 95 dB in the speech range) between the ages of 8 years and 11 years 11 months, 150 profoundly deaf students (hearing losses greater than 95 dB in the speech range) between the same ages, and 240 normally hearing subjects between the ages of 3 years and 5 years 11 months. The reliability coefficients were based on test–retest procedures for 20 hearing–impaired subjects retested after a 2-month interval and resulted in coefficients of .96 for the prompted (or production) task and .95 for the imitation task. Test–retest reliability for a sample of 26 children with normal hearing resulted in correlations of .82 for the prompted task and .81 for the imitation task. Statistical validity was demonstrated by correlations with external tests assessing both receptive and expressive skills. The correlations with tests assessing receptive skills ranged from .45 to .68. Correlations with tests assessing expressive skills ranged from .83 to .87. The tests utilized for validity purposes included subtests of the Illinois Test of Psycholinguistic Abilities, the Northwestern Syntax Screening Test, the

Peabody Picture Vocabulary Test, and the Test for Auditory Comprehension of Language.

Berko Morphology Test. The Berko Morphology Test (Berko, 1958) was designed to assess children's knowledge of the morphological structure of English. The test stimuli consist of 27 picture cards with accompanying sentences assessing the morphemes associated with plurals, singular and plural possessives, past tense, present progressive, and derivational morphemes. The test also contains 14 compound words for which the subjects were to provide an explanation. For example, students' would be presented with a stimulus such as "A birthday is called a birthday because ____ " and they would be expected to provide an explanation.

The 27 pictured stimuli are represented by the most frequently cited example of an item from the Berko test. The item consists of a picture of an animal with birdlike characteristics. Underneath the picture of one of these creatures is another picture depicting two of them. The examiner states "This is a wug. Now there is another one. There are two of them. There are two ____ ." The students are to provide the appropriate form of the missing nonsense word. The test stimuli were, therefore, closely controlled; the students were not however, constrained by a choice of words they should provide for their responses.

Berko did not publish any norms for her test; she did, however, provide percentages of correct responses for preschool and first-grade children. One could, therefore, compare a student's obtained results with these scores. The potential user of this assessment procedure should be aware that Berko's sample consisted only of 56 children unevenly divided among seven age levels ranging from 4 to 7 years in 6-month increments. There were, for example, only 14 subjects between the ages of 4 years and 5 years 6 months (preschool age) but 42 subjects between the ages of 6 and 7 years (first-grade age). Furthermore, one should be aware of the fact that as few as two test stimuli assess some of the morphological features identified as areas of interest by the test developer.

The Berko Test of Morphology was slightly modified and published as the Exploratory Test of Grammar (Berry & Talbot, 1966). The primary modifications consisted of increasing the number of pictorial stimuli from 27 to 30 and changing the age ranges assessed from 4–7 to 5–8 years. The limitations associated with the Berko test remain, however, with this test. Approximately 60% of the items on the Exploratory Test of Grammar assess plural nouns and past tense verb forms while only 40% of the items assess factors such as third-person singulars, possessives, derived adjectives, comparatives and superlatives, diminutives, and the progressive aspect.

Adaptations of these procedures have been used to assess hearing–impaired children's knowledge of the morphological rules of English. The adaptations consisted of presenting the linguistic stimuli in visual modes such as writing and forms of manual communication instead of orally. The results have been reported by Cooper (1967), Perlman (1973), and Raffin (1976).

Northwestern Syntax Screening Test. The Northwestern Syntax Screening Test, developed by Lee (1969) for use with children between the ages of 3 years and 7 years 11 months, contains items assessing children's expressive and receptive skills. Both parts of the test include items that assess prepositions, personal pronouns, noun–verb agreements, tense, possessives, present progressives, and Wh-questions. Items are also included that assess active and passive voice constructions. The expressive portion of the test is based on an imitation task. The subject is shown 20 pairs of contrasting pictures with accompanying sentences. For example, pictures of two babies, one awake and one sleeping, would be presented with the examiner stating "The baby is sleeping. The baby is not sleeping. Now, what's this picture?" At this point the examiner is pointing to one of the two pictures with the expectation that the subject will imitate the appropriate sentence associated with the picture. Failures to imitate the stimulus sentences, even though the student's responses may be grammatically correct, are counted as errors for the expressive portion of the test.

The receptive portion of the test consists of 20 items. Each item has four pictures with stimulus sentences designed to assess the structure under consideration. For prepositions, therefore, the examiner, with the appropriate pictures would say, "On one of these pictures the cat is behind the chair, on another, the cat is under the chair. Now show me The cat is behind the chair." This would be followed by having the student also point to the picture associated with the second stimulus sentence.

Although norms have been provided for children between the ages of 3 years and 7 years 11 months, it should be noted that approximately 47% of the subjects were in the 5-year-old age range and that the other 1-year age spans contained only 10 to 18% of the total sample. All of the subjects were selected from middle to upper income families from the midwest who used standard American dialects. Also, none of the subjects demonstrated any handicapping conditions. These limitations, in addition to the fact that the author did not address the issues of reliability and validity in the test manual, should be kept in mind by the test user. It should also be emphasized that Lee (1969) has strongly indicated that the instrument was designed to be used only for the screening of syntactic skills in young children and that, in order to gain more in depth knowledge of the students' syntactic skills or of other linguistic phenomena, one would need to employ other assessment instruments. The use of this test with hearing–impaired children has been discussed by Presnell (1973).

Test for Auditory Comprehension of Language. The Test for Auditory Comprehension of Language, originally developed by Carrow in 1968, is designed to measure the developmental comprehension of language structures when presented orally and to diagnose language comprehension deficits. The test consists of both an English and a Spanish version and contains 101 items each with three line drawings. The examiner reads the stimulus for the item to the examinee and the examinee is asked to point to the picture which depicts the stimulus spoken by the examiner. Although the test is not timed, Carrow (1973) estimates the time required for administration to be approximately 20 minutes. The test assesses children's comprehension of four broad language areas which include (1) vocabulary, (2) morphology, (3) grammar, and (4) syntax. The vocabulary section contains 52 items assessing nouns, adjectives, verbs, adverbs, demonstratives, prepositions, and interrogatives. The morphology section consists of nine items assessing the English derivational suffixes -er associated with nouns and verbs, the -er and -est associated with adjectives, and -ist, associated with nouns as in the word pianist. The grammar section includes 28 items that assess categories such as number, gender, tense, and voice as opposed to the syntax section which includes 12 items which assess imperatives, noun–verb agreement, complementation, modification, and coordination. The test has undergone five revisions since its original publication and the latest revision (Carrow, 1973) contains descriptive data on the use of the test with hearing–impaired children.

The fifth edition of the test (Carrow, 1973) was normed on 200 middle-class black, Anglo, and Mexican-American children between the ages of 3 and 6 years. The test manual indicates that the "results from the three ethnic groups were collapsed because studies comparing Test for Auditory Comprehension of Language performance of middle-class children from the three groups have indicated no significant differences among them" (p. 23). Carrow (1973) demonstrated the validity of the instrument in three ways. First, as the subjects increased in age they also increased in their performance on the test. Second, the test discriminates between individuals with known language disorders and those with no disorders, and third, individuals with language disorders also demonstrated positive changes in their performance as they increased in age.

The primary reliability data were collected in 1971 and were based on 51 students (25 were Mexican-American). The test–retest results for the English version yielded a reliability coefficient of .94. Thirty-two Mexican-American children were given the Spanish version of the test on two occasions resulting in a test–retest coefficient of .93. For both versions of the test the retest was given after an interval of 2 weeks. Carrow (1973) also reported on a study by Jones (1972) in which the Kuder–Richardson internal consistency reliability coefficient was calculated on the performances of middle and lower class black and Anglo children. The KR–20 reliability coefficient was .77.

Carrow Elicited Language Inventory. The Carrow Elicited Language Inventory utilizes an elicited imitation task to measure "a child's productive control of grammar" (Carrow, 1974, p. 4). The procedure is based on the idea that children's imitations of adult utterances will reflect the children's grammar if sufficient stress has been put on their immediate memory capabilities (Slobin & Welsh, 1973; Smith, 1970).

The test stimuli consist of 51 sentences and one phrase ranging in length from 2 to 10 words. Of the 51 sentences, 47 are presented in the active voice and 4 in the passive voice. Thirty-seven of the stimulus sentences are affirmative and fourteen are negative. Additionally, of the 51 sentences, 37 are declarative, 12 are interrogative, and two are imperative. The grammatical features assessed by the test include a wide variety of articles, adjectives, nouns, pronouns, verbs, negatives, contractions, adverbs, prepositions, demonstratives, and conjunctions. According to the test manual the Carrow Elicited Language Inventory should take one about 45 minutes to administer and score. The task involves the examinee's imitations of the stimulus sentences as spoken by the examiner. The examiner records all of the deviations from the stimulus sentences and categorizes them into five error types: substitutions, omissions, additions, transpositions, and reversals.

The CELI was standardized in 1973 on 475 white children attending day-care centers and church schools in Houston, Texas. The children were between the ages of 3 years and 7 years 11 months and came from middle socioeconomic homes where standard American English was the sole language spoken. Percentile ranks and stanine scores are provided for each age level. One should, however, cautiously interpret the normative scores for children who do not have the characteristics of the children in the normative sample.

Carrow (1974) demonstrated the reliability of the CELI using test–retest and interexaminer techniques. The test–retest procedure was based on 25 children (5 each at the ages of 3, 4, 5, 6, and 7) who were given the test again after a period of 2 weeks. The resulting correlation coefficient was .98. The two interexaminer tests resulted in coefficients of .98 and .99.

The validity of the CELI was demonstrated through concurrent and congruent validity procedures. The concurrent procedures consisted of demonstrating, first, that the scores of the standardization sample did significantly increase with age and, second, that the instrument does differentiate between children with normal language and those with disordered language. Congruent validity was demonstrated by comparing the CELI with the Developmental Sentence Scoring techniques reported by Lee and Canter (1971). Significant correlations were found between the two instruments.

It should be stressed again that, of the tests discussed in this section, only the TSA and the GAEL were normed on hearing–impaired populations. This is not to suggest that the other instruments should not be used; on the contrary, the information one can gain from using these techniques and methods may well be useful as one determines a particular child's manner in dealing with the linguistic principles being assessed by these tests. One does, however, need to be aware of the limitations in using the normative information on these tests with hearing–impaired children.

Free methods

All investigators of language behaviors are interested in those aspects of language that individuals will spontaneously produce. The data collection procedures usually incorporate the recording of a large corpus of utterances (at least 50 to 100) collected in as naturalistic a setting as possible. The data are then subjected to analyses by the examiner.

Strengths and limitations

The primary advantage of using these procedures lies in the fact that if a child consistently produces a language behavior one can legitimately assume that the child knows that aspect of language. This fact alone is sufficient rationale for utilizing free methods of data collection. There is, additionally, a general strength and weakness associated with analyses of spontaneously generated language samples—the data are analyzed from an idiosyncratic point of view. The strength lies in the fact that the interpretation is based on the student's own linguistic features in comparison with other students' language productions rather than with percentile or age and grade equivalent scores. The weakness lies in the small comparison sample from which one must make a decision. The comparison sample generally consists of only two or three subjects.

There are, additionally, several limitations associated with these techniques. A prime factor for consideration is the size of the language sample. If the corpus is small there is a distinct possibility that one will underestimate the child's actual language competence. If this should occur then the investigator has not measured what he or she intended to measure and, thus, cannot demonstrate the validity of the procedure. Second, it is more difficult to estimate the reliability of the measures utilizing free methods. It is obviously impossible to demonstrate reliability for these procedures with equivalent forms, test–retest, or internal consistency coefficients. Those who use these procedures have, therefore, developed the concepts of inter- and intrarater reliability coefficients. A third major factor involves the amount of subjectivity that could be present in analyses of the data. The danger of "reading into the data" those factors which one wants to find is much more present with these methods than for the more controlled methods. To alleviate this potential most analysis procedures require extensive training of those who will perform the analyses.

There are additional limitations associated with these techniques that are specific to their use with hearing impaired individuals. First, with many profoundly deaf individuals, an auditory recording of their utterances would not be sufficient. There is the likelihood that their speech would be unintelligible. The result would be, therefore, the absence of data to analyze. There is also the likelihood that their utterances would be conveyed through the medium of sign. It is suggested, therefore, that investigators use video recordings when working with hearing impaired individuals. Second, many investigators have substituted the collection of spoken or signed utterances by deaf individuals with collections of written language samples. Although one can learn much useful information through analyses of written productions, one is, in essence, examining different language behaviors. Also, the written productions of individuals (deaf or hearing) are generally more limited in scope than their spoken or signed utterances.

Traditional grammar analysis procedures

The analysis procedures discussed in this section of the chapter have been traditionally used to compare the written language of deaf students to that of hearing students. These procedures can be classified under five headings, first suggested by Cooper and Rosenstein in 1966. These headings are productivity, complexity, flexibility, distribution of parts of speech, and grammatical correctness.

Productivity. Two measures of productivity have been used by Heider and Heider (1940), Simmons (1963), and Myklebust (1960). The first measure, the average number of words written in an essay, failed to discriminate between the essays written by the deaf students and the hearing students. The second measure, the mean length of the sentences in the essays, did, however, discriminate between the two groups, with the deaf students writing shorter sentences.

Complexity. Three measures have been used as indices of the complexity of written language samples. Heider and Heider (1940) used two of these measures. The first is the ratio of simple sentences to compound, complex, and compound-complex sentences and is calculated simply by dividing the number of simple sentences by the number of compound sentences, followed by dividing the number of simple sentences by the number of complex sentences and then the number of compound-complex sentences. Heider and Heider (1940) reported, on the basis of these measures, that deaf students wrote more simple sentences than the hearing students. The second measure, the subordination ratio, (the number of subordinate clauses per main clause) produced the same general results—deaf children use fewer subordinate clauses than hearing children.

Hunt's (1965) index of complexity, the T-unit, was defined as "one main clause plus all the subordinate clauses attached to or embedded in it" (p. 141). Taylor (1969) utilized the measures associated with the T-unit and found that deaf children did show appreciable gains in their abilities to use the more complex structures of English as they increased in age. This, with the findings of Marshall and Quigley (1970), indicated that the T-unit was a good indicator of the development of linguistic complexity.

Flexibility. Simmons (1963) and Tervoort (1967) used the type–token ratio described by Templin (1957) as a measure of vocabulary diversity. This ratio is calculated by dividing the total number of different words by the total number of words from a 50-utterance sample. When this measure was applied to the written language samples of deaf and hearing children Simmons (1963) found that the ratio for the deaf children was significantly lower than that for the hearing children. Tervoort (1967) reported, however, that the type–token ratio increased with age indicating that deaf children, as they grow older, exhibit a greater degree of vocabulary diversity.

Distribution of parts of speech. Myklebust (1960) and Simmons (1963) measured students' usages of the different parts of speech by dividing the number of occurrences of a particular part of speech (nouns, for example) by the total number of words in an essay. Both studies indicated that the deaf subjects display a higher percentage of nouns and determiners in their essays than do hearing students. In like manner, they display a lower percentage of prepositions, adjectives, adverbials, and conjunctions.

Correctness. Two approaches have been used to describe what has been traditionally referred to as "errors" or "deviations" from standard English usage. The first approach has been of little use from an educational viewpoint and consists merely of frequency counts for the types of errors one encounters in the essays written by deaf students. This approach has been used by Thompson (1936), Myklebust (1960), and Perry (1968). Their results indicate that the most frequently occurring errors in the essays of deaf students consists of omissions of necessary words followed by substitutions of wrong words, additions of unnecessary words, and errors in word order.

The second approach, described by Taylor (1969), has been much more informative. She, like previous researchers, also reported on the frequencies of the types of errors made by the subjects in her sample. However, she also described "the rules violated in the production of any deviant or nongrammatical structures" (p. 45). As an example of her analysis procedures the results of her analyses of omissions of direct objects in the essays of deaf students at the third- , fifth- , seventh- , and ninth-grade levels are presented. She found, as had Thompson (1936), Myklebust (1960), and Perry (1968), that deaf students frequently omitted direct objects. However, when she analyzed this phenomenon in terms of the environments in which omissions of direct objects occurred at the different grade levels she found that the direct object omissions at the third-grade level consisted, primarily, in simple sentences containing transitive verbs. At the fifth- and seventh-grade levels, however, omissions of direct objects occurred most frequently in conjoined sentences. At the ninth-grade level the students produced fewer omissions of direct objects in conjoined sentences, but their use of more complicated structures led to omissions in complementized structures. Thus, even though the frequency of occurrence of direct object omissions did not decrease between the different grade levels, the analyses of the environments in which they occurred did indicate that the students' levels of syntactic complexity were increasing.

Current analysis procedures

More currently used analysis procedures for spontaneously generated language samples include the Mean Length of Utterance (Brown, 1973), Developmental Sentence Types (Lee, 1966; 1974), Developmental Sentence Scoring (Lee

& Canter, 1971), the Bloom and Lahey approach, (Bloom & Lahey, 1978), the Teacher Assessment of Grammatical Structure, (Moog & Kozak, 1983), and the Kretschmer Spontaneous Language Analysis procedure (1978). It should be emphasized again that each of these procedures was designed primarily for analyses of spoken utterances. The results obtained from analyses of written essays using these techniques should not, therefore, be taken as indicative of the students' primary expressive language skills.

Mean length of utterance. The MLU is calculated by determining the average number of morphemes per utterance in a sample of 100 utterances. A morpheme is, of course, the minimal unit of meaning in language. Thus, the word *cats* consists of two morphemes—the word *cat* and the *s* which indicates plurality. The procedures for calculating the MLU have been described in detail by Brown (1973); the following rules should, however, be followed in any determination of MLU.

1. All compound words and proper names count as single morphemes.
2. All irregular past tense verbs count as one morpheme.
3. All auxiliaries (can, must, should) and inflectional morphemes (possessives, plurals, third-person singulars, regular past tense verb endings, and progressive aspect endings) count as separate morphemes.

The MLU has been shown to be a good index of syntactic development for children with MLUs of five or less. In speech samples with MLUs greater than five, however, conjoined structures become more frequent and one could credit a child with a much higher MLU than his/her language development merited. Miller (1981) has reported on predicted chronological ages from the MLU for normally hearing children. One could, therefore, compare the results of MLU for deaf children with the data Miller has provided.

Blackwell et al. (1978) noted four problems associated with the use of the MLU. First, length of utterance measures obscure differences in syntactic and semantic complexity. Second, the MLU does not provide an investigator with any information regarding children's functional use of language. The third problem mentioned by Blackwell et al. (1978) relates specifically to the analysis of language samples from hearing–impaired children. Brown (1973) described qualitative syntactic and semantic differences associated with each of his five stages based on the MLU measure. One cannot, however, assume that a deaf child with a MLU of 2.3 (placing the child in Brown's Stage II) would display the same linguistic features as a normally hearing child at the same stage of development.

Developmental Sentence Types. The Developmental Sentence Types (DST) procedure was first proposed by Lee (1966) and revised in 1974 to assess the "pre-sentence" stage of language development. It is suggested for use only when less than 50% of a child's utterances contain both a subject and a predicate. If more than 50% of a child's utterances contain both a subject and a predicate then the Developmental Sentence Scoring system (Lee & Canter, 1971, Lee, 1974) should be used.

After the language sample has been collected (remember that spontaneously generated language samples should consist of at least 50 utterances) one can check the types of utterances produced by the child on a chart containing three horizontal dimensions and five vertical dimensions. The three horizontal levels consist of single words, two-word combinations, and multiword constructions. The vertical dimensions consist of noun phrases, designative phrases, predicative sentences, subject–verb sentences, and fragments. Kretschmer and Kretschmer (1978) have pointed out that a major shortcoming of the DST analysis procedures is that they are based on the unwarranted assumption that children first learn simple, active, affirmative, declarative sentences and then learn to apply transformations to these sentences.

Developmental Sentence Scoring. The Developmental Sentence Scoring (DSS) analysis procedures can be used, as previously stated, when more than 50% of a child's utterances contain a subject and a predicate. The procedures for the DSS analysis have been described in detail by Lee (1974) and Lee and Canter (1971). In general, however, 50 utterances are scored for eight grammatical categories including indefinite pronouns or noun modifiers, personal pronouns, main verbs, secondary verbs, negatives, conjunctions, interrogative reversals and Wh-questions. A scale of 1 to 8 points was developed to assess these eight categories. For example, first- and second-person pronouns are given a score of 1 and pronouns such as *oneself* are given a score of 7. The total number of points for the 50 sentences are then added and divided by 50 and the resultant score can be compared with norms for children between the ages of 2 to 6 years, 11 months. These procedures, like those of the Developmental Sentence Types, exclude pragmatic and semantic considerations.

Bloom and Lahey approach. This approach has been described in great detail by Bloom and Lahey in 1978. The procedures focus on semantic and syntactic (content and form) features. Bloom and Lahey (1978) identified 21 semantic features that interact in a hierarchical manner with 8 syntactic categories labeled as phases in the Bloom and Lahey protocol. Thus, Phases 1 and 2, which correspond roughly to one- and two-word utterances (Phase 1 utterances have MLU values of less than 1.2 and Phase 2 utterances have MLU values of less than 1.5), contain the semantic features of existence, nonexistence, recurrence, rejection, denial, attribution, possession, action, and locative action. Phase 3 utterances (MLU values less than 2.0) include the semantic features in Phase 1 and 2 and add the features of locative state, state, and quantity. Phase 4 utterances which correspond to MLU values of less than 2.5 add the semantic features of notice and time and Phase 5 utterances (MLU values of less than 3.0) add the features of coordinate, causality, dative, and specifier. Phases 6 through 8, while not corresponding to any specific MLU values, are identified as complex sentences, syntactic connectives, and modal verbs, and relative clauses, respectively. The semantic features added to Phase 6 through 8 include epistemic, mood, and antithesis. The reader is directed to Bloom and Lahey (1978) for descriptions and definitions of each of these 21 semantic categories.

Although the focus of this analysis procedure is primarily on content and form, the authors have also specified cognitive goals that are precursors of language development and pragmatic (use) goals that develop concurrently with the semantic and syntactic features. One can, therefore, utilizing these analytic procedures, gain a rather complete view of a child's language development. There is, however, one primary obstacle to these procedures—the time required for the collection of the language sample (Bloom & Lahey recommend a corpus of 200 utterances) and the time required for the subsequent analysis.

Teacher assessment of grammatical structures. These rating forms for analyzing spontaneous language productions of deaf children were developed by Moog and Kozak (1983) to serve as companions to the GAEL tests discussed in the section on Controlled Methods in this chapter. There are, therefore, Teacher Assessment of Grammatical Structures (TAGS) forms for the presentence level (TAGS-P), the simple sentence level (TAGS-S), and the complex sentence level (TAGS-C) to correspond with the equivalent levels for the GAEL tests. As the title indicates, teachers should be able to complete the rating forms for the students in their classrooms. The ratings suggested for use indicate whether the students have acquired or are in the process of acquiring the structures under consideration. Additionally, one can, using the rating format, specify which of the structures will serve as objectives for the teacher's language development program. The authors of the TAGS procedures have also specified levels of competence for each of the structures under consideration. With the exception of the presentence level, which also includes comprehension as a level of competence, each of the rating forms contains levels of imitated, prompted, and spontaneous productions.

Each of the TAGS procedures consists of analyses of six grammatical categories. The TAGS-P, which was designed for hearing–impaired children up to the age of 6 years, contains the grammatical categories of single words, two-word combinations, three-word combinations, Wh-questions, pronouns, and tense markers. The TAGS-S includes noun modifiers, pronouns, prepositions, adverbs, verbs, and questions as the grammatical categories for analysis. Each of these six categories is also broken down into six levels of development ranging from the simpler aspects of the structure to the more complex. The TAGS-S was designed for hearing–impaired children between the ages of 5 and 9 years. The TAGS-C was designed for hearing–impaired children beyond the age of 8 years and includes the grammatical categories of nouns, pronouns, verb inflections, secondary verbs, conjunctions, and questions. These six categories are also divided into six levels indicating increasing syntactic complexity.

Kretschmer spontaneous language analysis procedure. The most comprehensive analysis procedure developed to date for the purpose of investigating freely generated language samples of hearing–impaired students are those described by Kretschmer and Kretschmer (1978). These procedures can be used for spoken or signed utterances as well as with written language samples.

The technique is similar to that of the Bloom and Lahey approach previously described with these major exceptions. First, the Kretschmer analysis procedures are not dependent on the quantitative measure of MLU. Second, Kretschmer's treatment of semantic categories is more extensive, and third, the system provides one with strategies to describe atypical language performances of hearing–impaired individuals.

The analysis protocol consists of six sections. Section 1 provides the examiner with descriptive information on the preverbal level of the student. Section 2 provides information to help the examiner tally syntactic and semantic features for the one- and two-word stage. Section 3 provides syntactic and semantic descriptors for single prepositions and Section 4 provides syntactic descriptions for complex sentences. Section 5 of the analysis protocol focuses on the communication competence of the child and Section 6 assists the examiner in isolating those structures which differ from standard English usage.

Although one can provide a rather complete analysis of a child's language by using this technique, there are two primary limitations to its use. The first is the factor of time—it takes a considerable amount of time for one to analyze a child's language sample using this procedure. The second potential limitation is the amount of linguistic knowledge the examiner must possess to provide an adequate analysis. Many teachers, unfortunately, do not possess this knowledge. As Kretschmer and Kretschmer (1978) have indicated "The study of contemporary linguistics, psycholinguistics, and child language must be pursued in formal and informal settings with assistance from persons knowledgeable in language description. Anyone seriously interested in teaching deaf children or learning to productively analyse their language difficulties should follow this course" (p. 175).

INSTRUCTION PROCEDURES

Language assessment, as the previous section has indicated, should serve as the basis for the language goals and objectives one should pursue in the classroom. In the same way that assessment can be considered the cornerstone of an instructional program, the goals and objectives one pursues in a language program can be considered as the bricks (building blocks) of the program. This is especially true for profoundly, prelingually deaf individuals since their sensory deficits have largely deprived them of the means by which they can naturally develop their language and communication skills. Educators of hearing–impaired individuals have, therefore, an extraordinary challenge— the challenge to provide language instructional materials and techniques that will provide the building blocks for effective communication. In this section of the chapter are presented the results of a recent survey (King, 1983) which indicates the materials and techniques currently in use, and a brief description of those most often utilized. The reader should, however, refer to chapter 1 on Definitions and Historical Perspectives in this volume for a discussion of less recent techniques utilized for teaching language to deaf individuals for two reasons. First, the discussion on the uses of natural versus grammatical or structural methods which originated centuries ago (Schmitt, 1966) still persist, and second, some of the materials and techniques discussed in chapter 1 are still being used.

Survey of language methods and materials

In February of 1982 King (1983) sent questionnaires to 576 programs serving hearing–impaired students throughout the United States seeking information on the materials and techniques they use in their language programs. Although several investigators (Schmitt, 1966; Kretschmer & Kretschmer, 1978; Moores, 1978; Levine, 1981) have provided descriptions of the various methods and philosophies, King's survey is the first generally available report since 1949 describing the extent of their usage in classrooms throughout the country. The results of the survey discussed in this section focus on (1) general approaches to language instruction, (2) the use of metalinguistic symbol systems in language instruction, and (3) research needs as perceived by the respondents.

Approaches to language instruction

King (1983), in her questionnaire, asked the respondents to indicate whether their approaches to language instruction could be described as structural, natural, combined, or eclectic. The definitions she provided for these terms follow:

Structural approaches. The study of grammar and syntax is important in the teaching of language. Frequently, some symbol system is used to represent the structure of language. Other names for this method include scientific, formal, logical, analytical, and systematic.

Natural approaches. The emphasis is on the development of colloquial and idiomatic language. Symbol systems to represent the structure of language are not used. Other names for this method include mother tongue, informal, synthetic, and developmental.

Combined approaches. This approach combines aspects of the structural approaches and the natural approaches. The relative use of structural or natural methods varies from program to program.

Eclectic approaches. The approach to language instruction (structural, natural, or combined) is left to the individual teacher and may vary from classroom to classroom within the same program.

It is interesting to note that at all levels (preschool, primary, intermediate, junior high, and high school) combined approaches were used most frequently with percentages ranging from 36.3 at the preschool level to 55.9 at the intermediate level. However, it was only at the preschool level that a significant number of respondents indicated that natural approaches were used (34.1%). The percentage of programs reporting usage of natural approaches at the other levels ranged from 1.5 at the junior high level to 6.2 at the primary level.

Within the exclusion of the preschool level, the second most frequently reported approach was the eclectic approach with percentages ranging from 27.3 at the primary level to 39.4 at the high school level. It is also interesting to note, in light of this data, that only 53% of the respondents indicated that their programs had a stated philosophy regarding language instruction.

Use of metalinguistic symbol systems

The data provided above indicate that the majority of the programs utilize metalinguistic symbols for language instruction. Metalinguistic symbols refer to symbols such as NP, VP, subject, predicate, or other symbols and words to describe language. Further analyses of the responses to King's question-naire reveal that the average age at which children are introduced to a symbol system for the purposes of production of sentences is 6.65 years. The average age at which they are introduced to the systems for the purposes of sentence analysis and correction is 8.9 years.

In this category, as in the language approaches utilized, the preschool level programs differ from the other levels. Approximately 65% of the preschool programs indicated that they seldom (19.4%) or never (45.2%) used symbol systems in their language instruction. This is in contrast to a mean percentage rate of 57.4 for programs at the other levels that use symbol systems either very frequently or frequently. The most frequently reported symbol systems in use include sentence patterns (particularly the Apple Tree Sentence Patterns), parts of speech, names of syntactic structures, and the Fitzgerald key.

Research needs

The identification of research and materials development needs by educators reflects not only the needs of the profession but, also, the areas in which they believe their approaches are most lacking. The data collected by King in this area is unequivocal—the three most highly ranked areas (again, with the exception of the preschool level) were discourse (paragraph/story cohesion), turn-taking and conversational skills, and pragmatics. The three most highly ranked areas at the preschool level consisted of phonetics, discourse, and pragmatics.

Description of language methods and materials

In this portion of the chapter are presented descriptions of selected methods and materials developed for hearing–impaired students since 1970. It should be stressed that the language methods described herein should be considered as reflective of an overall philosophy toward language instruction. The language materials, on the other hand, were designed to meet specific goals and objectives of broader programs of instruction for hearing–impaired individuals. One should not, therefore, depend exclusively on any set of materials for one's language program. To illustrate this point, the author of Apple Tree (Anderson et al., 1980), which King's survey (1983) indicated was one of the most widely used set of materials, wrote in the Teacher's manual that "the program does not attend to all aspects of communication and should not be considered the sum total of the child's language needs. Any complete language program would encompass a natural language approach, using Apple Tree as an important part of classroom instruction" (p. vii). Similar statements have also been made by each of the authors of the other materials described in this chapter.

Language methods

Maternal reflective method. This method, described by van Uden (1977), is basically a natural approach toward language instruction with elements of the structural approach. It is natural in the sense that van Uden stresses development of the "mother tongue" ("the language first learnt by the speaker as a child" p. 93) through oral conversational methods based on children's experiences. He sharply criticizes the use of "constructive" methods which are characterized by contrived experiences and language patterning. Children, he would argue, do not learn questioning techniques by being given isolated sentences such as "The box is on the table" and being asked to produce Wh-questions based on those sentences. They do, however, learn language by participating in dialogue that is meaningful and by listening to the conversations of others. Teachers of deaf children should, therefore, not only engage in meaningful dialogue with their students but should, also, direct the attention of their students to the conversations of others.

One might assume, given this description of the maternal reflective method, that one needs only to talk with deaf children. The importance of talking with one's students should not be diminished; however, van Uden emphasizes that teachers must take advantage of conversational opportunities to direct the students' attention to linguistic principles they are endeavoring to teach. Additionally, there are definite structural aspects to van Uden's approach. These aspects constitute the reflective portion of the approach. Students should, for example, be able to identify the intonation patterns of sentences, their constituent structures, their underlying semantic propositions, the transformations involved in the analysis of the sentences, and errors which they may have made in the production of the sentences.

Rhode Island Curriculum. The Rhode Island Curriculum was designed by Blackwell et al. (1978) for students at the Rhode Island School for the Deaf. It is, primarily, a structural approach based on the assumptions of early transformational–generative grammar theory (Chomsky, 1957). In terms of linguistic principles, the students are first introduced to five sentence patterns (kernel sentences) as shown in Table 5. There are basically three levels of the curriculum. The first is designed for children at the preschool and kindergarten levels and consists of activities for exposure, recognition, comprehension, production, and writing of the linguistic principles. The second (simple sentence stage) and third (complex sentence stage) levels include activities for each of the areas identified for Level 1 with the addition of

TABLE 5. SENTENCE PATTERNS AND EXAMPLES FOR THE RHODE ISLAND CURRICULUM

Sentence Pattern	Example
NP + V	The bird flies.
NP_1 + V + NP_2	The bird eats worms.
NP + LV + Adjective	The bird is small.
NP + LV + NP	The bird is a sparrow.
NP + LV + Adverbial	The bird is in the nest.

activities for sentence analysis. Although syntax serves as the unifying factor of the linguistic portion of the curriculum it should be noted that Blackwell et al. (1978) have made provisions in their approach for the cognitive, semantic, and pragmatic development of students.

Blackwell and his associates have also made provision for the coordination of the language goals of the curriculum with their content area goals. Language is not, therefore, to be taught in isolation. Since language must be used to impart information in social studies, mathematics, science, health, and other content areas it is only natural that teachers should consider not only their students' abilities to understand the content but, also, their abilities to understand the language through which the information is transmitted. The way in which Blackwell et al. (1978) have coordinated these areas could serve as a model for other curriculum development projects.

Language materials

Two sets of materials, Apple Tree (Anderson et al., 1980) and the TSA Syntax Program (Quigley & Power, 1979) are described in this section. These were selected for inclusion since their scope is sufficiently broad that some institutions (despite admonitions to the contrary) will utilize them as sole components in a language curriculum.

Apple Tree. Apple Tree, which is an acronym for A Patterned Program of Linguistic Expansion through Reinforced Experiences and Evaluations, consists of six workbooks and a teacher's manual designed to teach the 10 sentence patterns depicted in Table 6. The authors, Anderson et al. (1980), have also developed a pre- and posttest booklet to accompany the materials. The exercises in the workbooks consist of comprehension, manipulation, substitution, production, and transformation activities. The only transformations that are presented, however, are negation and question forms. As a supplement to the basic Apple Tree materials a series of 30 short story books—three for each of the 10 sentence patterns have been developed. All of the stories are written

TABLE 6. SENTENCE PATTERNS AND EXAMPLES FOR APPLE TREE

Sentence Pattern	Example
$N_1 + V_{(be)} + \text{Adjective}$	The boy is short.
$N_1 + V_{(be)} + \text{Where}$	The girls are in school.
$N_1 + V_{(be)} + N_1$	I am a student.
$N_1 + V$	The boy is running.
$N_1 + V + \text{Where}$	The children are running to school.
$N_1 + V + \text{Where} + \text{When}$	Mother went to work this morning.
$N_1 + V + N_2$	The boy bought a car.
$N_1 + V + N_2 + \text{Where}$	The boys took their bats to the game.
$N_1 + V + N_2 + \text{Where} + \text{When}$	I will take my wife to the doctor tonight.
$N_1 + V + N_3 + N_2$	Bobby gave me a toy.

only in the sentence structures depicted in Table 6. There is, additionally, another set of 10 workbooks called *Fun Pages* which were designed to provide supplemental activities for each of the 10 sentence structures. This approach toward language instruction is, obviously, structural; in order to successfully complete the exercises contained in the workbooks the students must know and understand the metalinguistic terminology utilized throughout the materials.

TSA syntax program. This set of materials, edited by Quigley and Power (1979), was designed to aid students in the comprehension and production of the syntactic structures listed in Table 4. Included in the set are nine teacher's manuals (one for each of the major structures assessed by the TSA) and 20 workbooks (one for each of the linguistic components assessed by individual tests of the TSA). The teacher's guides provide descriptions of the structures, information on the acquisition of those structures by both deaf and hearing students, objectives for teaching the nine structures, diagnostic guides for assessing students' performances on the TSA, and suggestions for additional activities to reinforce the students' learning of the structures. The 20 workbooks consist of linear programmed activities for individual components of the structures. The students do not, however, need a knowledge of metalinguistic terminology to complete the exercises.

In addition to these materials Quigley and King (1981, 1982, 1983, 1984) have developed a set of reading materials (Reading Milestones) that systematically introduce increasingly difficult syntactic structures and vocabulary. The series consist of eight levels. Each level contains 10 readers, 10 workbooks, and a teacher's guide.

The TSA Syntax Program and Reading Milestones are based on a large body of information gained by research conducted by Quigley and his associates between 1968 and 1978. This is certainly one of the major strengths of these materials. One should, however, be aware of the limitations of the TSA Syntax Program. First, the activities of a programmed instruction format may not readily generalize to spontaneous productions of the same structures the student has been manipulating. For this reason, the authors of the materials suggested more natural activities in the teacher's guides which may assist in the generalization process. The second limitation is that the materials were designed only for the syntactic component of English. One should, therefore, use these materials, as Quigley and Power (1979) have indicated, only as supplements to language programs which are broader in scope.

SUMMARY

In this chapter the importance of establishing the critical concerns of reliability and validity for any assessment tool or technique has been emphasized. Although different procedures for ascertaining reliability and validity have been discussed for the different tests and techniques it is essential that examiners verify through the techniques most appropriate for their assessment procedures the precision of their instruments. If they find that they can, indeed, depend on the consistency of their measures then they must also verify through either statistical, content, or construct validity that they are indeed measuring what they intended to measure. In fact, if all evaluators would insist on verification of any test or technique they utilized two primary benefits would ensue. First, the information gained from the testing would always be useful and second, much unessential testing would be eliminated. In other words, evaluators would cease the practice of utilizing particular tests or techniques merely because they were available or because they had always been used.

Controlled and free methods of data collection were then discussed. The strengths and limitations of each were presented and representative samples of each type of test and technique were briefly described. It should be obvious to the reader that no one test or procedure can provide one with the comprehensive knowledge of students' language behaviors one desires. The controlled methods usually provide one with very detailed information on some aspect of language behavior as exemplified by the Test of Syntactic Abilities (Quigley et al., 1978). Tests such as these are frequently criticized because they do not provide the users with a global prespective of their students' language skills. It should be remembered, however, that the narrow focus of tests such as these makes it possible for the test users to isolate students' specific language problems associated with the variables of interest and thus plan very detailed remediation procedures.

The free methods discussed in this chapter provide one with the data to ascertain whether language behaviors are indeed part of the students' language competence. If a student fails to produce spontaneous utterances representative of particular language phenomena, one cannot assume that the student has not acquired that aspect of language. But, if the student consistently produces some aspect of language one knows that the student has acquired that aspect. Also, analysis procedures such as those designed by Kretschmer and Kretschmer (1978) do enable one to gain a more global view of the students' language since features of the students' syntactic, semantic, and pragmatic skills are part of the analysis protocol.

The central point, therefore, is that one should use combinations of controlled and free methods and a wide variety of tests and techniques. It is only by being knowledgeable about the types of information one can legitimately gain from each that assessment can truly serve its function as the cornerstone for effective and efficient educational practices.

Instructional methods and materials were discussed. Results from King's (1983) survey, which indicated that programs for hearing impaired students use combinations of natural and structural methods for language instruction were discussed and descriptions of selected methods and materials developed since 1970 were presented. These methods and materials were described as the bricks or building blocks of language programs. It is only through thoughtful consideration and application of both assessment and language instructional techniques that one can provide hearing-impaired children with the language and communication skills they need to function efficiently in the general society.

chapter 8

CONCLUSIONS

As stated in chapter 1, more attention needs to be paid to the definitions and classifications of hearing impairment, particularly to what is meant by the term, deaf. In recent years there has been a movement (Ross & Calvert, 1967) to eliminate the term and substitute a range of decibel classifications corresponding to a range of descriptive terms from mild to profound hearing impairment, with profound impairment corresponding roughly to what has been defined in chapter 1 as deaf. The movement is well intentioned in that it seeks to eradicate negative educational attitudes and expectations that have been associated with the term. It also has some research and clinical support in that very few hearing–impaired children fail to respond totally at every frequency and every decibel level in an audiometric examination. There is usually a response at some level to some frequency or frequencies. And a number of investigators (Hudgins, 1954; Ling, 1976; Ling & Ling, 1978) have shown that even very small remnants of hearing can be trained to be functional in speech reception and production. Although teachers of deaf children should be well prepared in these areas, realizing the full potential of amplification and residual hearing probably requires that a qualified audiologist be part of every educational program for deaf children to support and supplement the work of teachers in language and communication development.

Educational and clinical experience have shown, however, that beyond some level of hearing impairment (modified by the interaction of other factors such as IQ and SES) even the best amplification and utilization of residual hearing provide only extremely limited assistance in speech reading and equally limited feedback in speech production. Hearing impairment is certainly a continuum as measured on a decibel scale, but at some point on that continuum an individual ceases to be linked to the world of communication, to any useful extent, primarily by hearing and becomes linked to it primarily by vision. At this point, the term deaf can be usefully applied as distinguishing people who must process language by eye from the vast majority of hearing–

impaired people who can, with appropriate amplification and training, process it by ear. This is a critical distinction and it is not always made. There is an increasing tendency to regard children with hearing impairments from 70 to 90 dB as part of the deaf population when substantial clinical experience and research data show that such children can be trained to process language primarily by ear (Ling, 1976; Ling & Ling 1978).

A good case can be made that any child who can learn to acquire language by ear should be supplied with the program to do so. This is not to denigrate language by eye, but simply to recognize that reading and written language and the whole educational system of most countries are based on auditory language. Language by eye, either in the forms of MCE as a first language or ASL as a first language and an auditory based language such as English as a second language, might be the appropriate procedures for visually oriented (deaf) children, but they raise the difficult question of how the reading of the written language of the general society (any general society) can be taught. As discussed in chapter 4, new ways of teaching reading might have to be developed for deaf children who have MCE or ASL as first languages, since the methods now in use assume the existence of a spoken language.

The point of all this, and of the discussion of definitions of deafness in chapter 1, is that care is needed in classifying hearing–impaired children for educational purposes, and that the term deaf is still useful to distinguish children who must process language primarily by eye from those, whether normally hearing or hearing impaired, who can process it primarily by ear. Also, if spoken English and MCE as it is usually practiced are incompatible (Marmor & Pettito, 1979; Reich & Bick, 1977) for deaf children (roughly 90 dB+), it is likely they are also incompatible for hard-of-hearing children (roughly less than 90 dB). Yet, there has been an increasing tendency to use MCE with hearing–impaired children who are not deaf as defined in this book.

The study of cognitive processes with deaf individuals has produced various answers at various periods to the question of how deaf people perform in comparison to hearing people on a variety of cognitive tasks. The present-day answer seems to be that there is essentially equality of performance for most practical educational and occupational purposes (Furth, 1966b; Rosenstein, 1961; Vernon, 1967). This is somewhat puzzling, however, since close examination of the published research indicates that, whereas deaf individuals tend to exhibit similar developmental orders to hearing individuals on various cognitive tasks, there often is a substantial delay at each stage of development (Quigley & Kretschmer, 1982). Present thinking seems to be that the remaining differences still found would disappear if greater experimental control could be exerted over linguistic factors in supposedly nonverbal cognitive tasks. But the possibility that the differences are real must also be entertained. If the differences discussed in chapter 2 are real, they have obvious educational implications, since adequate language development, both primary and secondary, is dependent on adequate development of such cognitive abilities as perception, attention, and memory.

The cognitive research of most interest in recent years has been the work on the various forms used by deaf individuals for coding linguistic material in short-term memory and the relation of these coding forms to the memory spans and English language abilities of deaf individuals (Conrad, 1979; Lichtenstein, 1983). This work has significant implications for the development of primary and secondary language, and particularly for the development of reading. The research indicates that speech coding is the most efficient means of coding linguistic material in short-term memory and that it is importantly, perhaps essentially, related to the reading of connected discourse. Lichtenstein (1983), in particular, has pointed out the implications of this research for reading and written language and its relation to the repeated findings of lowered performances of deaf people in comparison to hearing people on tasks of temporal–sequential memory. A surprising finding has been that many deaf students who have unintelligible speech nonetheless use speech coding in reading. If speech coding is confirmed as an essential factor in the reading of deaf children, then methods of developing reading different from those presently in use will need to be devised for those deaf children who, for whatever reasons, are unable to develop a speech code. In fact, it might be that reading of the written word is not feasible for some deaf children.

One of the themes of this book is that the primary language development of deaf children can only be considered in terms of the communication form by which it is developed and through which it finds expression. This means that primary language development has to be considered in terms of OE, MCE (including PSE), and ASL. The material in chapter 3 on the primary language of deaf children is organized in this manner. It is obvious from the presentation that there is only a very limited amount of data on primary language development in any of the communication forms. There is also only very limited information on the educational effectiveness of the various communication forms. The most extensive information on that issue is a large-scale retrospective study by Ogden (1979) of the educational and occupational achievement of more than 600 former students of three private oral schools. Even though this was an elite group intellectually and socioeconomically, the educational and occupational achievements were impressive. The educational effectiveness of the other two approaches, MCE and ASL, has not yet been directly evaluated on as large a scale as the Ogden study.

The lack of substantial research evaluation of MCE approaches is surprising, since various forms of MCE are now the dominantly used approaches in the United States and have been for 10 to 15 years (Jordan et al., 1976). The few small-scale studies that have been reported are summarized in chapter 3 and more extensively in Quigley and Kretschmer (1982). The reported results to date have been disappointing. MCE approaches, and the rubric of total communication under which they have been advanced, have had the positive effect of providing many deaf children with a ready means of manual communication, but there is very little evidence that this has resulted in higher levels of literacy (reading and written language) than was previously the case.

Perhaps it is too soon to expect substantial progress in literacy skills; perhaps, too, such progress has been made and not yet documented; but the reported results to date are not promising.

Probably more books have been written on ASL as a language, and even as a culture and an educational philosophy, during the past decade than have been written in that period on all other aspects of the education of deaf people. Yet, there is an almost complete lack of research evaluation of the educational effectiveness of ASL in terms of literacy. It can be argued that skill in reading and writing the general language of a society should not be used as criteria for evaluating the educational effectiveness of ASL. It can also be argued that ASL has not been used extensively in any educational program and thus has not had a chance to be evaluated, formally or informally. There is justification for both arguments.

As discussed in chapter 4, methods for developing reading with deaf children are usually modeled after methods used with hearing children, and those methods assume the existence of a spoken language. They often assume, also, that children come to the beginning reading process with substantial cognitive and linguistic development (e.g., a lexicon, a syntax, a store of figurative language, and inferencing ability) which aid the top-down processes of reading. In fact, if these abilities are well developed, the primary task in learning to read is the bottom-up skill of decoding the printed or written word. In many hearing children, however, these abilities are not well developed, and much of beginning reading instruction is devoted to the development of cognitive and linguistic skills which are part of general language ability and not just of reading.

With deaf children these important requisites for learning to read are often present only in rudimentary form. The material in chapter 2 on cognitive development and in chapter 3 on primary language development demonstrate that most deaf children reach the beginning reading stage with inadequate development of the cognitive and linguistic skills that are requisites for learning to read. Thus, the process of learning to read becomes also a language learning process for them (Quigley & King, 1981). The inadequate development of reading and its related written language are extensively documented in chapters 4 and 5, although some investigators (e.g., Ewoldt, 1981; McGill-Franzen & Gormley, 1980) claim that the reading levels of deaf children are better than indicated by the studies cited in those chapters.

If deaf children have been prepared for the beginning reading process primarily by OE, then it is possible that the methods commonly used to teach reading with hearing children can be used with them also. In spite of controversies in the field of reading, this usually involved an eclectic approach using an emphasis on meaning and elements of both the phonics and the look–say (whole word) techniques. But if deaf children have been prepared by MCE approaches, the situation is different. Although it is claimed for this approach that it provides deaf children with English in manual form as a first language, the claim is in doubt. Marmor and Pettito, (1979) and Reich and Bick (1977) have been cited as demonstrating that strict adherence to English structure is difficult with various MCE approaches, and perhaps rare, so that many MCE users are probably using a form of PSE. And, as discussed previously, there is very little hard evidence of positive effects of MCE on reading. Also, although OE might certainly provide deaf children with the speech coding which Conrad (1979) and Lichtenstein (1983) indicate might be a critical factor in reading skill, it is not clear that this would be true with MCE.

The issue of reading for deaf children who have been exposed primarily to ASL prior to beginning school is even more puzzling. (It should be remembered that these children usually are children of ASL-using deaf parents and as such have other positive early life experiences besides ready communicative interaction with their parents. For example, the parents probably do not experience the trauma that hearing parents often do at the birth of a deaf child and probably are more able to provide an emotionally healthy and intellectually stimulating early environment.) ASL is not only a different communication form from OE (manual rather than oral) but also a different language. Theoretically, this should make the development of reading doubly difficult for ASL-using children as compared to OE- or MCE-using ones. Yet, a number of studies discussed in chapters 3 and 4, have reported that deaf children of deaf parents (probably mostly ASL-using) score higher on reading achievement tests on the average than comparison groups of deaf children of hearing parents. As Quigley and Kretschmer (1982) have indicated, however, there is considerable doubt as to whether these higher scores resulted primarily from exposure to ASL or from other positive factors in the early environment.

It seems reasonable to at least wonder how the transition can be made from ASL, a visual/manual non-English language, to reading, which is based on auditory/vocal English. It would seem that new methods of teaching reading might have to be developed for ASL-using deaf children, and perhaps for many other deaf children also who lack speech coding ability. What those methods might be is not clear, but studies of highly skilled deaf readers who are children of ASL-using deaf parents might determine in what ways they acquired their skill in reading.

As reported in chapter 5, written language is probably the most intensively studied aspect of the language of deaf children. Extensive investigations are cited ranging from the traditional grammar-oriented study of Thompson (1936) to the transformational–generative-grammar-oriented studies of Quigley, Wilbur, Power, Montanelli, and Steinkamp (1976). A large body of knowledge has been accumulated about the vocabulary and syntax of the written language of deaf children which should be useful to researchers and practitioners alike. It seems likely, too, that extensive information on the written language of deaf individuals based on discourse theory will be accumulated during the present decade. Unfortunately, as is the case with reading, all of this knowledge has not resulted in any demonstrated improvement in the written language of deaf children in general. Comparisons of data in published reports on the reading and written language of deaf children over the past 50 years reveal no differences in general performance.

A development of interest during the past decade has been the increasing number of proposals that English be taught to deaf children as a second language (ESL) after ASL has been developed as a first language (Bockmiller, 1981; Erting, 1981; Stokoe, 1975). These proposals are related to the large increase in bilingual and ESL programs that have been established during the past 20 years for minority culture hearing children (Hornby, 1980; Troike, 1981). The survey in chapter 6 indicated that there are substantial similarities between the educational situations of deaf children and minority culture hearing children. The controversies over goals and procedures in the field of bilingualism and ESL with minority culture hearing students are highly reminiscent of those concerning whether deaf children should be educated to function largely in the general society and whether ASL or English should be the initial and primary language for them.

As Quigley and Paul (1984) have reported, the literature on bilingualism and ESL indicates that positive effects (e.g., development of the majority language) are most likely to appear in programs known as developmental maintenance models in which the goal is to develop a high level of competence in both languages (Eddy, 1978). According to Quigley and Paul (1984), research also indicates that there must be a well-established first language before English can be developed successfully as a second language, and teachers need to establish a bilingual environment where equal attention and status are accorded to both languages in order to have a successful program. This seems to require that teachers be bilingual, and with teachers of deaf children this seems to require that they be proficient in ASL and in manually coded and oral English.

Quigley and Paul (1984) have presented a case for programs of ASL and ESL for deaf children as have others (Bockmiller, 1981; Erting, 1981; Stokoe, 1975; Wilbur, 1979). Quigley and Paul have also proposed that these programs be tried carefully and experimentally at first, and that deaf children of ASL-using parents be the ones to whom those programs are first made available. It seems likely that there will be considerable activity with the ASL/ESL approach during the next decade. Its effectiveness awaits evaluation.

Chapter 7 contains extensive information on assessment and instruction. As stated there, assessment is the cornerstone of good instruction and reliability and validity are essentials to good assessment. Jones describes the strengths and limitations of the controlled and free methods of language assessment and concludes that each has a place and that comprehensive assessment requires the use of both approaches. Various modern instructional approaches used with deaf children are described and are related to the historical treatment of instructional methods presented in chapter 1. A survey by King (1983) is cited as reporting that the language instruction approach most widely used at present with deaf students in the United States is the Apple Tree Program

(Anderson et al., 1980). Natural methods of instruction prevail in the early school years, but structural methods are soon added and the most common method seems to be some eclectic combination of these two.

An obvious conclusion from work in the language and communication development of deaf children is that those children cannot be considered as a single population. This is not a trite restatement of the doctrine of individual differences, but a recognition that the development of language in a deaf child is a direct product of the form of communication which is used initially and consistently with the child. Thus, there are several major groupings of deaf children for language study purposes: (1) those who acquired language initially and consistently through oral English (OE); (2) those who acquired it through some form of manually coded English (MCE); and (3) those who acquired it through American Sign Language (ASL). A case could also be made for a fourth grouping of children whose primary early exposure was to pidgin sign English (PSE).

It follows from this first conclusion that language studies of, and language programs for, deaf children need to describe specifically the communication form being used by and with the children, *not as they have been prescribed or defined but as they are actually practiced.* Given the tendency for MCE systems to evolve into PSE, it is possible there are only three major systems, and three groupings of deaf children: OE, PSE, and ASL. The existence of these several possible approaches to language development presents the persons who are primarily responsible for a deaf child's language development with the dilemma of choosing one in the absence of any clear directions from research of their relative effectiveness (Quigley & Kretschmer, 1982). But even though research (which is in its infancy in this field) has produced limited results in studies of the educational effectiveness of the various communication approaches it has helped to clarify the issues involved and has, as researchers want to say when they are confused, created an awareness of the problem. It has also at least indicated that there presently is no "true path" to language development for all deaf children (Quigley & Kretschmer, 1982).

REFERENCES

Aaronson, D., & Rieber, R. (Eds.) *Psycholinguistic research: Implications and applications.* Hillsdale, NJ: Erlbaum, 1979.

Adams, M. Models of word recognition. *Cognitive Psychology,* 1979, *112,* 133–176.

Adams, M. *What good is orthographic redundancy?* (Tech. Rep. No. 192). Urbana: University of Illinois, Center for the Study of Reading, 1980.

American National Standards Institute. *American National Standard Specifications for Audiometers* (ANSI S3.6-1969). New York: American National Standards Institute, 1969.

Anderson, R. *A proposal to continue a center for the study of reading* (Tech. Proposal, 4 vols.). Urbana: University of Illinois, Center for the Study of Reading, February, 1981.

Anderson, M., Boren, N., Caniglia, J., Howard, W., & Krohn, E. *Apple Tree.* Beaverton, OR: Dormac, 1980.

Anderson, R., & Freebody, P. *Vocabulary knowledge* (Tech. Rep. No. 136). Urbana: University of Illinois, Center for the Study of Reading, 1979 (ERIC Document Reproduction Service No. ED 177 480).

Anken, J., & Holmes, D. Use of adapted "Classics" in a reading program for deaf students. *American Annals of the Deaf,* 1977, *122,* 8–14.

Anthony, D. *Seeing essential English.* Unpublished master's thesis, Eastern Michigan University, Ypsilanti, 1966.

Antinucci, F., & Parisi, D. Early language acquisition: A model and some data. In C. Ferguson & D. Slobin (Eds.), *Studies of child language development.* New York: Holt, Rinehart & Winston, 1973.

Armbruster, B., Echols, C., & Brown, A. The role of metacognition in reading to learn. *Volta Review,* 1982, *84,* 45–56.

Babb, R. *A study of the academic achievement and language acquisition levels of deaf children of hearing parents in an educational environment using Signing Exact English as the primary mode of manual communication.* Unpublished doctoral dissertation, University of Illinois, Urbana, 1979.

Baddeley, A. Working memory and reading. In H. Bouma (Ed.), *Processing of visible language* (Vol. 1). New York: Plenum Press, 1979.

Baddeley, A., & Hitch, G. Working memory. In G. H. Bower (Ed.), *The psychology of learning and motivation. Advances in research and theory* (Vol. 8). New York: Academic Press, 1974.

Baker, C., & Cokely, D. *American Sign Language: A teacher's resource on grammar and culture.* Silver Spring, MD: T. J. Publishers, 1980.

Baker, C., & Padden, C. Focusing on the nonmanual components of American Sign Language. In P. Siple (Ed.), *Understanding language through sign language research.* New York: Academic Press, 1978.

Bakker, D. *Temporal order in disturbed reading.* The Netherlands: Rotterdam University, 1972.

Baron, T. Phonemic stage not necessary for reading. *Quarterly Journal of Experimental Psychology*, 1973, *25*, 241–246.

Barry, K. *The five-slate system. A system of objective language teaching.* Philadelphia: Sherman & Co., Printers, 1899.

Bates, E. Pragmatics and sociolinguistics in child language. In D. Morehead & A. Morehead (Eds.), *Normal and deficient child language.* Baltimore, MD: University Park Press, 1976.(a)

Bates, E. *Language and context: The acquisition of pragmatics.* New York: Academic Press, 1976.(b)

Battison, R. Phonological deletion in American Sign Language. *Sign Language Studies*, 1974, *5*, 1–19.

Beck, I., Omanson, R., & McKeown, M. An instructional redesign of reading lessons: Effects on comprehension. *Reading Research Quarterly*, 1982, *17*, 462–481.

Bell, A. Upon a method of teaching language to a very young congenitally deaf child. *American Annals of the Deaf*, 1883, *28*, 124–139.

Bellugi, U., & Fischer, S. A comparison of sign language and spoken language. *Cognition*, 1972, *1*, 173–200.

Bellugi, U., & Klima, E. The roots of language in the sign talk of the deaf. *Psychology Today*, 1972, *6*, 61–76.

Bellugi, U., Klima, E., & Siple, P. Remembering in signs. *Cognition*, 1974, *3*, 93–125.

Belmont, J., & Karchmer, M. Deaf people's memory: There are problems testing special populations. In M. Gruneberg, P. Morris, & R. Sykes (Eds.), *Practical aspects of memory.* New York/London: Academic Press, 1978.

Belmont, J., Karchmer, M., & Pilkonis, P. Instructed rehearsal strategies influence on deaf memory processing. *Journal of Speech and Hearing Research*, 1976, *19*, 36–47.

Bender, R. *The conquest of deafness.* Cleveland: Press of Case Western Reserve, 1960.

Ben-Zeev, S. The influence of bilingualism on cognitive strategy and cognitive development. *Child Development*, 1977, *48*, 1009–1018.

Berko, J. The child's learning of English morphology. *Word*, 1958, *14*, 150–177.

Bernero, R., & Bothwell, H. *Relationship of hearing impairment to educational needs.* Springfield: Illinois Department of Public Health and Office of the Superintendent of Public Instruction, 1966.

Berry, M., & Talbot, R. *Exploratory test for grammar.* Rockford, IL: Berry & Talbot, 1966.

Best, B., & Roberts, G. Early cognitive development in hearing impaired children. *American Annals of the Deaf*, 1976, *121*, 560–564.

Bever, T., Fodor, J., & Weksel, W. On the acquisition of syntax: A critique of "contextual generalization." *Psychological Review*, 1965, *72*, 467–482.(a)

Bever, T., Fodor, J., & Weksel, W. Is linguistics empirical? *Psychological Review*, 1965, *72*, 493–500.(b)

Biemiller, A. Relationship between oral reading rates for letters, words, and simple text in the development of reading achievement. *Reading Research Quarterly*, 1977–78, *13*, 223–253.

Black, J. Psycholinguistic processes in writing. In S. Rosenberg (Ed.), *Handbook of applied psycholinguistics.* Hillsdale, NJ: Erlbaum, 1982.

Blackwell, P., Engen, E., Fischgrund, J., & Zarcadoolas, C. *Sentences and other systems.* Washington, D.C.: Alexander Graham Bell Association for the Deaf, 1978.

Blair, F. A study of the visual memory of deaf and hearing children. *American Annals of the Deaf,* 1957, *102,* 254–263.

Bloom, L. *Language development: Form and function in emerging grammars.* Cambridge, MA: MIT Press, 1970.

Bloom, L. *One word at a time: The use of single-word utterances before syntax.* The Hague: Mouton, 1973.

Bloom, L., & Lahey, M. *Language development and language disorders.* New York: Wiley, 1978.

Bloom, L., Lightbown, P., & Hood, L. Structure and variation in child language. *Monographs of the Society for Research on Child Development,* 1975, *40,* No. 2.

Bloom, L., Miller, P., & Hood, L. Variation and reduction as aspects of competence in language development. In A. Pick (Ed.), *Minnesota Symposia on Child Psychology* (Vol. 9). Minneapolis: University of Minnesota Press, 1975.

Bloomfield, L. *Language.* New York: Holt, Rinehart & Winston, 1933.

Blumenthal, A. *Language and psychology: Historical aspects of psycholinguistics.* New York: Wiley, 1970.

Bobrow, D., & Norman, D. Some principles of memory schemata. In D. Bobrow & A. Collins (Eds.), *Representation and understanding: Studies in cognitive science.* New York: Academic Press, 1975.

Bockmiller, P., Hearing impaired children: Learning to read a second language. *American Annals of the Deaf,* 1981, *126,* 810–813.

Bode, L. Communication of agent, object, and indirect object in signed and spoken languages. *Perceptual and Motor Skills,* 1974, *39,* 1151–1158.

Bonet, J. *Reducion de las letras y arte para ensenar a hablar los mudos.* Madrid: Francisco Arbaco de Angelo, 1620.

Bornstein, H. A description of some current sign systems designed to represent English. *American Annals of the Deaf,* 1973, *118,* 454–463.

Bornstein, H. Signed English: A manual approach to English language development. *Journal of Speech and Hearing Disorders,* 1974, *39,* 330–343.

Bornstein, H. Towards a theory of use for Signed English: From birth through adulthood. *American Annals of the Deaf,* 1982, *127,* 26–31.

Bornstein, H., Saulnier, K., & Hamilton, L. Signed English: A first evaluation. *American Annals of the Deaf,* 1980, *125,* 467–481.

Bornstein, H., & Saulnier, K. Signed English: A brief follow-up to the first evaluation. *American Annals of the Deaf,* 1981, *126,* 69–72.

Bowd, A. Linguistic background and non-verbal intelligence: A crosscultural comparison. *The Journal of Educational Research,* 1974, *68,* 26–27.

Bowen, J. Linguistic perspectives on bilingual education. In B. Spolsky & R. Cooper (Eds.), *Frontiers of bilingual education.* Rowley, MA: Newbury House, 1977.

Bowerman, M. Structural relationships in children's utterances: Syntactic or semantic? In T. Moore (Ed.), *Cognitive development and the acquisition of language.* New York: Academic Press, 1973.

Bowerman, M. Cross-linguistic similarities at two stages of syntactic development. In E. H. Lenneberg & E. Lenneberg (Eds.), *Foundation of language development: A multidisciplinary approach* (Vol. 1). New York: Academic Press, 1975.

Bowerman, M. Semantic factors in the acquisition of rules for word use and sentence construction. In D. Morehead & A. Morehead (Eds.), *Normal and deficient child language.* Baltimore: University Park Press, 1976.

Bragg, B. Ameslish—Our American heritage: A testimony. *American Annals of the Deaf,* 1973, *118,* 672–674.

Braine, M. The ontogeny of English phrase structure: The first phase. *Language,* 1963, *39,* 1–13.(a)

Braine, M. On learning the grammatical order of words. *Psychological Review,* 1963, *70,* 323–348.(b)

Braine, M. On two types of models of the internalization of grammars. In D. Slobin (Ed.), *The ontogenesis of grammar.* New York: Academic Press, 1971.

Brannon, J. Linguistic word classes in the spoken language of normal, hard-of-hearing, and deaf children. *Journal of Speech and Hearing Research,* 1968, *11,* 279–287.

Brasel, K., & Quigley, S. The influence of certain language and communication environments in early childhood on the development of language in deaf individuals. *Journal of Speech and Hearing Research,* 1977, *20,* 95–107.

Brewer, W. Memory for ideas: Synonym substitution. *Memory & Cognition,* 1975, *3,* 458–464.

Brimer, A. *Wide-span reading test.* London: Nelson, 1972.

Brown, A. Metacognitive development and reading. In R. Spiro, B. Bruce, & W. Brewer (Eds.), *Theoretical issues in reading comprehension.* Hillsdale, NJ: Erlbaum, 1980.

Brown, A., & Day, J. *Strategies and knowledge for summarizing texts: The development of expertise.* Unpublished manuscript, 1980.

Brown, A., Campione, J., & Day, J. Learning to learn: On training students to learn from texts. *Educational Researcher,* 1980.

Brown, R. *Words and things.* Glencoe, IL: Free Press, 1958.

Brown, R. *A first language: The early stages.* Cambridge, MA: Harvard University Press, 1973.

Brown, R., Cazden, C., & Bellugi, U. The child's grammar from I to III. In C. Ferguson & D. Slobin (Eds.), *Studies of child language development.* New York: Holt, Rinehart & Winston, 1973.

Bruner, J. From communication to language: A psychological perspective. *Cognition,* 1974–75, *3,* 255–287.

Bruner, J. The ontogenesis of speech acts. *Journal of Child Language,* 1975, *2,* 1–19.

Bruner, J., & Bruner, B. On voluntary action and its hierarchial structure. *International Journal of Psychology,* 1968, *3,* 239–255.

Caccamise, F., & Drury, A. A review of current terminology in education of the deaf. *Deaf American,* 1976, *29,* 7–10.

Carroll, J., Davies, P., & Richman, B. *The American heritage word frequency book.* (Boston: Houghton Mifflin) New York: American Heritage, 1971.

Carrow, E. *Test for auditory comprehension of language.* Lamar, TX: Learning Concepts, 1973.

Carrow, E. *Carrow elicited language inventory.* Austin, TX: Learning Concepts, 1974.

Cathcart, W. Effects of a bilingual instructional program on conceptual development in primary school children. *The Alberta Journal of Educational Research,* 1982, *28,* 31–43.

Cattell, J. The time it takes to see and name objects. *Mind,* 1886, *11,* 63–65.

Cazden, C. The acquisition of noun and verb inflections. *Child Development,* 1968, *39,* 433–448.

Chafe, W. *Meaning and the structure of language.* Chicago: University of Chicago Press, 1970.

Chall, J. *Learning to read: The great debate.* New York: McGraw–Hill, 1967.

Charrow, V. A psycholinguistic analysis of deaf English. *Sign Language Studies,* 1975, *7,* 139–150.

Charrow, V., & Charrow, R. *Let the rewriter beware.* Washington, D.C.: American Institute for Research, 1979.

Charrow, V., & Fletcher, J. English as the second language of deaf children. *Developmental Psychology,* 1974, *10,* 463–470.

Chen, K. Acoustic image in visual detection for deaf and hearing college students. *Journal of General Psychology,* 1976, *94,* 243–246.

Chomsky, N. *Syntactic structures.* The Hague: Mouton, 1957.

Chomsky, N. *Aspects of the theory of syntax.* Cambridge, MA: MIT Press, 1965.

Chomsky, N. *Language and mind.* New York: Harcourt, Brace & World, 1968.

Chomsky, N. *Reflections on language.* New York: Pantheon Books, 1975.

Chomsky, N., & Halle, M. *The sound pattern of English.* New York: Harper & Row, 1968.

Chun, J. A survey of research in second language acquisition. *The Modern Language Journal,* 1980, *64,* 287–296.

Cicourel, A., & Boese, R. Sign language acquisition and the teaching of deaf children, Part I. *American Annals of the Deaf,* 1972, *117,* 27–33.(a)

Cicourel, A., & Boese, R. Sign language acquisition—Conclusion. *American Annals of the Deaf,* 1972, *117,* 403–411.(b)

Clark, E. What's in a word? On the child's acquisition of semantics in his first language. In T. Moore (Ed.), *Cognitive development and the acquisition of language.* New York: Academic Press, 1973.

Clark, H., & Clark, E. *Psychology and language: An introduction to psycholinguistics.* New York: Harcourt Brace Jovanovich, 1977.

Clarke, B., Rogers, W., & Booth, J. How hearing-impaired children learn to read: Theoretical and practical issues. In R. E. Kretschmer (Ed.), Reading and the hearing-impaired individual. *Volta Review,* 1982, *84*(5), 57–69.

Clarke, B., & Ling, D. The effects of using cued speech: A follow-up study. *Volta Review,* 1976, *78,* 23–35.

Clarke, M. Reading in Spanish and English: Evidence from adult ESL students. *Language Learning,* 1979, *29,* 121–150.

Clarke School for the Deaf. *Curriculum series on reading.* Northampton, MA, 1972.

Clerc, L. Some hints to the teachers of the deaf and dumb. *Proceedings of the Second Convention of American Instructors of the Deaf and Dumb* (pp. 64–75). Hartford, CN: Press of Case, Tiffany, 1851.

Cohen, A. The case for partial or total immersion education. In A. Simoes (Ed.), *The bilingual child: Research and analysis of existing educational themes.* New York: Academic Press, 1976.

Cohen, A., & Swain, M. Bilingual education: The "Immersion" model in the North American context. *TESOL Quarterly,* 1976, *10,* 45–53.

Cokely, D. When is a pidgin not a pidgin? An alternate analysis of the ASL-English contact situation. *Sign Language Studies,* 1983, *38,* 1–23.

Coley, J., & Bockmiller, P. Teaching reading to the deaf: An examination of teacher preparedness and practices. *American Annals of the Deaf,* 1980, *125,* 909–915.

Collins-Ahlgren, M. Teaching English as a second language to young deaf children: A case study. *Journal of Speech and Hearing Disorders,* 1974, *39,* 486–500.

Collins-Ahlgren, M. Language development of two deaf children. *American Annals of the Deaf,* 1975, *120,* 524–539.

Conley, J. Role of idiomatic expressions in the reading of deaf children. *American Annals of the Deaf,* 1976, *121,* 381–385.

Conrad, R. Acoustic confusion in immediate memory. *British Journal of Psychology,* 1964, *55,* 75–84.

Conrad, R. Short-term memory processes in the deaf. *British Journal of Psychology,* 1970, *61,* 179–195.

Conrad, R. The effect of vocalizing on comprehension in the profoundly deaf. *British Journal of Psychology,* 1971, *62,* 147–150.(a)

Conrad, R. The chronology of the development of covert speech in children. *Developmental Psychology,* 1971, *5,* 398–405.(b)

Conrad, R. Short-term memory in the deaf: A test for speech coding. *British Journal of Psychology,* 1972, *63,* 173–180.

Conrad, R. Internal speech in profoundly deaf children. *The Teacher of the Deaf,* 1973, *71,* 384–389.

Conrad, R. *The deaf school child.* London: Harper & Row, 1979.

Conrad, R., Freeman, P., & Hull, A. Acoustic factors versus language factors in short-term memory. *Psychonomic Science,* 1965, *3,* 57–58.

Conrad, R., & Rush, M. On the nature of short-term memory encoding by the deaf. *Journal of Speech and Hearing Disorders,* 1965, *30,* 336–343.

Cooper, C., Cherry, R., Gerber, R., Fleischer, S., Copley, B., & Sartisky, M. *Writing abilities of regularly-admitted freshmen at SUNY/Buffalo.* Unpublished manuscript, University Learning Center, State University of New York, Buffalo, 1979.

Cooper, R. The ability of deaf and hearing children to apply morphological rules. *Journal of Speech and Hearing Research,* 1967, *10,* 77–86.

Cooper, R., & Rosenstein, J. Language acquisition of deaf children. *Volta Review,* 1966, *68,* 58–67.

Cordasco, F. (Ed.) *Bilingualism and the bilingual child: Challenges and problems.* New York: Arno Press, 1978.

Cornett, O. Cued speech. *American Annals of the Deaf,* 1967, *112,* 3–13.

Cornett, O. In answer to Dr. Moores. *American Annals of the Deaf,* 1969, *114,* 27–33.

Corson, H. *Comparing deaf children of oral deaf parents and deaf parents using manual communication with deaf children of hearing parents on academic, social, and communication functioning.* Unpublished doctoral dissertation, University of Cincinnati, OH, 1973.

Crandall, K. Inflectional morphemes in the manual English of young hearing impaired children and their mothers. *Journal of Speech and Hearing Research,* 1978, *21,* 372–386.

Crittenden, J. Categorization of cheremic errors in sign language reception. *Sign Language Studies,* 1975, *5,* 64–71.

Croker, G., Jones, M., & Pratt, M. *Language stories and drills. Books I, II, III, and IV. Manuals.* Brattleboro, VT: The Vermont Printing Co. 1920, 1922, 1928.

Cromer, R. The development of language and cognition: The cognition hypothesis. In B. Foss (Ed.), *New perspectives in child development.* Harmondsworth, England: Penguin, 1974.

Cromer, R. The cognitive hypothesis of language acquisition and its implications for child language deficiency. In D. Morehead & A. Morehead (Eds.), *Normal and deficient child language.* Baltimore: University Park Press, 1976.

Crutchfield, P. Prospects for teaching English Det + N structures to deaf students. *Sign Language Studies,* 1972, *1,* 8–14.

Cruttenden, A. A phonetic study of babbling. *British Journal of Disorders of Communication,* 1970, *5,* 110–117.

Cruttenden, A. *Language in infancy and childhood: A linguistic introduction to language acquisition.* New York: St. Martin's Press, 1979.

Crystal, D., & Craig, E. Contrived sign language. In I. Schlesinger & L. Namir (Eds.), *Sign language of the deaf: Psychological, linguistic, and social perspectives.* New York: Academic Press, 1978.

Cummins, J. Cognitive factors associated with the attainment of intermediate levels of bilingual skill. *The Modern Language Journal,* 1977, *61,* 3–12.

Cummins, J. Educational implications of mother tongue maintenance in minority-language groups. *Canadian Modern Language Review,* 1978, *34,* 395–416.

Dale, P. *Language development: Structure and function* (2nd ed.). New York: Holt, Rinehart & Winston, 1976.

Dalgleish, B. Communication preference and the social conditions of language learning in the deaf. *American Annals of the Deaf,* 1975, *120,* 70–77.

Daneman, M., & Carpenter, P. Individual differences in working memory and reading. *Journal of Verbal Learning and Verbal Behavior,* 1980, *19,* 450–466.

Davis, H., & Silverman, R. *Hearing and deafness* (3rd ed.). New York: Holt, Rinehart & Winston, 1978.

Day, J. *Training summarization skills: A comparison of teaching methods.* Unpublished doctoral dissertation, University of Illinois, 1980.

DeLand, F. *The story of lipreading.* Washington, D.C.: The Volta Bureau, 1931.

Denton, D. Remarks in support of a system of total communication for deaf children. In *Communication Symposium,* Maryland School for the Deaf, Frederick, 1970.

de Villiers, J., & de Villiers, P. *Language acquisition.* Cambridge, MA: Harvard University Press, 1978.

DiFrancesca, S. *Academic achievement test results of a national testing program for hearing impaired students, United States, Spring, 1971* (series D, No. 9). Washington, D.C.: Gallaudet College, Office of Demographic Studies, 1972.

DiStefano, P., & Valencia, S. The effects of syntactic maturity on comprehension of graded reading passages. *Journal of Educational Research,* 1980, *73,* 247–251.

Diver, W. Phonology as human behavior. In D. Aaronson & R. Rieber (Eds.), *Psycholinguistic research: Implications and applications.* Hillsdale, NJ: Erlbaum, 1979.

Dixon, K., Pearson, P., & Ortony, A. *Some reflections on the use of figurative language in children's textbooks.* Paper presented at the annual meeting of the National Reading Conference, San Diego, 1980.

Dodd, B. The phonological systems of deaf children. *Journal of Speech and Hearing Disorders,* 1976, *41,* 185–198.

Doehring, D., Bonnycastle, D., & Ling, A. Rapid reading skills of integrated hearing impaired children. *Volta Review,* 1978, *80,* 399–409.

Dore, J. A pragmatic description of early language development. *Journal of Psycholinguistic Research,* 1974, *3,* 343–350.

Dore, J. Holophrases, speech acts, and language universals. *Journal of Child Language,* 1975, *2,* 21–40.

Dore, J., Franklin, M., Miller, R., & Ramer, A. Transitional phenomena in early language acquisition. *Journal of Child Language,* 1976, *3,* 13–28.

Durkin, D. *Children who read early.* New York: Teachers College Press, 1966.

Durkin, D. *Teaching them to read* (3rd ed.). Boston: Allyn & Bacon, 1978.

Eddy, P. Does foreign language study aid native language development? *ERIC/CLL News Bulletin,* 1978, *1,* 1–2.

Edwards, H., Fu, L., McCarrey, H., & Doutriaux, C. Partial French immersion for English-speaking pupils in elementary school: The Ottawa Roman Catholic Separate School Board study in grades one to four. *Canadian Modern Language Review,* 1981, *37,* 283–296.

Eimas, P. Linguistic processing of speech by young infants. In R. Schiefelbusch & L. Lloyd (Eds.), *Language perspectives: Acquisition, retardation, and intervention.* Baltimore: University Park Press, 1974.

Eimas, P., Siqueland, E., Jusczyk, P., & Vigorito, J. Speech perception in infants. *Science,* 1971, *171,* 303–306.

Ellenberger, R., & Staeyert, M. A child's representation of action in American Sign Language. In P. Siple (Ed.), *Understanding language through sign language research.* New York: Academic Press, 1978.

Erting, C. An anthropological approach to the study of the communicative competence of deaf children. *Sign Language Studies,* 1981, *32,* 221–238.

Ervin-Tripp, S. Is Sybil there? The structure of some American English directives. *Language in Society,* 1976, *5,* 25–66.

Ervin-Tripp, S., & Mitchell-Kernan, C. (Eds.) *Child discourse.* New York: Academic Press, 1977.

Ewoldt, C. A psycholinguistic description of selected deaf children reading in Sign Language. *Reading Research Quarterly,* 1981, *17,* 58–89.

Farrar, A. *Arnold on the education of the deaf: A manual for teachers* (2nd ed.). Derby: Francis, Cartes, 1923.

Feldman, C., & Shen, M. Some language-related cognitive advantages of bilingual five-year-olds. *Journal of Genetic Psychology,* 1971, *118,* 235–244.

Ferguson, C. Diglossia. *Word,* 1959, *15,* 325–340.

Ferguson, C. Linguistic theory. In *Bilingual education: Current perspectives, Volume 2.* Arlington, VA: Center for Applied Linguistics, 1977.

Ferguson, C., & Farwell, C. Words and sounds in early language acquisition: English consonants in the first 50 words. *Language,* 1975, *51,* 419–439.

Ferguson, C., & Garnica, O. Theories of phonological development. In E. H. Lenneberg & E. Lenneberg (Eds.), *Foundation of language development: A multidisciplinary approach* (Vol. 1). New York: Academic Press, 1975.

Fillmore, C. The case for case. In E. Bach & R. Harms (Eds.), *Universals in linguistic theory.* New York: Holt, Rinehart & Winston, 1968.

Fischer, S. Influences on word order change in American Sign Language. In C. Li (Ed.), *Word order and word order change.* Austin: University of Texas Press, 1975.

Fischer, S., & Gough, B. Verbs in American Sign Language. *Sign Language Studies,* 1978, *18,* 17–48.

Fitzgerald, E. *Straight language for the deaf.* (Staunton, VA: McClure, 1929), Washington, D.C.: The Volta Bureau, 1949.

Flesch, R. *Why Johnny can't read and what you can do about it.* New York: Harper, 1955.

Freedle, F., & Fine, F. Prose comprehension in natural and experimental settings: The theory and its practical implications. In S. Rosenberg (Ed.), *Handbook of applied psycholinguistics.* Hillsdale, NJ: Erlbaum, 1982.

Friedman, L. The manifestation of subject, object, and topic in American Sign Language. In C. Li (Ed.), *Subject and topic.* New York: Academic Press, 1976.

Friedman, L. (Ed.) *On the other hand.* New York: Academic Press, 1977.

Fries, C. *The structure of English.* New York: Harcourt, Brace, 1952.

Fromkin, V., & Rodman, R. *An introduction to language* (2nd ed.). New York: Holt, Rinehart & Winston, 1978.

Furth, H. Conservation of weight in deaf and hearing children. *Child Development,* 1964, *35,* 143–150.

Furth, H. A comparison of reading test norms of deaf and hearing children. *American Annals of the Deaf,* 1966, *111,* 461–462.(a)

Furth, H. *Thinking without language: Psychological implications of deafness.* New York: Free Press, 1966.(b)

Furth, H. A review and perspective on the thinking of deaf people. In J. Hellmuth (Ed.), *Cognitive Studies: Volume 1.* New York: Brunner/Mazel, 1970.

Furth, H. *Deafness and learning: A psychosocial approach.* Belmont, CA: Wadsworth, 1973.

Furth, H., & Youniss, J. Formal operations and language: A comparison of deaf and hearing adolescents. *International Journal of Psychology,* 1971, *6,* 49–64.

Furth, H., & Youniss, J. The influence of language and experience on discovery and use of logical symbols. *British Journal of Psychology,* 1965, *56,* 381–390.

Fusaro, J., & Slike, S. The effect of imagery on the ability of hearing impaired children to identify words. *American Annals of the Deaf,* 1979, *124,* 829–832.

Fusfeld, I. The academic program of schools for the deaf. *Volta Review*, 1955, *57*, 63–70.

Gaines, R., Mandler, J., & Bryant, P. Immediate and delayed story recall by hearing and deaf children. *Journal of Speech and Hearing Research*, 1981, *24*, 463–469.

Gamez, G. Reading in a second language: Native language approach vs. direct method. *The Reading Teacher*, 1979, *32*, 665–670.

Geers, A., & Moog, J. Syntactic maturity of spontaneous speech and elicited imitations of hearing impaired children. *Journal of Speech and Hearing Disorders*, 1978, *43*, 380–391.

Gelman, R. Cognitive development. *Annual Review of Psychology*, 1978, *29*, 297–332.

Genesee, F. Acquisition of reading skills in immersion programs. *Foreign Language Annals*, 1979, *12*, 71–77.

Gilman, L., Davis, J., & Raffin, M. Use of common morphemes by hearing impaired children exposed to a system of manual English. *Journal of Auditory Research*, 1980, *20*, 57–69.

Giorcelli, L. *The comprehension of some aspects of figurative language by deaf and hearing subjects.* Unpublished doctoral dissertation, University of Illinois, Urbana, 1982.

Goetzinger, C., & Rousey, C. Educational achievement of deaf children. *American Annals of the Deaf*, 1959, *104*, 221–231.

Goldberg, J., & Bordman, P. English language instruction for the hearing impaired: An adaptation of ESL methodology. *TESOL Quarterly*, 1974, 263–270.

Goldberg, J., & Bordman, M. The ESL approach to teaching English to hearing-impaired students. *American Annals of the Deaf*, 1975, *120*, 22–27.

Goodman, K. Reading: A psycholinguistic guessing game. *Journal of the Reading Specialist*, 1967, *6*, 126–135.

Goodman, K. Behind the eye: What happens in reading. In H. Singer & R. Ruddell (Eds.), *Theoretical models and processes in reading*. Newark, DE: International Reading Association, 1976.

Goodman, L. Meeting children's needs through materials modification. *Teaching Exceptional Children*, 1978, *10*, 92–94.

Gormley, K., & McGill-Franzen, A. Why can't the deaf read? Comments on asking the wrong question. *American Annals of the Deaf*, 1978, *123*, 542–547.

Graesser, A., Hoffman, N., & Clark, L. Structural components of reading time. *Journal of Verbal Learning and Verbal Behavior*, 1980, *19*, 135–151.

Greenberger, D. The natural method. *American Annals of the Deaf*, 1878, *23*, 107–116; 1879, *24*, 33–38.

Greenfield, P., & Smith, J. *The structure of communication in early language development.* New York: Academic Press, 1976.

Griswold, E., & Cummings, J. The expressive vocabulary of preschool deaf children. *American Annals of the Deaf*, 1974, *119*, 16–28.

Groht, M. *Natural language for deaf children.* Washington, D.C.: A. G. Bell Association for the Deaf, 1958.

Gruber, H., & Vonéche, J. (Eds.) *The essential Piaget: An interpretive reference and guide.* New York: Basic Books, 1977.

Guberina, P. Verbotonal method and its application to the rehabilitation of the deaf. In *Proceedings of the International Congress on Education of the Deaf* (pp. 279–293). Washington, D.C.: U.S. Govt. Printing Office, 1964.

Gumperz, J., & Hymes, D. (Eds.) *Directions in sociolinguistics: The ethnography of communication.* New York: Holt, Rinehart & Winston, 1972.

Gustason, C., Pfetzing, D., & Zawolkow, E. *Signing exact English.* Silver Spring, MD: Modern Signs Press, 1972.

Gustason, G., Pfetzing, D., & Zawolkow, E. *Signing exact English* (Rev. ed.). Rossmor, CA: Modern Signs Press, 1975.

Guszak, F. Teacher questioning and reading. *Reading Teacher,* 1967, *21,* 227–234.

Hakuta, K., & Cancino, H. Trends in second-language-acquisition research. *Harvard Educational Review,* 1977, *47,* 294–316.

Halliday, M. *Learning how to mean: Explorations in the development of language.* New York: Elsevier/North Holland, 1975.

Hammermeister, F. Reading achievement in deaf adults. *American Annals of the Deaf,* 1971, *116,* 25–28.

Hansen, J., & Pearson, P. *The effects of inference training and practice on young children's comprehension* (Tech. Rep. No. 166). Urbana: University of Illinois, Center for the Study of Reading, 1980 (ERIC Document Reproduction Service No. ED 186 839).

Hanson, V. Short-term recall by deaf signers of American Sign Language: Implications of encoding strategy for order recall. *Journal of Experimental Psychology: Learning, Memory, and Cognition,* 1982, *8,* 572–583.

Hardyck, C., & Petrinovich, L. Subvocal speech and comprehension level as a function of the difficulty level of reading material. *Journal of Verbal Learning and Verbal Behavior,* 1970, *9,* 647–652.

Harrell, L., Jr. A comparison of oral and written language in school age children. *Monographs of the Society for Research in Child Development,* 1957, 22(3).

Hart, B. *Teaching reading to deaf children* (The Lexington School for the Deaf Education Series, Book IV). Washington, D.C.: Alexander Graham Bell Association for the Deaf, 1963.

Hasenstab, M., & McKenzie, C. A survey of reading programs used with hearing-impaired students. *Volta Review,* 1981, *83,* 383–388.

Hatcher, C., & Robbins, N. *The development of reading skills in hearing-impaired children.* Cedar Falls: University of Northern Iowa, 1978 (ERIC Document Reproduction Service No. ED 167 960).

Hatfield, N., Caccamise, F., & Siple, P. Deaf students' language competency: A bilingual perspective. *American Annals of the Deaf,* 1978, *123,* 847–851.

Haugen, E. *Bilingualism in the Americas: A bibliography and a research guide.* Montgomery: University of Alabama Press, 1956.

Hawes, M., & Danhauer, J. Perceptual features of the manual alphabet. *American Annals of the Deaf,* 1978, *123,* 464–474.

Hayes, D., & Tierney, R. *Increasing background knowledge through analogy: Its effects upon comprehension and learning* (Tech. Rep. No. 186). Urbana: University of Illinois, Center for the Study of Reading, 1980.

Heider, F., & Heider, G. A comparison of sentence structure of deaf and hearing children. *Psychological Monographs,* 1940, *52,* 42–103.

Heine, M. *Comprehension of high and low level information in expository passages: A comparison of deaf and hearing readers.* Unpublished doctoral dissertation, University of Pittsburgh, 1981.

Higgins, E. An analysis of the comprehensibility of three communication methods used with hearing impaired students. *American Annals of the Deaf,* 1973, *118,* 46–49.

Hirsh-Pasek, K., & Treiman, R. Recoding in silent reading: Can the deaf child translate print into a more manageable form? In R. E. Kretschmer (Ed.), Reading and the hearing-impaired individual. *Volta Review,* 1982, *84,* 71–82.

Hoffmeister, R. *The influential point.* Philadelphia, PA: Temple University, 1978.

Hoffmeister, R., & Wilbur, R. The acquisition of sign language. In H. Lane & F. Grosjean (Eds.), *Recent perspectives on American Sign Language.* Hillsdale, NJ: Erlbaum, 1980.

Hornby, P. Achieving second language fluency through immersion education. *Foreign Language Annals,* 1980, *13,* 107–114.

Howe, C. Interpretive analysis and role semantics a ten-year mésalliance? *Journal of Child Language,* 1981, *8,* 439–456.

Houck, J. *The effects of idioms on reading comprehension of hearing impaired students.* Unpublished doctoral dissertation, University of Northern Colorado, 1982 (Abstract).

Hudgins, C. Auditory training—Its possibilities and limitations. *Volta Review,* 1954, *56,* 339-349.

Huey, E. *The psychology and pedagogy of reading.* New York: Macmillan, 1908. (Reprinted, Cambridge, MA: MIT Press, 1968.)

Humphries, T., Padden, C., & O'Rourke, T. *A basic course in American Sign Language.* Silver Spring, MD: T. J. Publishers, 1980.

Hunt, K. *Grammatical structures written at three grade levels.* Champaign, IL: National Council of Teachers of English, 1965.

Huttenlocher, J. The origins of language comprehension. In R. Solso (Ed.), *Theories in cognitive psychology.* Hillsdale, NJ: Erlbaum, 1974.

Hymes, D. *Foundations in sociolinguistics.* Philadelphia: University of Pennsylvania Press, 1974.

Ianco-Worrall, A. Bilingualism and cognitive development. *Child Development,* 1972, *43,* 1390–1400.

Ingram, D. Current issues in child phonology. In D. Morehead & A. Morehead (Eds.), *Normal and deficient language.* Baltimore: University Park Press, 1976.

Ingram, R. Theme, rheme, topic, and comment in the syntax of American Sign Language. *Sign Language Studies,* 1978, *20,* 193–218.

Iran-Nejad, A., Ortony, A., & Rittenhouse, R. The comprehension of metaphorical uses of English by deaf children. *Journal of Speech and Hearing Research,* 1981, *24,* 551–556.

Israelite, N. *Direct antecedent context and comprehension of reversible passive voice sentences by deaf readers.* Unpublished doctoral dissertation, Pennsylvania State University, 1981.

Ivimey, G., & Lachterman, D. The written language of deaf children. *Language and Speech*, 1980, *23*, 351–377.

Jakobson, R. *[Child language aphasia and phonological universals]* (A. Keiler, trans.). The Hague: Mouton, 1968.

Jarvella, R. Syntactic processing of connected speech. *Journal of Verbal Learning and Verbal Behavior*, 1971, *10*, 409–416.

Jarvella, R. Immediate memory and discourse processing. In G. Bower (Ed.), *The psychology of learning and motivation*. New York: Academic Press, 1979.

Jarvella, R., & Lubinsky, J. Deaf and hearing children's use of language describing temporal order among events. *Journal of Speech and Hearing Research*, 1975, *18*, 58–73.

Jeffers, J., & Barley, M. *Speechreading (lipreading)*. Springfield, IL: Thomas, 1971.

Jensema, C. *The relationship between academic achievement and the demographic characteristics of hearing-impaired children and youth*. Washington, D.C.: Gallaudet College, Office of Demographic Studies, 1975.

Johnson, P. Effects on reading comprehension of language complexity and cultural background of a text. *TESOL Quarterly*, 1981, *15*, 169–181.

Johnson, L., & Otto, W. Effects of alternations in prose style on the readability of college text. *Journal of Educational Research*, 1982, *75*, 222–229.

Johnson, D., Toms-Bronowski, S., & Pittelman, S. Vocabulary development. In R. E. Kretschmer (Ed.), Reading and the hearing-impaired individual. *Volta Review*, 1982, *84*(5), 11–24.

Jones, B. *A study of oral language comprehension of black and white, middle and lower class, pre-school children using standard English and Black dialect in Houston, Texas, 1972*. Unpublished doctoral dissertation, University of Houston, 1972.

Jones, P. Negative interference of signed language in written English. *Sign Language Studies*, 1979, *24*, 273–279.

Jones, W. A critical study of bilingualism and non-verbal intelligence. *British Journal of Educational Psychology*, 1960, *30*, 71–77.

Jones, W., & Stewart, W. Bilingualism and verbal intelligence. *British Journal of Psychology (Statistical Section)*, 1951, *4*, 3–8.

Jordan, I., Gustason, G., & Rosen, R. An update on communication trends at programs for the deaf. *American Annals of the Deaf*, 1979, *124*, 350–357.

Jordan, I., Gustason, G., & Rosen, R. Current communication trends in programs for the deaf. *American Annals of the Deaf*, 1976, *121*, 527–532.

Jordan, K. A referential communication study of signers and speakers using realistic referents. *Sign Language Studies*, 1975, *6*, 65–103.

Just, M., & Carpenter, P. A theory of reading: From eye fixations to comprehension. *Psychological Review*, 1980, *4*, 329–354.

Kachuk, B. Relative clauses may cause confusion for young readers. *The Reading Teacher*, 1981, *34*, 372–377.

Kantor, R., The acquisition of classifiers in American Sign Language. *Sign Language Studies*, 1980, *28*, 193–208.

Kantor, R. Communicative interaction: Mother modification and child acquisition of American Sign Language. *Sign Language Studies*, 1982, *36*, 233–282.

Kaplan, E., & Kaplan, G. The prelinguistic child. In J. Eliot (Ed.), *Human development and cognitive processes*. New York: Holt, Rinehart & Winston, 1971.

Karchmer, M., Milone, M., & Wolk, S. Educational significance of hearing loss at three levels of severity. *American Annals of the Deaf*, 1979, *124*, 97–109.

Kates, S. *Language development in deaf and hearing adolescents*. Northampton, MA: Clarke School for the Deaf, 1972.

Kavanagh, J., & Cutting, J. (Eds.) *The role of speech in language*. Cambridge: MIT Press, 1975.

Kavanagh, J., & Mattingly, I. (Eds.) *Language by ear and by eye: The relationship between speech and reading*. Cambridge, MA: MIT Press, 1972.

Keep, J. On the best method of teaching language to the higher classes in our institutions for the deaf and dumb. *Proceedings of the Third Convention of American Instructors of the Deaf and Dumb*, Columbus, OH: Steam Press of Smith & Cox, 1853, 15–31.

King, C. *An investigation of similarities and differences in the syntactic abilities of deaf and hearing children learning English as a first or second language*. Unpublished doctoral dissertation, University of Illinois, 1981.

King, C. *Survey of language methods and materials used with hearing impaired students in the United States*. Paper presented at Entre Amis '83, Convention of ACEHI, CAID, and CEASD, Winnipeg, Manitoba, June 1983.

King, C., & Quigley, S. *Reading and Deafness*. San Diego: College-Hill Press, in press.

Kintsch, W., & van Dijk, T. Toward a model of text comprehension and production. *Psychological Review*, 1978, *85*, 363–394.

Klare, G. A second look at the validity of readability formulas. *Journal of Reading Behavior*, 1976, *8*, 129–152.

Kleiman, G. Speech recoding in reading. *Journal of Verbal Learning and Verbal Behavior*, 1975, *14*, 323–339.

Klima, E., & Bellugi, U. *The signs of language*. Cambridge, MA: Harvard University Press, 1979.

Kluwin, T. The grammaticality of manual representations of English in classroom settings. *American Annals of the Deaf*, 1981, *126*, 417–421.

Krashen, S. Lateralization, language learning, and the critical period: Some new evidence. *Language Learning*, 1973, *23*, 63–74.

Kretschmer, R. E. *Judgments of grammaticality by 11, 14, and 17 year old hearing and hearing impaired youngsters*. Unpublished doctoral dissertation, University of Kansas, 1976.

Kretschmer, R. E. Reading and the hearing-impaired individual: Summation and application. In R. E. Kretschmer (Ed.), Reading and the hearing-impaired individual. *Volta Review*, 1982, *84*(5), 107–122.

Kretschmer, R. R., & Kretschmer, L. *Language development and intervention with the hearing impaired*. Baltimore, MD: University Park Press, 1978.

Kyle, J. Reading development of deaf children. *Journal of Research in Reading*, 1980, *3*, 86–97.

LaBerge, D., & Samuels, S. Toward a theory of automatic information processing in reading. *Cognitive Psychology*, 1974, *6*, 293–323.

Labov, W. The logic of non-standard English. In F. Williams (Ed.), *Language and poverty*. Chicago: Markham, 1970.

Labov, W. *Language in the inner city: Studies in the black English vernacular.* Philadelphia: University of Pennsylvania Press, 1972.

Lake, D. Syntax and sequential memory in hearing impaired children. In H. Reynolds & C. Williams (Eds.), *Proceedings of the Gallaudet conference on reading in relation to deafness.* Washington, D.C.: Gallaudet College, 1980.

Lambert, W. Culture and language as factors in learning and education. In A. Wolfgang (Ed.), *Education of immigrant students.* Toronto: Ontario Institute for Studies in Education, 1975.

Lambert, W., & Tucker, G. *Bilingual education of children: The St. Lambert experiment.* Rowley, MA: Newbury House, 1972.

Lamendella, J. General principles of neurofunctional organization and their manifestation in primary and nonprimary language acquisition. *Language Learning,* 1977, *27,* 155–196.

Lane, H., & Baker, D. Reading achievement of the deaf: Another look. *Volta Review,* 1974, *76,* 489–499.

Lane, H., Boyes-Braem, P., & Bellugi, U. Preliminaries to a distinctive feature analysis of handshapes in American Sign Language. *Cognitive Psychology,* 1976, *8,* 263–289.

Lane, H., & Grosjean, F. (Eds.) *Recent perspectives on American Sign Language.* Hillsdale, NJ: Erlbaum, 1980.

Laughton, J. Nonlinguistic creative abilities and expressive syntactic abilities of hearing-impaired children. *Volta Review,* 1979, *81,* 409–420.

Layton, T., Holmes, D., & Bradley, P. A description of pedagogically imposed signed semantic–syntactic relationships in deaf children. *Sign Language Studies,* 1979, *23,* 137–160.

Lee, D. Are there signs of diglossia? Re-examining the situation. *Sign Language Studies,* 1982, *35,* 127–152.

Lee, L. Developmental sentence types: A method for comparing normal and deviant syntactic development. *Journal of Speech and Hearing Disorders,* 1966, *31,* 311–330.

Lee, L. Northwestern Syntax Screening Test. Evanston, IL: Northwestern University Press, 1969.

Lee, L. Developmental Sentence Analysis. Evanston, IL: Northwestern University Press, 1974.

Lee, L., & Canter, S. Developmental sentence scoring: A clinical procedure for estimating syntactic development in children's spontaneous speech. *Journal of Speech and Hearing Disorders,* 1971, *36,* 315–340.

Legarreta, D. The effects of program models on language acquisition by Spanish speaking children. *TESOL Quarterly,* 1979, *13,* 521–534.

Lenneberg, E. Biological foundations of language. New York: Wiley, 1967.

Levine, E. *The ecology of early deafness: Guides to fashioning environments and psychologial assessments.* New York: Columbia University Press, 1981.

Levy, B. Reading: Speech and meaning processes. *Journal of Verbal Learning and Verbal Behavior,* 1977, *16,* 623–638.

Lewis, D. Bilingualism and non-verbal intelligence: A further study of test results. *British Journal of Educational Psychology*, 1959, *29*, 17–22.

Liberman, I., Shankweiler, D., Liberman, A., Fowler, C., & Fischer, F. Phonetic segmentation and recoding in the beginning reader. In A. Reber & D. Scarborough (Eds.), *Towards a psychology of reading: The proceedings of the C.U.N.Y. conferences.* Hillsdale, NJ: Erlbaum, 1977.

Lichtenstein, E. *The relationships between reading processes and English skills of deaf students.* Rochester, NY: National Technical Institute for the Deaf, 1983.

Liddell, S. *Restrictive relative clauses in American Sign Language.* San Diego, CA: Salk Institute and University of California, 1975.

Liddell, S. *American Sign Language syntax.* The Hague: Mouton, 1980.

Lindberg, C. Is the sentence a unit of speech production and perception? In J. Mey (Ed.), *Pragmalinguistics: Theory and practice.* The Hague: Mouton, 1979.

Lindfors, J. *Children's language and learning.* Englewood Cliffs, NJ: Prentice–Hall, 1980.

Ling, D. *Speech and the hearing impaired child: Theory and practice.* Washington, D.C.: A. G. Bell Association for the Deaf, 1976.

Ling, D., & Clarke, B. Cued speech: An evaluative study. *American Annals of the Deaf,* 1975, *120*, 480–488.

Ling, D., Leckie, D., Pollack, D., Simser, J., & Smith, A. Syllable reception by hearing impaired children trained from infancy in auditory–oral programs. *Volta Review*, 1981, *83*, 451–457.

Ling, D., & Ling, A. *Aural habilitation: The foundations of verbal learning in hearing-impaired children.* Washington, D.C.: A. G. Bell Association for the Deaf, 1978.

Loban, W. *The language of elementary school children.* Champaign, IL: National Council of Teachers of English, 1963.

Locke, J. Phonemic effects in the silent reading of hearing and deaf children. *Cognition*, 1978, *6*, 175–187.

Locke, J., & Fehr, F. Subvocal rehearsal as a form of speech. *Journal of Verbal Learning and Verbal Behavior*, 1970, *9*, 495–498.

Locke, J., & Locke, V. Deaf children's phonetic, visual, and dactylic coding in a grapheme recall task. *Journal of Experimental Psychology*, 1971, *89*, 142–146.

Looney, P., & Rose, S. The acquisition of inflectional suffixes by deaf youngsters using written and fingerspelled modes. *American Annals of the Deaf*, 1979, *124*, 765–769.

Lucas, E. *Semantic and pragmatic language disorders: Assessment and remediation.* Rockville, MD: Aspen Systems, 1980.

Luetke, B. Questionnaire results from Mexican-American parents of hearing impaired children in the United States. *American Annals of the Deaf*, 1976, *121*, 565–568.

Luetke-Stahlman, B. A philosophy for assessing the language proficiency of hearing impaired students to promote English literacy. *American Annals of the Deaf*, 1982, *127*, 844–851.

Luetke-Stahlman, B., & Weiner, F. Assessing language and/or system preferences of Spanish-deaf preschoolers. *American Annals of the Deaf*, 1982, *127*, 789–796.

Macnamara, J. *Bilingualism and primary education: A study of Irish experience.* Chicago: Aldine, 1966.

Mandler, J. A code in the node: The use of a story schema in retrieval. *Discourse Processes,* 1978, *1,* 14–35.

Mandler, J., & Johnson, N. Remembrance of things parsed: Story structure and recall. *Cognitive Psychology,* 1977, *9,* 111–151.

Marmor, G., & Pettito, L. Simultaneous communication in the classroom: How well is English grammar represented? *Sign Language Studies,* 1979, *23,* 99–136.

Marshall, W., & Quigley, S. *Quantitative and qualitative analysis of syntactic structure in the written language of deaf students.* Urbana: University of Illinois, Institute for Research on Exceptional Children, 1970.

Mason, J., & Kendall, J. Facilitating reading comprehension through text structure manipulation. *Alberta Journal of Educational Psychology,* 1979, *24,* 68–76.

Mason, J., Osborn, J., & Rosenshine, B. *A consideration of skill hierarchy approaches to the teaching of reading.* Tech. Rep. No. 42, Center for the Study of Reading, University of Illinois, 1977.

Mavilya, M., & Mignone, B. *Educational strategies for the youngest hearing impaired children, 0–5 years of age.* New York: Lexington School for the Deaf, Educatino Series, Book 10, 1977.

Max, L. An experimental study of the motor theory of consciousness: Action-current responses in deaf-mutes during sleep, sensory stimulation, and dreams. *Journal of Comparative Psychology,* 1935, *19,* 469–486.

McCawley, J. The role of semantics in a grammar. In E. Bach & R. Harms (Eds.), *Universals in linguistic theory.* New York: Holt, Rinehart & Winston, 1968.

McConkie, G. Some perceptual aspects of reading. In R. E. Kretschmer (Ed.), Reading and the hearing-impaired individual. *Volta Review,* 1982, *84*(5), 35–43.

McConkie, G., & Zola, D. Language constraints and the functional stimulus in reading. In A. Lesgold & C. Perfetti (Eds), *Interactive processes in reading.* Hillsdale, NJ: Erlbaum, 1981.

McGill-Franzen, A., & Gormley, K. The influence of context on deaf readers' understanding of passive sentences. *American Annals of the Deaf,* 1980, *125,* 937–942.

McIntire, M. The acquisition of American Sign Language hand configurations. *Sign Language Studies,* 1977, *16,* 247–266.

McKee, N. Etymology and syntax in a school for the deaf. *Proceedings of the Fourteenth Convention of American Instructors of the Deaf,* Flint: Michigan School for the Deaf, 1895, 66–89.

McKee, P., Harrison, M., McCowen, A., Lehr, E., & Durr, W. *Reading for meaning* (4th ed.). Boston: Houghton Mifflin, 1966.

McLaughlin, B. *Second-language acquisition in childhood.* Hillsdale, NJ: Erlbaum, 1978.

McLaughlin, B. Second-language learning and bilingualism in children and adults. In S. Rosenberg (Ed.), *Handbook of applied psycholinguistics.* Hillsdale, NJ: Erlbaum, 1982.

McNeill, D. *The acquisition of language: The study of developmental psycholinguistics.* New York: Harper & Row, 1970.

McNeill, D. Speech and thought. In I. Markova (Ed.), *The social context of language.* New York: Wiley, 1978.

Meadow, K. Early manual communication in relation to the deaf child's intellectual, social, and communicative functioning. *American Annals of the Deaf,* 1968, *113,* 29–41.

Menn, L. Child language as a source of constraints for linguistic theory. In L. Obler & L. Menn (Eds.), *Exceptional language and linguistics.* New York: Academic Press, 1982.

Menyuk, P. A preliminary evaluation of grammatical capacity in children. *Journal of Verbal Learning and Verbal Behavior,* 1963, *2,* 429–439.

Menyuk, P. The role of distinctive features in children's acquisition of phonology. *Journal of Speech and Hearing Research,* 1968, *11,* 138–146.

Menyuk, P. Early development of receptive language: From babbling to words. In R. Schiefelbusch & L. Lloyd (Eds.), *Language perspectives: Acquisition, retardation, and intervention.* Baltimore: University Park Press, 1974.

Menyuk, P. *Language and maturation.* Cambridge, MA: MIT Press, 1977.

Mey, J. *Pragmalinguistics: Theory and practice.* The Hague: Mouton, 1979.

Miller, G., & Johnson-Laird, P. *Language and perception.* Cambridge, MA: Harvard University Press, 1976.

Miller, J. *Assessing language production in children.* Baltimore, MD: University Park Press, 1981.

Modiano, N. National or mother language in beginning reading: A comparative study. *Research in the Teaching of English,* 1968, *2,* 32–43.

Moerk, E. *Pragmatic and semantic aspects of early language development.* Baltimore: University Park Press, 1977.

Mohay, H. The effects of cued speech on the language development of three deaf children. *Sign Language Studies,* 1983, *38,* 25–47.

Monsen, R. The production of labial occlusives in young hearing-impaired children. *Language and Speech,* 1979, *22,* 311–318.

Moog, J., & Geers, A. Grammatical analysis of elicited language: Simple Sentence Level. St. Louis, MO: Central Institute for the Deaf, 1979.

Moog, J., & Geers, A. Grammatical Analysis of Elicited Language: Complex Sentence Level. St. Louis, MO: Central Institute for the Deaf, 1980.

Moog, J., & Kozak, V. *Teacher assessment of grammatical structures.* St. Louis, MO: Central Institute for the Deaf, 1983.

Moog, J., Kozak, V., & Geers, A. Grammatical Analysis of Elicited Language: Pre-Sentence Level. St. Louis, MO: Central Institute for the Deaf, 1983.

Moores, D. *Applications of "cloze" procedures to the assessment of psycholinguistic abilities of the deaf.* Unpublished doctoral dissertation, University of Illinois, 1967.

Moores, D. *Educating the deaf: psychology, principles, and practices.* Boston: Houghton Mifflin, 1978.

Morehead, D., & Morehead, A. From signal to sign: A Piagetian view of thought and language during the first two years. In R. Schiefelbusch & L. Lloyd (Eds.), *Language perspectives: Acquisition, retardation, and intervention.* Baltimore: University Park Press, 1974.

Morgan, E. Bilingualism and non-verbal intelligence: A study of test results. Pamphlet No. 4, Collegiate Faculty of Education, Aberystwyth, 1957.

Morgan, J., & Sellner, M. Discourse and linguistic theory. In R. Spiro, B. Bruce, & W. Brewer (Eds.), *Theoretical issues in reading comprehension*. New York: Erlbaum, 1980.

Morkovin, B. Experiment in teaching deaf preschool children in the Soviet Union. *Volta Review*, 1960, *62*, 260–268.

Morse, P. Infant speech perception: A preliminary model and review of the literature. In R. Schiefelbusch & L. Lloyd (Eds.), *Language perspectives: Acquisition, retardation, and intervention*. Baltimore: University Park Press, 1974.

Moskowitz, B. On the status of vowel shift in English. In T. Moore (Ed.), *Cognitive development and the acquisition of language*. New York: Academic Press, 1973.

Moulton, R., & Beasley, D. Verbal coding strategies used by hearing impaired individuals. *Journal of Speech and Hearing Research*, 1975, *18*, 559–570.

Myklebust, H. *The psychology of deafness*. New York: Grune & Stratton, 1960.

Myklebust, H. *The psychology of deafness* (2nd ed.). New York: Grune & Stratton, 1964.

Namir, L., & Schlesinger, I. The grammar of sign language. In I. Schlesinger & L. Namir (Eds.), *Sign language of the deaf: Psychological, linguistic, and sociological perspectives*. New York: Academic Press, 1978.

Nelson, K. Structure and strategy in learning to talk. *Monographs of the Society for Research in Child Development*, 1973, *38*, (Serial No. 149).

Nelson, K. The nominal shift in semantic–syntactic development. *Cognitive psychology*, 1975, *7*, 461–479.

Nelson, M. The evolutionary process of methods of teaching language to the deaf with a survey of the methods now employed. *American Annals of the Deaf*, 1949, *94*, Pt. I, 230–294; Pt. II, 354–396; Pt. III, 491–499.

Newport, E., & Ashbrook, E. The emergence of semantic relations in American Sign Language. *Papers and Reports on Child Language Development*, 1977, *13*, 16–21.

Nicholls, G. *Cued speech and the reception of spoken language*. Unpublished master's thesis, McGill University, Montreal, Canada, 1979.

Odom, P., Blanton, R., & McIntyre, C. Coding medium and word recall by deaf and hearing subjects. *Journal of Speech and Hearing Research*, 1970, *13*, 54–58.

O'Donnell, R., Griffin, W., & Norris, R. *Syntax of kindergarten and elementary school children: A transformational analysis*. Champaign, IL: National Council of Teachers of English, 1967.

Ogden, P. *Experiences and attitudes of oral deaf adults regarding oralism*. Unpublished doctoral dissertation, University of Illinois, 1979.

Oller, D., Jensen, H., & Lafayette, R. The relatedness of phonological processes of a hearing-impaired child. *Journal of Communication Disorders*, 1978, *11*, 97–105.

Omanson, R., Warren, W., & Trabasso, T. Goals, inferential comprehension, and recall of stories by children. *Discourse Processes*, 1978, *1*, 337–354.

O'Neill, M. *The receptive language competence of deaf children in the use of the base structure rules of transformational generative grammar.* Unpublished doctoral dissertation, University of Pittsburgh, PA, 1973.

O'Rourke, T. *A basic course in manual communication.* Silver Spring, MD: National Association of the Deaf, 1973.

Otheguy, R., & Otto, R. The myth of static maintenance in bilingual education. *The Modern Language Journal,* 1980, *64,* 350–356.

Ottem, E. An analysis of cognitive studies with deaf subjects. *American Annals of the Deaf,* 1980, *125,* 564–575.

Owens, R., Haney, M., Giesow, V., Dooley, L., & Kelly, R. Language test content: A comparative study. *Language Speech & Hearing Services in Schools,* 1983, *14,* 7–21.

Padden, C. Some arguments for syntactic patterning in American Sign Language. *Sign Language Studies,* 1981, *32,* 239–259.

Page, S. *The effect of idiomatic language in passages on the reading comprehension of deaf and hearing students.* Unpublished doctoral dissertation, Ball State University, 1981 (Abstract).

Parisi, D., & Antinucci, F. *Essentials of grammar.* New York: Academic Press, 1976.

Paulston, C. Ethnic relations and bilingual education: Accounting for contradictory data. In J. Alatis & K. Twaddell (Eds.), *English as a second language in bilingual education.* Washington, D.C.: TESOL, 1976.

Payne, J. *A study of the comprehension of verb–particle combinations among deaf and hearing subjects.* Unpublished doctoral dissertation, University of Illinois, 1982.

Peal, E., & Lambert, W. The relation of bilingualism to intelligence. *Psychological Monographs: General and Applied,* 1962, *76,* 1–23.

Pearson, P., & Johnson, D. *Teaching reading comprehension.* New York: Holt, Rinehart & Winston, 1978.

Peet, H. The order of the first lessons in language for a class of deaf mutes. *Proceedings of the Sixth Convention of the American Instructors of the Deaf,* Washington, D.C.: U.S. Govt. Printing Office, 1869, 19–26.

Peet, H. *Course of instruction for the deaf and dumb. Part Third* (7th ed.). New York: Egbert, Crawford, & King, Printers, 1870.

Perlman, C. *An investigation of deaf and hearing children's ability to apply morphological rules to lexical and nonsense items.* Unpublished master's thesis, University of Cincinnati, 1973.

Perry, F. The psycholinguistic abilities of deaf children: An exploratory investigation—II. *The Australian Teacher of the Deaf,* 1968, *9,* 153–160.

Pettifor, J. The role of language in the development of abstract thinking: A comparison of hard-of-hearing and normally hearing children on levels of conceptual thinking. *Canadian Journal of Psychology,* 1968, *22*(3), 139–156.

Piaget, J. *[Play, dreams and imitation in childhood]* (C. Gattegno & F. Hodgson, trans.). New York: Norton, 1951 (originally published, 1945).

Piaget, J. *[The construction of reality in the child]* (M. Cook, trans.). New York: Basic Books, 1954 (originally published, 1937).

Piaget, J. *The language and thought of the child.* New York: Meridian Books, 1955.

Piaget, J. Language and thought from the genetic point of view. In D. Elkind (Ed.), *Six psychological studies.* New York: Random House, 1967.

Piaget, J. *[Biology and knowledge: An essay on the relations between organic regulations and cognitive processes]* (B. Walsh, trans.). Chicago: University of Chicago Press, 1971 (originally published, 1967).

Pintner, R., Eisenson, J., & Stanton, M. *The psychology of the physically handicapped.* New York: Crofts, 1941.

Pintner, R., & Patterson, D. A measurement of the language ability of deaf children. *Psychological Review,* 1916, *23,* 413–436.

Pintner, R., & Reamer, J. A mental and educational survey of schools for the deaf. *American Annals of the Deaf,* 1920, *65,* 451–472.

Pollack, D. Acoupedics: A uni-sensory approach to auditory training. *Volta Review,* 1964, *66,* 400–409.

Power, D., & Quigley, S. Deaf children's acquisition of the passive voice. *Journal of Speech and Hearing Research,* 1973, *16,* 5–11.

Powers, A., & Wilgus, S. Linguistic complexity in the written language of deaf children. *Volta Review,* 1983, *85,* 201–210.

Presnell, L. Hearing-impaired children's comprehension and production of syntax in oral language. *Journal of Speech and Hearing Research,* 1973, *16,* 12–21.

Pugh, G. Summaries from appraisal of the silent reading abilities of acoustically handicapped children. *American Annals of the Deaf,* 1946, *91,* 331–349.

Quigley, S. The influence of fingerspelling on the development of language, communication, and educational achievement in deaf children. Urbana, IL: Institute for Research on Exceptional Children, 1969.

Quigley, S. Reading achievement and special reading materials. In R. E. Kretschmer (Ed.), Reading and the hearing-impaired individual. *Volta Review,* 1982, *84*(5), 95–106.

Quigley, S., & Frisina, R. *Institutionalization and psychoeducational development of deaf children.* CEC Research Monograph, Washington, D.C.: Council on Exceptional Children, 1961.

Quigley, S., & King, C. *Reading milestones.* Beaverton, OR: Dormac, 1981, 1982, 1983, 1984.

Quigley, S., & King, C. Language development of deaf children and youth. In S. Rosenberg (Ed.), *Handbook of applied psycholinguistics.* Hillsdale, NJ: Erlbaum, 1982.

Quigley, S., & Kretschmer, R. E. *The education of deaf children.* Baltimore: University Park Press, 1982.

Quigley, S., & Paul, P. ASL and ESL? *Topics in Early Childhood Special Education,* 1984.

Quigley, S., & Power, D. *TSA syntax program.* Beaverton, OR: Dormac, 1979.

Quigley, S., Power, D., & Steinkamp, M. The language structure of deaf children. *Volta Review,* 1977, *79,* 73–83.

Quigley, S., Smith N., & Wilbur, W. Comprehension of relativized sentences by deaf students. *Journal of Speech and Hearing Research,* 1974, *17,* 325–341.

Quigley, S., Steinkamp, M., Power, D., & Jones, B. Test of Syntactic Abilities. Beaverton, OR: Dormac, 1978.

Quigley, S., Wilbur, R., & Montanelli, D. Question formation in the language of deaf students. *Journal of Speech and Hearing Research,* 1974, *17,* 699–713.

Quigley, S., Wilbur, R., & Montanelli, D. Complement structures in the language of deaf students. *Journal of Speech and Hearing Research,* 1976, *19,* 448–457.

Quigley, S., Wilbur, R., Power, D., Montanelli, D., & Steinkamp, M. *Syntactic structures in the language of deaf children.* Urbana: University of Illinois, Institute for Child Behavior and Development, 1976.

Raffin, M. *The acquisition of inflectional morphemes by deaf children using Seeing Essential English.* Unpublished doctoral dissertation, University of Iowa, 1976.

Raffin, M., Davis, J., & Gilman, L. Comprehension of inflectional morphemes by deaf children exposed to a visual English sign system. *Journal of Speech and Hearing Research,* 1978, *21,* 387–400.

Rainer, J., Altschuler K., & Kallman, F. (Eds.) *Family and mental health problems in a deaf population.* Springfield, IL: Thomas, 1969.

Rawlings, B., & Jensema, C. *Two studies of the families of hearing impaired children.* Washington, D.C.: Gallaudet College, Office of Demographic Studies, Series R, No. 5, 1977.

Rayner, K., McConkie, G., & Zola, D. Integrating information across eye movements. *Cognitive Psychology,* 1980, *12,* 206–226.

Reich, P., & Bick, M. How visible is visible English? *Sign Language Studies,* 1977, *14,* 59–72.

Reynolds, R., & Ortony, A. Some issues in the measurement of children's comprehension of metaphorical language. *Child Development,* 1980, *51,* 1110–1119.

Richards, J. A non-contrastive approach to error analysis. In J. Richards (Ed.), *Error analysis: Perspectives on second language acquisition.* London: Longman, 1974.

Rittenhouse, R. *Horizontal decalage: The development of conservation in deaf students and the effect of the task instructions on their performance.* Unpublished doctoral dissertation, University of Illinois, 1977.

Robbins, N., & Hatcher, C. The effects of syntax on the reading comprehension of hearing-impaired children. *Volta Review,* 1981, *83,* 105–115.

Robins, R. *General linguistics: An introductory survey* (3rd ed.). London: Longman, 1980.

Robinson, W. A new device for teaching language. *American Annals of the Deaf,* 1898, *43,* 78–87; 170–183.

Rogers, W., Leslie, P., Clarke, B., Booth, J., & Horvath, A. Academic achievement of hearing impaired students: Comparison among selected sub-populations. *British Columbia Journal of Special Education,* 1978, *2,* 183–213.

Rosenstein, J. Cognitive abilities of deaf children. *Journal of Speech and Hearing Research,* 1960, *3,* 108–119.

Rosenstein, J. Perception, cognition, and language in deaf children. *Exceptional Children,* 1961, *27,* 276–284.

Rosier, P., & Farella, M. Bilingual education at Rock Point—Some early results. *TESOL Quarterly,* 1976, *10,* 379–388.

Ross, M., & Calvert, D. The semantics of deafness. *Volta Review,* 1967, *69,* 644–649.

Rumelhart, D. Toward an interactive model of reading. In S. Dornic (Ed.), *Attention and performance VI.* New York/London: Academic Press, 1977.

Russell, J. *Reversal and nonreversal shift in deaf and hearing kindergarten children.* Unpublished master's thesis, Catholic University of America, Washington, D.C., 1964.

Russell, W., Quigley, S., & Power, D. *Linguistics and deaf children.* Washington, D.C.: A. G. Bell Association for the Deaf, 1976.

Saer, D. The effects of bilingualism on intelligence. *British Journal of Psychology,* 1923, *14,* 25–38.

Salzinger, K. Ecolinguistics: A radical behavior theory approach to language behavior. In D. Aaronson & R. Rieber (Eds.), *Psycholinguistic research: Implications and applications.* Hillsdale, NJ: Erlbaum, 1979.

Sapir, E. Language and environment. In D. Mandelbaum (Ed.), *Selected writings of Edward Sapir in language, culture, and personality.* Berkeley: University of California, 1958.

Schlesinger, H. The acquisition of signed and spoken language. In L. Liben (Ed.), *Deaf children: Developmental perspectives.* New York: Academic Press, 1978.

Schlesinger, H., & Meadow, K. *Sound and sign: Childhood deafness and mental health.* Berkeley: University of California Press, 1972.

Schlesinger, I. The role of cognitive development and linguistic input in language acquisition. *Journal of Child Language,* 1977, *4,* 153–169.

Schlesinger, I. *Steps to language: Toward a theory of native language acquisition.* Hillsdale, NJ: Erlbaum, 1982.

Schlesinger, I., & Namir, L. (Eds.) *Sign language of the deaf.* New York: Academic Press, 1978.

Schmitt, P. Language instruction for the deaf. In S. P. Quigley (Ed.), *Language acquisition. Volta Review,* 1966 (Reprint No. 852).

Schmitt, P. *Deaf children's comprehension and production of sentence transformations and verb tenses.* Unpublished doctoral dissertation, University of Illinois, 1969.

Schulze, B. An evaluation of vocabulary development by thirty-two deaf children over a three year period. *American Annals of the Deaf,* 1965, *110,* 424–435.

Scouten, E. The Rochester method: An oral multi-sensory approach for instructing prelingual deaf children. *American Annals of the Deaf,* 1967, *112,* 50–55.

Searle, J. *Speech acts.* Cambridge: Cambridge University Press, 1969.

Searle, J. Indirect speech acts. In M. Cole & J. Morgan (Eds.), *Syntax and semantics* (Vol. 3). New York: Academic Press, 1975.

Selinger, H. Implications of a multiple critical periods hypothesis for second language learning. In W. Ritchie (Ed.), *Second language acquisition research.* New York: Academic Press, 1978.

Shankweiler, D., Liberman, I., Mark, L., Fowler, C., & Fischer, F. The speech code and learning to read. *Journal of Experimental Psychology: Human Learning and Memory,* 1979, *5,* 531–545.

Shipley, E., Smith, C., & Gleitman, L. A study in the acquisition of language; free responses to commands. *Language,* 1969, *45,* 322–342.

Simmons, A. A comparison of the type–token ratio of spoken and written language of deaf children. *Volta Review,* 1962, *64,* 417–421.

Simmons, A. *Comparison of written and spoken language from deaf and hearing children at five age levels.* Unpublished doctoral dissertation, Washington University, 1963.

Sinclair-de Zwart, H. Language acquisition and cognitive development. In T. Moore (Ed.), *Cognitive development and the acquisition of language.* New York: Academic Press, 1973.

Siple, P. (Ed.) *Understanding language through sign language research.* New York: Academic Press, 1978.

Siple, P. Signed language and linguistic theory. In L. Obler & L. Menn (Eds.), *Exceptional language and linguistics.* New York: Academic Press, 1982.

Siple, P., Fischer, S., & Bellugi, U. Memory for nonsemantic attributes of American Sign Language signs and English words. *Journal of Verbal Learning and Verbal Behavior,* 1977, *16,* 561–574.

Skarakis, E., & Prutting, C. Early communication: Semantic function and communicative intentions in the communications of the preschool child with impaired hearing. *American Annals of the Deaf,* 1977, *122,* 382–391.

Skinner, B. *About behaviorism.* New York: Knopf, 1974.

Slobin, D. *Psycholinguistics* (2nd ed.). Glenview, IL: Scott, Foresman, 1979.

Slobin, D. Comments on developmental psycholinguistics. In F. Smith & G. Miller (Eds.), *The genesis of language: A psycholinguistic approach.* Cambridge, MA: MIT Press, 1966.

Slobin, D., & Welsh, C. Elicited imitation as a research tool in developmental psycholinguistics. In C. Ferguson & D. Slobin (Eds.), *Studies of child language development.* New York: Holt, Rinehart & Winston, 1973.

Smith, C. An experimental approach to children's linguistic competence. In J. Hayes (Ed.), *Cognition and the development of language.* New York: Wiley, 1970.

Smith, F. *Comprehension and learning: A conceptual framework for teachers.* New York: Holt, Rinehart & Winston, 1975a.

Smith, F. The role of prediction in reading. *Elementary English,* 1975b, *52,* 305–311.

Smith, F. *Understanding reading* (rev. ed.). New York: Holt, Rinehart & Winston, 1978.

Snow, C. The development of conversation between mothers and babies. *Journal of Child Language,* 1977, *4,* 1–22.

Snow, C., & Ferguson, C. (Eds.) *Talking to children: Language input and acquisition.* Cambridge: Cambridge University Press, 1977.

Sokolov, A. *Inner speech and thought.* New York: Plenum Press, 1972.

Spiro, R. Remembering information from text: Theoretical and empirical issues concerning the "State of Schema" reconstruction hypothesis. In R. Anderson, R. Spiro, & W. Montague (Eds.), *Schooling and the acquisition of knowledge.* Hillsdale, NJ: Erlbaum, 1977.

Staats, A. Linguistic–mentalistic theory versus an explanatory S–R learning theory of language development. In D. Slobin (Ed.), *The ontogenesis of grammar.* New York: Academic Press, 1971.

Stanovich, K. Toward an interactive-compensatory model of individual differences in the development of reading fluency. *Reading Research Quarterly,* 1980, *16,* 32–71.

Stanovich, K., & West, R. Mechanisms of sentence context effects in reading: Automatic activation and conscious attention. *Memory and Cognition,* 1979, *7,* 77–85.

Stokoe, W., Jr. *Sign language structure: An outline of the visual communication systems of the American deaf.* Studies in Linguistics, Occasional Paper No. 8, 1960. (Reissued Washington, D.C.: Gallaudet College, 1971.)

Stokoe, W., Jr. *Semiotics and human sign languages.* The Hague: Mouton, 1972.

Stokoe, W., Jr. The use of sign language in teaching English. *American Annals of the Deaf,* 1975, *120,* 417–421.

Stowitschek, J., Gable, R., & Hendrickson, J. *Instructional materials for exceptional children: Selection, management, and adaptation.* Germantown, MD: Aspen Systems, 1980.

Streng, A. *Reading for deaf children.* Washington, D.C.: Alexander Graham Bell Association for the Deaf, 1965.

Stuckless, E. R., & Birch, J. The influence of early manual communication on the linguistic development of deaf children. *American Annals of the Deaf,* 1966, *111,* 452–460, 499–504.

Stuckless, E. R., & Hurwitz, A. Recording speech in real-time print: Dream or reality? *The Deaf American,* 1982, *34,* 10–15.

Stuckless, E. R., & Marks, C. *Assessment of the written language of deaf students.* Pittsburgh, PA: University of Pittsburgh, School of Education, 1966.

Stuckless, E. R., & Matter, J. *Word accuracy and error in steno/computer transliteration of spoken lectures into real-time graphic display.* Rochester NY: National Technical Institute for the Deaf, RTGD Working Paper No. 1, 1982.

Stuckless, E. R., & Pollard, G. Processing of fingerspelling and print by deaf students. *American Annals of the Deaf,* 1977, *122,* 475–479.

Swain, M. Linguistic expectations: Core, extended and immersion programs. *Canadian Modern Language Review,* 1981, *37,* 486–497.

Taylor, L. *A language analysis of the writing of deaf children.* Unpublished doctoral dissertation, Florida State University, Tallahassee, 1969.

Templin, M. *Certain language skills in children, their development and interrelationships.* Institute of Child Welfare Monograph Service, 26. Minneapolis: University of Minnesota Press, 1957.

Tervoort, B. *Analysis of communicative structure patterns in deaf children.* (Final Report, Project No. R. D. 467-64-65), Washington, D.C.: United States Department of Health, Education, and Welfare, Vocational Rehabilitation Administration, 1967.

Tervoort, B. Bilingual interference. In I. Schlesinger & L. Namir (Eds.), *Sign language of the deaf: Psychological, linguistic, and sociological perspectives.* New York: Academic Press, 1978.

Thompson, W. An analysis of errors in written compositions by deaf children. *American Annals of the Deaf,* 1936, *81,* 95–99.

Thorndike, R. Reliability. In E. Lindquist (Ed.), *Educational Measurement.* Washington, D.C.: American Council on Education, 1951.

Thorndike, R., & Hagen, E. *Measurement and evaluation in psychology and education* (2nd ed.). New York: Wiley, 1961.

Trabasso, T. On the making and assessment of inferences during reading. In J. Guthrie (Ed.), *Reading comprehension and education.* Newark, DE: International Reading Association, 1980.

Troike, R. Research evidence for the effectiveness of bilingual education. *NABE Journal,* 1978, *3,* 13–24.

Troike, R. Synthesis of research on bilingual education. *Educational Leadership,* 1981, *38,* 498–504.

Truax, R. Reading and language. In R. R. Kretschmer & L. Kretschmer (Eds.), *Language development and intervention with the hearing impaired.* Baltimore: University Park Press, 1978.

Trybus, R., & Karchmer, M. School achievement scores of hearing impaired children: National data on achievement status and growth patterns. *American Annals of the Deaf Directory of Programs and Services,* 1977, *122,* 62–69.

Tucker, G. The linguistic perspective. In *Bilingual education: Current perspectives, Vol. 2.* Arlington, VA: Center for Applied Linguistics, 1977.

Turner, R. (Ed.) *Ethnomethodology.* Harmondsworth, England: Penguin, 1974.

Tweeney, R., Hoeman, H., & Andrews, C. Semantic organization in deaf and hearing subjects. *Journal of Psycholinguistic Research,* 1975, *4,* 61–73.

Tyack, D., & Gottesleben, R. *Language sampling, analysis, and training: A handbook for teachers and clinicians.* Palo Alto, CA: Consulting Psychologist's Press, 1974.

Van der Geest, T. *Evaluation of theories on child grammars.* The Hague: Mouton, 1974.

van Uden, A. *A world of language for deaf children, Part I. Basic principles.* Amsterdam, Holland: Swets & Zeitlinger, 1977.

Vellutino, F. Theoretical issues in the study of word recognition: The unit of perception controversy reexamined. In S. Rosenberg (Ed.), *Handbook of applied psycholinguistics,* (pp. 33–197). NJ: Erlbaum, 1982.

Venezky, R. *Theoretical and experimental base for teaching reading.* The Hague: Mouton, 1976.

Ventry, I., & Schiavetti, N. *Evaluating research in speech pathology and audiology: A guide for clinicians and students.* Menlo Park, CA: Addison–Wesley, 1980.

Vernon, M. Relationship of language to the thinking process. *Archives of General Psychiatry,* 1967, *16,* 325–333.

Vernon, M. Multiply handicapped deaf children: Medical, educational and psychological considerations. Washington, D.C.: *Council for Exceptional Children Research Monograph,* 1969.

Walter, G. Lexical abilities of hearing and hearing-impaired children. *American Annals of the Deaf,* 1978, *123,* 976–982.

Wardrop, J. *Standardized testing in the schools: Uses and roles.* Monterey, CA: Brookes/Cole, 1976.

Wheeler, D. Processes in word recognition. *Cognitive Psychology,* 1970, *1,* 59–85.

White, A., & Stevenson, V. The effects of total communication, manual communication, oral communication and reading on the learning of factual information in residential school deaf children. *American Annals of the Deaf*, 1975, *120*, 48–57.

Wilbur, R. An explanation of deaf children's difficulty with certain syntactic structures in English. *Volta Review*, 1977, *79*, 85–92.

Wilbur, R. *American sign language and sign systems.* Baltimore: University Park Press, 1979.

Wilbur, R. The linguistic description of American Sign Language. In H. Lane & F. Grosjean (Eds.), *Recent perspectives on American Sign Language.* Hillsdale, NJ: Erlbaum, 1980.

Wilbur, R., Fraser, J., & Fruchter, A. *Comprehension of idioms by hearing impaired students.* Paper presented at the American Speech–Language–Hearing Association Convention, Los Angeles, 1981.

Wilson, K. *Inference and language processing in hearing and deaf children.* Unpublished doctoral dissertation, Boston University, 1979.

Wing, G. The theory and practice of grammatical methods. *American Annals of the Deaf*, 1887, *32*, 84–92.

Winitz, H. *Articulatory acquisition and behavior.* New York: Appleton–Century–Crofts, 1969.

Winner, E., Engel, M., & Gardner, H. Misunderstanding metaphor: What's the problem? *Journal of Experimental Child Psychology*, 1980, *30*, 22–32.

Withrow, F. Immediate memory span of deaf and normally hearing children. *Exceptional Children*, 1968, *35*, 33–41.

Wolff, P. The natural history of crying and other vocalizations in early infancy. In B. Foss (Ed.), *Determinants of infant behavior* (Vol. 4). London: Methuen, 1969.

Woodward, J. Some characteristics of pidgin sign English. *Sign Language Studies*, 1973, *3*, 39–46.

Woodward, J. Historical bases of American Sign Language. In P. Siple (Ed.), *Understanding language through sign language research.* New York: Academic Press, 1978.

Woodward, J. Sociolinguistic research on ASL: An historical perspective. In C. Baker & R. Battison (Eds.), *Sign language and the deaf community: Essays in honor of William C. Stokoe.* Silver Spring, MD: National Association of the Deaf, 1980.

Woodward, J., & Markowicz, H. *Some handy new ideas on pidgins and creoles: Pidgin sign languages.* International Conference on Pidgins and Creole Languages, Honolulu, 1975.

Wrightstone, J., Aronow, M., & Moskowitz, S. Developing reading test norms for deaf children. *American Annals of the Deaf*, 1963, *108*, 311–316.

Youniss, J., & Furth, H. Prediction of causal events as a function of transitivity and perceptual congruency in hearing and deaf children. *Child Development*, 1966, *37*, 73–81.

Yussen, S., & Santrock, J. *Child development.* Dubuque: W. C. Brown, 1978.

Zola, D. *The effect of redundancy on the perception of words in reading* (Tech. Rep. No. 216). Urbana: University of Illinois, Center for the Study of Reading, 1981.

AUTHOR INDEX

SUBJECT INDEX